A. Surbone · F. Peccatori · N. Pavlidis (Eds.)

Cancer and Pregnancy

With 25 Figures and 53 Tables

Springer

Antonella Surbone, MD, PhD, FACP
Head, Teaching, Research and
Development Department
European School of Oncology
Via del Bollo 4
20123 Milan
Italy

and

Associate Professor of Clinical Medicine
New York Medical School
New York University
New York, NY 10016
USA

Fedro Peccatori, MD, PhD
Department of Medicine
Division of Hematology and Oncology
Istituto Europeo di Oncologia
Via Ripamonti 435
20141 Milan
Italy

Nicholas Pavlidis, MD
Professor of Medical Oncology
Department of Medical Oncology
Medical School
University of Ioannina
451 10 Ioannina
Greece

ISSN 0080-0015
ISBN 978-3-642-09036-3 e-ISBN 978-3-540-71274-9

Springer is a part of Springer Science+Business Media
springer.com

Editor: Dr. Ute Heilmann, Heidelberg
Desk editor: Dörthe Mennecke-Bühler, Heidelberg
Production editor: Anne Strohbach, Leipzig
Cover design: Frido Steinen-Broo, eStudio Calamar, Spain

Recent Results in Cancer Research 178

Foreword

The European School of Oncology is delighted to see that the faculty of its course on cancer and pregnancy has succeeded—and in a remarkably short time—in producing this greatly stimulating book.

Very few human and clinical situations encompass such opposite extremes as pregnancy and cancer, hope and fear, sometimes life and death.

Any health professional who has been confronted with this issue knows how difficult it is from the clinical viewpoint but also how challenging it is on the emotional side.

In recent years the success of cancer medicine has increased the number of survivors and the length of their survival, thus increasing the number of female former cancer patients expected to have a successful pregnancy.

Another group of individuals that deserves our attention are women who have survived a childhood cancer and who should be managed by a multidisciplinary specialist team. Fortunately, many studies are underway and we hope to soon have new insights into this extraordinarily complex issue.

The European School of Oncology is grateful to Dr. A. Surbone for her successful coordination of our teaching course and for having taken the initiative to publish this book. We hope that it will contribute to helping many children have their mother cured of her cancer and be able to love them forever.

Alberto Costa, MD
Director
European School of Oncology

Contents

List of Contributors

Stefan Aebi, MD
Associate Professor of Medical Oncology
University Hospital Bern
Inselspital
Breast and Gynecologic Cancer Center
3010 Bern
Switzerland

Judith Alder, PhD
University Women's Hospital Basel
Spitalstrasse 21
4031 Basel
Switzerland

Volmar Belisario-Filho, MD
IOSI, Oncology Institute of Southern Switzerland
6500 Bellinzona
Switzerland

Giulia Bellettini, MD
Pediatrician, IBCLC (International Board Certified Lactation Consultant)
Via Giuseppe Sapeto 2
20123 Milan
Italy

Johannes Bitzer, MD
University Women's Hospital Basel
Spitalstrasse 21
4031 Basel
Switzerland

Saverio Cinieri, MD
Co-Director, Hematology–Oncology Division
European Institute of Oncology
Via Giuseppe Ripamonti 435
20141 Milan
Italy

Mandish K. Dhanjal, BSc, MBBS, MRCP, MRCOG
Consultant Obstetrician and Gynaecologist
Queen Charlotte's and Chelsea Hospital
Du Cane Road
London W12 0NN
UK

Martin F. Fey, MD
Professor of Medical Oncology
Department of Medical Oncology
Inselspital and University
3010 Bern
Switzerland

Patrizia Froesch, MD
IOSI, Oncology Institute of Southern Switzerland
6500 Bellinzona
Switzerland

Oreste Gentilini, MD
Breast Surgery
European Institute of Oncology
Via Ripamonti 435
20141 Milan
Italy

Bianca Gibelli, MD
Thyroid Unit, Head and Neck Department
European Institute of Oncology
Via Ripamonti 435
20141 Milan
Italy

Harald J. Hoekstra, MD, PhD
Division of Surgical Oncology
University Medical Center Groningen
University of Groningen
P.O. Box 30001
9700 RB Groningen
The Netherlands

Sean Kehoe, MD
Professor of Gynaecological Cancer
The Women's Centre
John Radcliffe Hospital
Headly Way
Headington
Oxford OX3 9DU
UK

Vesna Kesic, MD, PhD
Institute of Obstetrics and Gynecology
Clinical Center of Serbia
Visegradska 26
11000 Belgrade
Serbia

Stella Kyriakides
Europa Donna
The European Breast Cancer Coalition
Cyprus Forum
71 Acropolis Avenue
2012 Nicosia
Cyprus

Marko Lens, MD, PhD, FRCS
King's College
Genetic Epidemiology Unit
St. Thomas' Hospital
Lambeth Palace Road
London SE1 7EH
UK

Michael Lishner, MD
Department of Internal Medicine A
Meir Medical Center
Kfar Sava 44281
Israel

Sibylle Loibl, MD
Assistant Professor of Gynecology
and Obstetrics
Department of Gynecology and Obstetrics
Johann Wolfgang Goethe University
Theodor-Stern-Kai 7
60590 Frankfurt am Main
Germany

Giovanni Lucignani, MD
Chair of Nuclear Medicine
University of Milan
Head of Nuclear Medicine Unit
Ospedale San Paolo
Via Di Rudini 8
20142 Milan
Italy

Michela Maur, MD
Oncologia Medica
Centro Oncologico Modenese
Policlinico Modena
Largo del Pozzo 71
41100 Modena
Italy

Sotiris Mitrou, MD
SpR in Obstetrics and Gynaecology
John Radcliffe Hospital
Headly Way
Headington
Oxford OX3 9DU
UK

Kutluk Oktay, MD
Department of Obstetrics and Gynecology
Joan and Sanford I. Weill Medical College
of Cornell University
505 East 70th Street
HT-340
New York, NY 10021
USA

Roberto Orecchia, MD
Chair of Radiation Therapy
University of Milan
Head of Radiation Therapy Department
European Institute of Oncology
Via Ripamonti 435
20141 Milan
Italy

Laura Orlando, MD
Assistant, Oncology Division
European Institute of Oncology
Via Giuseppe Ripamonti 435
20141 Milan
Italy

Nicholas Pavlidis, MD
Professor of Medical Oncology
Department of Medical Oncology
Medical School
University of Ioannina
451 10 Ioannina
Greece

Fedro Peccatori, MD, PhD
Department of Medicine
Division of Hematology and Oncology
Istituto Europeo di Oncologia
Via Ripamonti 435
20141 Milan
Italy

George Pentheroudakis, MD
Consultant in Medical Oncology
Department of Medical Oncology
Ioannina University Hospital
451 10 Ioannina
Greece

David Pereg, MD
Department of Internal Medicine A
Meir Medical Center
Kfar Sava 44281
Israel

Cristiana Sessa, MD, PhD
Ospedale San Giovanni
IOSI, Oncology Institute of Southern
Switzerland
6500 Bellinzona
Switzerland

Murat Sönmezer, MD
Department of Obstetrics and Gynecology
Ankara University
School of Medicine
06100 Ankara
Turkey

Daniel Surbek, MD
Professor of Obstetrics and Gynaecology
Women's Hospital
Inselspital and University
3010 Bern
Switzerland

Antonella Surbone, MD, PhD, FACP
Head, Teaching, Research and Development
Department
European School of Oncology
Via del Bollo 4
20123 Milan
Italy
and
Associate Professor of Clinical Medicine
New York Medical School
New York University
New York, NY 10016
USA

Giampiero Tosi, PhD
Head of Medical Physics
European Institute of Oncology
Via Ripamonti 435
20141 Milan
Italy

N. Tradati, MD
Head of Thyroid Unit
Head and Neck Department
European Institute of Oncology
Via Ripamonti 435
20141 Milan
Italy

P. Zamperini, MD
Consultant Obstetrican and Gynaecologist
European Institute of Oncology
Via Ripamonti 435
20141 Milan
Italy

E. Zucca, MD
Head, Lymphoma Unit
Medical Oncology Department
IOSI, Oncology Institute of Southern
Switzerland
6500 Bellinzona
Switzerland

1 Why Is the Topic of Cancer and Pregnancy So Important? Why and How to Read this Book

A. Surbone, F. Peccatori, N. Pavlidis

Recent Results in Cancer Research, Vol. 178

Cancer during pregnancy represents a philosophical and biological paradox. To be confronted with the diagnosis of cancer during a pregnancy is certainly one of the most dramatic events in a woman's life and in the life of her partner and family. The diagnostic and therapeutic management of the pregnant mother with cancer is especially difficult because it involves two persons, the mother and the fetus. Although treatment modalities and timing should be individualized, both obstetricians and oncologists should offer at the same time optimal maternal therapy and fetal well-being. The approach to these particular patients should be undertaken by a dedicated multidisciplinary team.

This book is the result of an advanced course that we organized on behalf of the European School of Oncology on the different aspects of cancer during pregnancy. During the 2 years of preparation for the course and through the 3-day presentations of our outstanding colleagues and the interactive discussion with highly qualified participants, we shared knowledge and first-hand clinical expertise on diagnosing, treating, and following women with different cancers during pregnancy. This is a field in which the published literature is still scanty, and we have decided to prepare this collection of chapters with the aim of reviewing the existing medical data on cancer during pregnancy and also of providing insight into the many ethical and psychosocial aspects involved. While each chapter provides general suggestions on diagnosis, treatment, and follow-up of young women who face the concomitance of cancer and pregnancy, this book is not intended as a practical guideline. Rather, the scope of this book is to present a comprehensive overview of the subject in all its complexity. Each chapter contains separate references on published literature and on online sources, where physicians can find additional information on referral centers and on ongoing clinical trials and registries.

Through the different chapters of this book, we see that the exact incidence of cancer in pregnancy is yet to be determined, but it is estimated that cancer occurs in 1 in 1,000 pregnancies and accounts for one-third of maternal deaths during gestation. The most common cancers in pregnancy are those with a peak incidence during the woman's reproductive period such as cancer of the breast and cervix, melanomas, lymphomas, and leukemias. As the trend for delaying pregnancy into the later reproductive years continues, this rare association is likely to become more common. Special registries are ongoing, and more should be established, to identify the real epidemiology of this coexistence, as well as the outcome of the offspring.

Diagnostic and staging work-up with radiological imaging should limit exposure to ionizing radiation and should be restricted to those methods that do not endanger fetal health. Especially during the first trimester of pregnancy, only absolutely necessary radiological investigations are justified. Other diagnostic procedures such as excisional or incisional biopsies, endoscopies, and lumbar puncture or bone marrow biopsies can be safely performed with the appropriate caution.

The therapeutic management of pregnant women with cancer requires specific "optimal gold standards". The medical personnel involved should try to benefit the mother's life, to treat the mother's curable cancers, to protect the fetus and the newborn from harmful effects of treatment, and to retain the mother's reproductive system intact, when possible, for future gestations.

Some chemotherapeutic agents can be safely administered during the second and third trimesters, whereas radiotherapy is better avoided throughout gestation. Surgery under general anesthesia is feasible during all trimesters.

Accumulating evidence suggests that pregnancy is not an independent poor prognostic variable for patients' survival. Survival appears to be similar between pregnant and nonpregnant cancer patients.

The mother's cancer cells can be transmitted vertically to the placenta or fetus—a rare phenomenon most commonly described in malignant melanoma. Macroscopic and histopathologic examination of the placenta as well as cytological examination of the umbilical cord blood should be performed routinely.

Cancer diagnosed during pregnancy is a dramatic event with profound impact on the life of the patient, offspring, family, and physician. Several medical, psychological, religious, social, and ethical issues contribute to the final decision, and establishing a trustful patient–doctor–family relationship is essential. The management of pregnant cancer patients is also highly emotionally charged for the physicians and all members of the oncology team, and support should also be offered to them.

As the number of cancer survivors increases worldwide and many women tend to postpone childbearing until later in their reproductive life, the morbidity related to reproductive sequelae of oncologic therapies may negatively affect the physical, psychological, and social dimensions of their lives. Treatment-related reproductive dysfunctions, often superimposed on independent factors, should be addressed with all young cancer patients at the time of diagnosis and treatment planning. Adequate information and education should be provided about means to preserve and enhance fertility in young women undergoing therapies for different cancers.

2 Prenatal Irradiation and Pregnancy: The Effects of Diagnostic Imaging and Radiation Therapy

R. Orecchia, G. Lucignani, G. Tosi

Recent Results in Cancer Research, Vol. 178

2.1 Introduction

The discoveries of X-rays and radioactivity at the end of the nineteenth century represented major events for medicine that have paved the way for extraordinary diagnostic and therapeutic techniques whose potential has still not been fully exploited. Nowadays, radiation is used in medicine for diagnosis and treatment of many diseases. It has been estimated that each year, worldwide, about 2 billion radiological and diagnostic procedures are performed while about 5.5 million patients are treated with radiation therapy for cancer.

Shortly after the introduction of different types of radiation as techniques for diagnosis and therapy, it became clear that there were not only beneficial effects derived from the possibility of imaging the body and its functions, but also detrimental biological effects from excessive exposure to these extremely powerful forms of energy. These hazards and potential damaging effects became evident long before the physical laws and the biochemical mechanisms underlying radiation-induced biological damage could be understood. With the increased use of radiation in diagnostic and therapeutic applications, concern for the biological effects continues to grow. The need to avoid unwanted radiation exposures has led to the development of the sciences of radiobiology and health physics. By combining knowledge in the fields of physics, biology, chemistry, statistics and instrumentation, sets of rules and guidelines for the protection of individuals and populations from the effects of radiation in all its forms have been developed.

Radiation is essentially a form of very fast-moving energy. Types of radiation include electromagnetic radiation, such as visible light, radio, and television waves, ultraviolet (UV) radiation, microwaves and X- and gamma rays. These types of electromagnetic waves may cause ionisation of atoms when they carry enough energy to separate molecules or remove tightly bound electrons from their orbits around atoms. Whereas electromagnetic non-ionising radiation (radio waves, microwaves, radar and low-energy light) disperse energy through heat and increased molecular movement, electromagnetic ionising radiation (X- and gamma rays) can separate molecules or remove electrons from atoms. Other forms of ionising radiation include subatomic particles, such as alpha particles, protons and beta particles, that is, electrically charged particles, and neutrons.

Ionisation is only the initial step in the breaking of chemical bonds, the production of free radicals, biochemical change and molecular damage such as mutations, chromosome aberrations, protein denaturation and eventually disruption of biological processes including missing or abnormal reproductive capacity and cell killing.

Radiation can be distinguished on the basis of different characteristics including origin, physical properties and energy. The effects of radiation will also depend on the physical mass of the target and on the number and frequency of hits on the target. Also, the intrinsic properties of the target determine the outcome of the irradiation. When an entire organism is hit, the effects vary depending on the maturation stage of the components of the organism.

Finally, while the biochemical effects due to irradiation initiate at the time of the interaction of radiation with the biological target, the full appearance of the consequent effects may be delayed for as much as several years.

Normal exposure to radiation can occur as a result of environmental exposure, due to natural and man-made background radiation, and after medical exposure. It can occur as a result of diagnostic procedures, by X-ray or nuclear medicine examination, entailing the use of radiopharmaceuticals emitting mainly gamma rays, and either as a result of radiation therapy with X-rays and electron beams produced by accelerators or after the administration of radioactive elements emitting mainly beta radiation.

2.2 Types of Radiation and Interactions Between Radiation and Matter

Ionising radiation consists of particles and electromagnetic radiation. The particles are electrons, protons, neutrons and alpha particles (composed of 2 protons and 2 neutrons). Electromagnetic radiation includes X- and gamma rays. The interaction of radiation with biological matter entails the dispersion of radiation energy by deposition in the matter. The pattern of distribution of energy in tissues and cells affects the extent of biological damage following the irradiation. The quantity of energy which is deposited into the tissue depends on the linear energy transfer (LET), that is, the amount of energy deposited per unit of path (normally expressed in keV/μm of water). Large amounts of energy can be deposited along a short track, in a few cells, by high-LET radiation, such as the alpha particles (whose LET is on the order of 100 keV/μm), which hardly penetrate tissues. Conversely, a small amount of energy is deposited along the path by low-LET (approximately 3.5 keV/μm), highly penetrating electromagnetic radiation, including X- and gamma rays. In the case of low-LET radiation the energy deposition occurs in points that are distant from each other and only a few ionisations result from a single X- or gamma ray. In biological terms it is concluded that high-LET radiation causes more molecular damage per unit of dose than low-LET radiation. This appears to be related to the higher concentration of energy depositions from a single particle in a single cell and also to so-called bystander effects, namely, the response of cells which are not directly hit by radiation but in which there is a gene induction by adjacent irradiated cells and the production of genetic changes which are potentially carcinogenic.

A very conservative approach assumes no dose threshold for the occurrence of biological effects of radiation and assumes that even exposure to background radiation can have a biological effect. Current radiation risk estimates and radiation protection standards and practices are based on the "linear no-threshold (LNT) hypothesis" based mainly on epidemiological data of human subjects exposed to high doses and dose rates, which maintains that any exposure to radiation, even at very low doses, may be harmful and extrapolates low-dose effects from known high-dose effects. This hypothesis states that risk is linearly proportional to dose, without a threshold. It is therefore assumed that every dose, no matter how low, carries with it some risk, that risk per unit dose is constant, additive and can only increase with dose and that biological responses, when apparent, are independent of the dose.

There is no complete agreement about the validity of the "LNT hypothesis" Alternative models in which thresholds do exist have been developed. This view maintains that some doses of radiation do not produce harmful health effects. One definition of low dose is a dose below which it is not possible to detect adverse health effects. This level has been hypothesised to be at 100 mSv (10,000 mrem). Others suggest that such a level is much too high and a more conservative definition of low dose is the level of radiation from the natural background, around or below 4 mSv. Low-dose studies are currently being conducted to investigate the response of cells and molecules. Current knowledge seems to suggest that health risks are either too small to be observed or are nonexistent for doses below 50–100 mSv and that radiation doses that are of a magnitude similar to those received from natural sources encompass a range of hypothetical outcomes, including a lack of adverse health effects. Finally, after exposures to low levels of ionising radiation it is not possible to detect a change in cancer incidence. This is related to the many factors which can produce cancer, the high incidence of cancers in the general population, and the high variable background levels of radiation exposure in the population.

The first physical event for the induction of biochemical alterations following radiation exposure is the ionisation of atoms encountered by radiation along their path. The removal of the electron by ionising radiation entails the formation of ions which tend to react with surrounding atoms and molecules to reach a stable state and the formation of free radicals, that is, unstable and highly reactive molecules, bearing an atom with an unpaired electron, which reacts with a variety of organic structures. Free radicals, in the form of potent oxidising agents such as hydroxyl and hydroperoxyl groups, can originate from the interaction of ionising radiation with water. Thus ionising radiation acts either directly with the biochemical structures in tissue, including proteins, DNA and other molecules, or indirectly by causing the formation of free radicals, from interaction with water, which in turn break the structure of proteins and DNA or any other critical part of the cell. DNA damage is the most critical event in the case of irradiation of the cell and large amounts of DNA damage are caused by free radicals soon after single, acute exposures to high radiation doses. This damage occurs in multiple sites in individual cells. It is not repaired easily, may be incorrectly repaired and can induce mutations and cancer.

There are different outcomes following the exposure of cells to radiation. First, cells may be undamaged by the irradiation. This is the case after ionisations which lead to the formation of substances that in some cases alter the structure of the cells, but such alterations may be the same as those which occur naturally in the cell and may have no negative effect. Second, cells may be damaged but operate normally after the repair of the damage. This process occurs when the ionising event produces abnormal substances not usually found in the cell which may break down the cell components. In this case repair is possible if the damage is limited. Chromosome damage is usually repaired constantly by effective mechanisms. Third, cells may be damaged and operate abnormally after failure to repair or defective repair of the damage. This means that they will be unable to perform their function correctly or completely. This may result in a limited damage to cell performance or in damage to other cells. Cell damage may result in a defective reproduction, including uncontrolled reproduction rate and cancer. Fourth, cells may die as a result of the damage. If a cell is extensively damaged by radiation, or damaged in such a way that reproduction is affected, the cell may die.

Radiation damage to cells may depend on how sensitive the cells are to radiation. Cells are not equally sensitive to radiation. In general, cell populations which divide rapidly and/or are relatively non-specialised tend to produce effects at lower doses of radiation than those which are less rapidly dividing and more specialised. Examples of the more sensitive cells are those of the haematopoietic system; in fact, the most sensitive biological indicator of radiation exposure is the effect of radiation on this system.

As is well known, the exposure of human beings to ionising radiation can produce two types of biological effects, depending on the dose: deterministic and stochastic effects. The deterministic effects are those produced by the reduction or the loss of functionality of an organ or a tissue. They are caused by severe cellular damage or even by the death of the cells and are characterised by a "threshold dose" and by a severity which increases with increasing dosage. The stochastic effects, on the other hand, are those caused by radiation-induced modifications of cells, which maintain their capability for replication. In the course of time, these modified cells can undergo a transformation into malignant cells. These stochastic effects do not have a threshold dose, but the probability of their appearance—though not their severity—depends on the dose, according to a simple model recognised by ICRP (ICRP Publication 60, 1991). A no-threshold linear relation between the dose and the probability of appearance of the effects is assumed. This means that even very small doses can give rise to very severe effects, both somatic and genetic, although the probability is very small (Fig. 2.1).

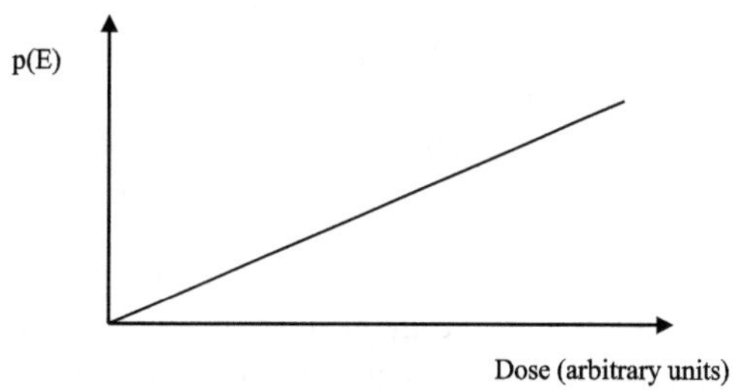

Fig. 2.1 LNT (linear no-threshold) model for stochastic effects

2.3 Radiation Effects on the Embryo/Foetus

The irradiation of the embryo/foetus during pregnancy can, in principle, cause the death of the embryo or increase the risk of somatic effects in the newborn child, such as an increase of leukaemia in children irradiated in the uterus. These possible effects were demonstrated by some pioneering epidemiological studies (Stewart 1956; Mac Mahon 1962). In recent years, however, a study performed in Sweden, comparing 652 children exposed to diagnostic X-ray examinations during their mother's pregnancy and diagnosed with leukaemia between 1973 and 1989 with an equivalent group of healthy children, did not reveal a statistically significant risk of childhood leukaemia in the irradiated children (Helmrot et al. 2007).

Depending on the damage produced by the irradiation on the cell components—DNA versus non-DNA, type of cell irradiated (i.e., somatic versus germinal) and timing of exposure (i.e., before or after conception)—the following effects can occur: somatic, genetic, and teratogenic. Somatic effects are those produced in the individual who undergoes the irradiation. Genetic effects are those produced in the offspring of the individuals who have undergone the irradiation before the conception of the offspring. Teratogenic effects are those produced in the offspring of the individual who has undergone irradiation after conception, that is, during the gestation period.

While no diagnostic procedure based on the use of low-dose ionising radiation is threatening to the well-being of the embryo and foetus, possible adverse effects on the embryo and foetus may derive from high doses of ionising radiation delivered to women being treated with radiation therapy for cancer. However, these doses are much higher than those used for diagnostic purposes. Congenital birth defects all seem to have a threshold dose of about 100 mGy (equivalent to 100 mSv) below which there are no measurable effects.

Almost always, if a diagnostic radiology examination is medically justified, the risk to the mother of not undergoing the procedure is greater than the risk of potential harm to the foetus. Foetal doses below 100 mGy should not be considered a reason for terminating a pregnancy. At foetal doses above this level, informed decisions should be made based upon individual circumstances. Termination of pregnancy is an individual's decision, affected by many factors.

As the sensitivity of a tissue to radiation is broadly proportional to its rate of proliferation, the human embryo/foetus which is in the stage of fast growth rate is more sensitive to radiation than the completely formed organism. Any type of diagnostic and therapeutic irradiation requires a careful evaluation of the risks and also extremely careful planning. It is possible to examine the effects of the exposure to ionising radiation of the foetus and embryo according to the type of procedure, either diagnostic or therapeutic, based on the classification of the effects of radiation as deterministic or stochastic.

Doses reached with properly executed diagnostic procedures (i.e. below 100 mGy) do not entail increased risk of deterministic effects, including either prenatal death or malformation or mental retardation compared to the background incidence of these entities (Naumburg 2001). However, with doses below 100 mGy stochastic effects are possible, though improbable.

Therapeutic doses instead may result in deterministic and stochastic effects. It is therefore important to ascertain whether a patient is pregnant before radiotherapy, and in case of pregnancy the risk of radiotherapy for the foetus must then be assessed based on gestational age and dose to the foetus. The latter largely depends on the region being irradiated by an external beam or by the biodistribution of the radiotracer when the irradiation occurs after the administration of a radiopharmaceutical for radio-metabolic therapy.

In human subjects, the main deleterious effects of embryonic and foetal irradiation at therapeutic doses consist of deterministic effects—foetal wastage (miscarriage), teratogenicity, mental retardation, intra-uterine growth retardation—and stochastic effects—the induction of cancers (such as leukaemia) which appear in childhood. The risk of occurrence of the above varies in relation to the timing of exposure during gestation.

During the early stages of foetal development

radiation exposure results in the death of cells which are critical to normal development. Loss of these cells results in the death of the foetus. Thus exposure during early foetal development does not result in defects but causes an increase in early spontaneous abortions. Between the 8th and the 25th week of gestation, the most concerning risk of foetal irradiation is the damage of the central nervous system and foetal doses higher than 100 mGy may result in mental retardation. The central nervous system is most sensitive between the 8th and the 15th week of gestation; during this time a foetal dose of 1,000 mGy entails the risk of severe mental retardation, that is, an IQ reduction of 30 points, or approximately 40%. Mental retardation may also occur between the 16th and 25th weeks with doses higher than 1,000 mGy, since below this threshold this risk is very low.

Stochastic effects, including the risks of developing various types of cancers, may follow the exposure of the embryo/foetus. It has been estimated that the absolute risk for fatal cancer in the age range 0–15 years after intra-uterine irradiation could be 0.006%/mGy, and for the entire life span the risk could be approximately 0.015%/mGy.

2.4 Diagnostic Imaging: Radiology and Nuclear Medicine

The problem of the newborn's risk due to diagnostic X-ray and nuclear medicine examinations during pregnancy was thoroughly examined by Directive MED 100 of the European Commission (European Commission 1999). Article 3 of this Directive states that all medical exposure of individuals must be justified, in view of the specific diagnostic objectives, taking into account the availability of previous diagnostic information and the possible use of alternatives to exposure of the patient to ionising radiation. In the case of the use of ionising radiation, the examination must be optimised, so as to obtain the requested diagnostic information with a dose "as low as reasonably achievable". In cases where pregnancy cannot be excluded, particular attention must be given to the justification, with particular regard to its urgency. After an estimate of the dose and of the corresponding risk by a medical physicist, the mother must be carefully informed about benefits and risk and she must decide whether or not to undergo the examination.

2.4.1 "Rules of Behaviour" for Patients of Fertile Age

In most radiological examinations in which the uterus and the pelvis are not exposed directly to the X-ray beam the dose to the uterus, and to the foetus in case of pregnancy, due partly to the leakage radiation from the X-ray tube housing and partly to the internally scattered radiation, is lower than 1 mSv (Wachsmann and Drexler 1976). In these situations no specific procedure for radiological protection is generally necessary. However, shielding of the abdomen with a lead-rubber apron, having an equivalent thickness of 0.5 mm Pb, can significantly reduce the dose received due to leakage radiation from the X-ray tube housing, but not the dose due to the scattered radiation inside the patient's body (Fig. 2.2). Use of the apron is not recommended for dental examination, where the tube is far from the abdomen.

In the case of radiological examinations in which the uterus is exposed to the primary beam or in which the uterus itself can receive a dose higher than 1 mSv, it is mandatory for a female patient aged between 12 and 50 years to be explicitly asked whether she is pregnant or is not sure she is not pregnant. It is advisable, for medico-legal purposes, to register the result of this enquiry and to ask the patient to sign it. If the patient is not sure of not being pregnant a pregnancy test could be prescribed or, if the examination is not urgent and can be deferred, the examination could be postponed until immediately after the subsequent menstruation. In general, only in the case of examinations delivering a high dose to the uterus can it be recommended to apply the so-called "10 days rule" according to which these examinations can be performed within the first 10 days after the beginning of menstruation, when pregnancy, in most cases, can be excluded. In very rare cases, however, there is the possibility of a "false menstruation" or an initial pregnancy.

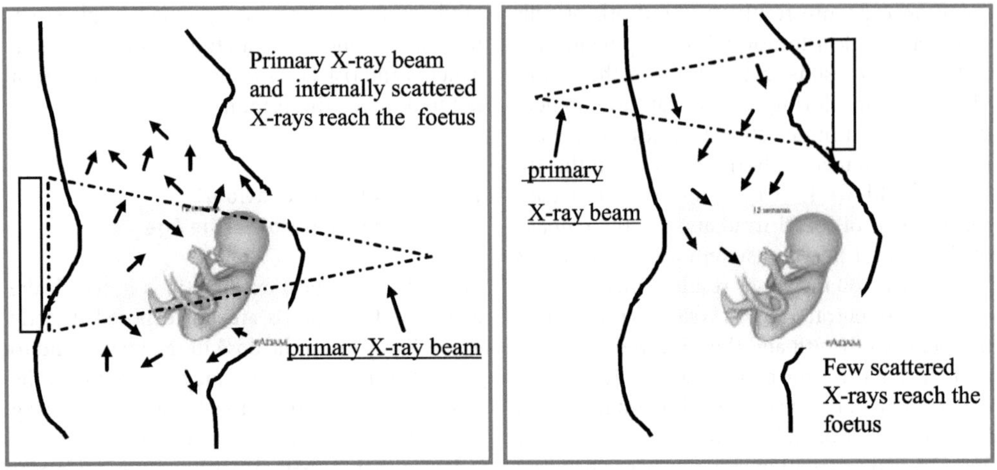

Fig. 2.2 Source of dose to the foetus during radiological examinations during pregnancy

Irradiation of the foetus from maternal intake of radiopharmaceuticals may be due to radiopharmaceuticals that do not cross the placenta and remain in the mother's circulation. Under this circumstance irradiation of the foetus occurs if the radiation penetrates through tissues, as is the case for most commonly used diagnostic radiopharmaceuticals. Alternatively, the foetus can be irradiated by radiopharmaceuticals that cross the placenta and enter into the foetal circulation. In this case they may either distribute uniformly or concentrate in the foetal organs according to their kinetics and to the state of maturation of the different organs.

Among the radiopharmaceuticals that cross the placenta are radiostrontium, radioiodine, radioiron, inert gases, gallium and technetium pertechnetate, whereas many other technetium-labelled compounds may or may not cross the placenta.

Nuclear medicine procedure entails an absorbed dose which derives from the external irradiation from the radiotracer in the circulation of the mother's body plus the dose due to the foetal uptake of radiotracer. Depending upon the timing and route of excretion (urinary system, gallbladder and intestine, lungs, etc.), irradiation from these sources may vary a great deal, being highest for radiotracers which are cleared via the urinary system mostly because of accumulation of radioactivity in the bladder. One particular case is represented by the irradiation by radioactive iodine; in fact, this element crosses the placenta and accumulates in the foetal thyroid after the 12th week of gestation. Therapeutic doses of radioiodine entail a significant risk of foetal thyroid damage after the 12th week of gestation. Hydration and voiding along with the administration of potassium iodide may keep the total foetal absorbed dose below 100 mGy.

2.4.2 "Rules of Behaviour" for Pregnant Patients

If a radiological examination involving the direct irradiation of the embryo or of the foetus is requested, it is recommended that the radiologist follow the procedures listed below:

- Evaluate the possibility of obtaining the required diagnostic information by means of other techniques not involving the use of ionising radiation, such as ultrasonography or MR.
- If other techniques are not able to give the requested information and if the diagnosis is not immediately and urgently indispensable, put off the execution of the examination until after birth.
- In the case when immediate examination is indispensable (such as in case of a suspected

malignant tumour or after a serious car crash) proceed as follows:

- Take all possible technical measures to reduce the dose.
- Ask a medical physicist to make a preliminary evaluation of the dose to the foetus.
- Give the mother exhaustive and convincing information about the dose and the corresponding risk.
- If the mother is unable to decide because of her clinical condition but requires immediate action, follow the recommendations of the responsible physician. In these cases, an accurate evaluation of the dose and a consequent estimation of the risk are highly recommended.
- If possible, measure the dose during the examination and register its value on the report.

2.4.3 Radiological Protection of the Unborn Child

When an examination or an interventional procedure directly involving the abdomen/the foetus, which is exposed both to the primary beam and to the internally scattered radiation, is indispensable, the following measures can significantly reduce the dose.

2.4.3.1 Fluoroscopy

- Reduce, as much as possible, the duration of observation.
- Use equipment able to deliver pulsed fluoroscopy.
- Reduce the X-ray tube current (mA) to the minimum value able to give an acceptable image contrast.
- Reduce the beam's cross section to the minimum value compatible with effective imaging of the region.

2.4.3.2 Radiography

- Use, if available, digital systems, setting the milliampere values at the minimum level.
- Reduce the beam's cross section, as in the case of fluoroscopy.
- Select radiographic projections able, if possible, to avoid the greatest part of the body of the foetus.
- Take the minimum number of radiographic images.

2.4.3.3 Computed Tomography

Computed tomography (CT) is a high-dose X-ray procedure. It is possible to reduce the dose:

- By avoiding, if possible, the acquisition of images after the injection of contrast medium.
- By using, with MSCT equipment, low-dose protocols, based on "dose modulation".
- By reducing as much as possible the number of acquired slices, that is, the extension of the acquired volume in the cranial-caudal direction.

2.4.3.4 Nuclear Medicine Procedures

The absorbed dose derives from the irradiation due to the radiotracer in the circulation of the mother's body plus the dose due to the foetal uptake of radiotracer. It is possible to reduce the dose:

- By avoiding radiopharmaceuticals that concentrate in the pelvis, abdomen and bladder.
- By choosing the radionuclide that results in the lowest dose.
- For tracers that are eliminated via the kidneys, by forcing fluids and inducing bladder emptying.
- By avoiding radiopharmaceuticals that cross the placental barrier.
- By distinguishing between indicated, elective, urgent and unwarranted studies, in particular in the case of pulmonary thromboembolism.

2.4.3.5 Radiological Examination Accidentally Performed on a Pregnant Woman

Cases of radiological examinations performed on women whose pregnancy was unknown are not rare. In this situation, the patient, upon becoming aware of her pregnancy, is frequently very anxious for her child and reverts immediately to the physician (the gynaecologist more frequently than the radiologist) for advice. The gynaecologist (or any other physician consulted by the patient) should ask the radiologist together with a medical physicist to immediately evaluate the dose to the foetus. If the uterus was not in the primary X-ray beam, or if the evaluated dose was less than 1 mSv, no particular measure must be taken regardless of the period of pregnancy, and the patient should be completely reassured.

On the other hand, if the dose is higher than 1 mSv but less than 50 mSv, the patient should be informed that the radiation risk is as low as the "natural" risk of having a child with some minor or major abnormality (approximately equal to 3%).

For doses between 50 and 100 mSv the risk is small, but not negligible, while for doses to the foetus higher than 100 mSv, particularly if received during the first 3 months of pregnancy, a deterministic effect can take place. In any case, this situation is extremely rare (an exception is CT of the abdominal-pelvic region with and without contrast medium), and the decision on abortion should be left to the patient and taken only in extreme cases.

2.4.3.6 Dosimetric Quantities

The most important dosimetric quantity used in the radiological protection is the *absorbed dose* (D), defined as the mean energy dε imparted by an ionising radiation to a quantity of matter of mass dm.

$$D = d\varepsilon / dm$$

In the SI, its unit is joules per kilogram (J/kg). The special name of this unit is *gray* (Gy):

$$1 \text{ Gy} = 1 \text{ J/kg}$$

The biological effects produced in tissues and organs by exposure to ionising radiation are linked not only to the absorbed dose (which is a mere physical quantity) but also to the type of radiation: In other words, some radiation is more effective than others, at equal dose, in producing biological effects. For this reason, another dosimetric quantity has been introduced, named the *equivalent dose* (H_T) and defined as the mean energy absorbed in a tissue or in an organ T, multiplied by a dimensionless weighting factor w_R, whose value depends on the type and energy of the radiation:

$$H_T = W_R \times D$$

The unit of equivalent dose is named the *sievert* (Sv):

$$1 \text{ Sv} = 1 \text{ Gy} \times W_R = 1 \text{ J/kg} \times W_R$$

For the X-rays employed in diagnostic radiology, the weighting factor w_R is equal to 1. Therefore, the numerical values of the absorbed dose and the equivalent dose are the same. However, in the field of radiological protection, in order to have the possibility of comparing and, if necessary, of adding the doses due to different sources of exposure, it is usual to express all the doses in sieverts (Sv).

In modern radiological equipment a "dosimetric device" to measure a "dose descriptor" is installed as shown in Fig. 2.3, allowing easy evaluation of the dose to the patient and, if necessary, to the foetus.

The dose-area product (*DAP*) is defined as the product of the dose by the cross-sectional area of the beam along its path at the distance of measurement and is usually expressed in grays times square centimeter. The value of this "dose descriptor", measured by a transmission ionisation chamber transparent to the light, does not depend on the distance between the chamber and the focus of the X-ray tube. In fact, the dose at a point at a given distance *d* from the focus is inversely proportional to the square of the distance, while the cross-sectional area of the beam is directly proportional to the square of the distance itself. The product of the two quantities therefore remains constant along the whole beam's path. For practical reasons, the DAP camera, which is able to integrate the DAP during a whole radiological examination, is mounted after the diaphragms, in correspondence with the exit window of the beam from the X-ray tube housing.

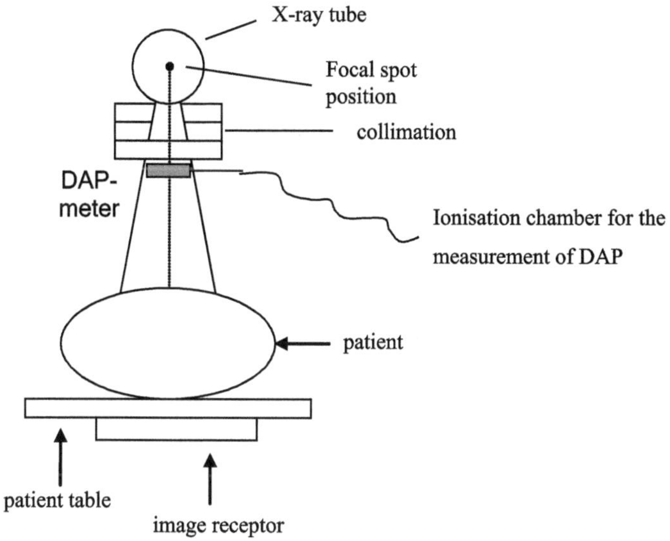

Fig. 2.3 DAP meter

This quantity is a very good and reliable "dose descriptor" since it takes into account both the dose and the area of the beam.

In CT, in order to allow the evaluation of the dose to the patient, a specific "dose descriptor" has been defined. It is called the computed tomography dose index (*CTDI*) and is defined as:

$$CTDI = \int_{-50\,mm}^{+50\,mm} \frac{D(z)}{N \times T} dz$$

that is, as the integral of the dose profile, from -50 mm to +50 mm, produced in a single axial scanning, along a line perpendicular to the tomographic plane, divided by the product of the number of tomographic sections N by the nominal slice thickness. The unit of CTDI is the gray (Gy). According to the IEC standards (IEC 2004), the value of the CTDI for each protocol of CT acquisitions must be displayed on the control panel of the equipment.

Many computer programs are available (CT Expo V.1.5 2001–2005), allowing the evaluation of the dose to the uterus and/ or foetus, starting from the value of the CTDI and from other technical parameters of the CT examination.

The *output of the X-ray tubes*, or the "amount of radiation" produced by an X-ray tube, substantially depends on the following parameters:

- X-ray tube voltage (kV);
- X-ray tube current (mA);
- Duration of exposure (s);
- Filtration of the X-ray beam (mm Al).

Because of the divergence of the beam, the intensity of the X-ray beam at a given distance *d* from the focus of the tube (expressed for instance in mGy/min) is inversely proportional to the square of the distance. In Table 2.1, the corresponding values at two different distances (SSD = 50 and 100 cm) are reported. Starting from these data and taking into account the exposure data used for the examination, the dose to the uterus/foetus can be easily calculated (see, for instance, NCPRP Report No. 54 1977).

In modern radiological equipment, where a DAP meter is installed, it is very easy to evaluate the dose to the foetus D_f by using an appropriate conversion factor C_{conv}, according to the following relation:

$$D_f = C_{conv} \times DAP$$

Table 2.2 shows the dose to the uterus/foetus evaluated starting from the DAP value (Helmrot et al. 2007).

In Table 2.3 an estimate of the dose to the foetus in the more common radiological examination is reported (De Maria et al. 1999).

Table 2.1 Output of X-ray tubes as a function of the following parameters: X-ray tube voltage, total filtration, distance from focus

SSD (cm)	Total Filtration (mm Al)	Dose rate in air (cGy/mA.min) X-ray tube voltage (kV) 60	80	100	120	150
50	2.0	0.92	1.92	2.98	5.08	9.86
	2.5	0.76	1.68	2.67	4.54	8.45
	3.0	0.64	1.42	2.40	4.02	7.04
100	2.0	0.23	0.48	0.74	1.27	2.46
	2.5	0.19	0.42	0.67	1.13	2.11
	3.0	0.16	0.36	0.60	1.00	1.76

Table 2.2 Dose to the uterus/foetus evaluated starting from the DAP value

Examination	DAP (Gy cm²)	Calculated uterus dose (PCXMC) (mGy)	Calculated uterus dose (WinDOS) (mGy)	Measured uterus dose (mGy)	Conversion factor, C_{conv} (foetus age <3 months) [mGy/(Gycm²)]	Conversion factor, C_{conv} (foetus age <9 months) [mGy/(Gycm²)]
Abdomen	0.79	0.40	0.38	0.44	0.56	1.1
Abdomen lower frontal single view	0.254	0.25	0.31	0.31	1.22	1.2
Abdomen	1.28	0.84	0.92	0.63	0.49	1.6
Chest bed side (AP)	0.028	<0.001	<0.001	<0.001	<0.04	0.4
Chest (PA + LAT)	0.086	<0.001	<0.001	0.001	0.01	1.0
Hip frontal	0.43	0.02	0.3	0.12	0.28	0.6
Lumbar spine	2.71	1.49	2.08/1.38[(a)]	1.38	0.51	1.5
L5 frontal single view	0.682	0.54	1.01/0.31[(a)]	0.91	1.33	3.8
Lumbar spine	4.15	2.01	1.51	1.75	0.42	1.2
Pelvis	1.22	0.67	0.9	0.72	0.59	0.8
Pelvis	1.28	0.85	1.06	0.66	0.52	1.2
Urography	6.01	4.0	4.6	2.8	0.47	2.5
Barium enema	20.2	12.3[(b)]	13.0[(b)]	7.8	0.39	1.3

In nuclear medicine procedures the dose depends on biological factors, including biological half-life and fraction of total taken up by each organ, and physical factors, including amount, type and physical half-life. Each organ (including the foetus) is irradiated by the radioactive source inside the organ itself plus the dose from the surrounding irradiating organs.

Table 2.3 Dose to the foetus in the more common radiological examinations

Dose to the foetus (mSv)		
Type of examination	Mean value/probability of induction of a lethal tumour	Max value
Skull	<0.01/–	
Lungs	<0.01/–	<0.01
Abdomen (only AP)	$1.40/7.1 \times 10^{-5}$	<0.01
Barium enema	$6.80/3.4 \times 10^{-4}$	4.2
Thoracic spine	<0.01/–	24
Lumbar spine	$1.70/8.3 \times 10^{-5}$	<0.01
Digestive tract	$1.10/5.5 \times 10^{-5}$	5.8
Pelvis	$1.10/5.5 \times 10^{-5}$	4.0
Urography enhanced nephrographic/pielographic	$1.70/8.3 \times 10^{-5}$	10
CT	$15.00/7.5 \times 10^{-4}$	50
Brain and skull	<0.005/–	<0.005
Lung and thorax	0.06/–	0.96
Pelvis	$25/1.25 \times 10^{-3}$	79
Abdomen	$8/4 \times 10^{-4}$	49

Table 2.4. Fetal whole body dose from common nuclear medicine examinations in early pregnancy and at term

Radiopharmaceutical	Procedure	Administered activity (MBq)	Early (mGy)	9 months (mGy)
^{99m}Tc	Bone scan (phosphate)	750	4.6–4.7	1.8
^{99m}Tc	Lung perfusion (MAA)	200	0.4–0.6	0.8
^{99m}Tc	Lung ventilation (aerosol)	40	0.1–0.3	0.1
^{99m}Tc	Thyroid scan (pertechnetate)	400	3.2–4.4	3.7
^{99m}Tc	Red blood cell	930	3.6–6.0	2.5
^{99m}Tc	Liver colloid	300	0.5–0.6	1.1
^{99m}Tc	Renal DTPA	750	5.9–9.0	3.5
^{67}Ga	Abscess/tumour	190	14–18	25
^{123}I	Thyroid uptake	30	0.4–0.6	0.3
^{131}I	Thyroid uptake	0.55	0.03–0.04	0.15
^{131}I	Metastases imaging	40	2.0–2.9	11.0

DTPA, diethylenetriamine pentaacetic acid; *MAA*, macroaggregated albumin

The radiation absorbed by a region, organ or foetus is the sum of the contributions from all sources around it and not only from the target organ. Foetal whole body doses from common nuclear medicine examinations in early pregnancy and at term are reported in Table 2.4.

2.5 Radiotherapy

During pregnancy, cancers which are remote from the pelvis usually can be adequately treated with radiotherapy, based on careful planning. This is not the case for cancers located in the pelvis, which cannot be irradiated without severe or, more probably, lethal consequences for the foetus.

2.5.1 Before Treatment

Since foetal doses in radiotherapy can be high, it is important to ascertain whether a female patient is pregnant before radiotherapy.

Pregnancy status may be ascertained on the basis of history, patient age and prior surgery (such as a hysterectomy or tubal ligation) or through the use of a pregnancy test. Even if a radiotherapy patient is not pregnant, she should be counselled to avoid pregnancy until the potentially harmful radiotherapeutical treatment or other treatment modalities are concluded and the tumour is cured or adequately controlled. If a patient is found to be pregnant, the decision relative to the treatment course should be an informed one made by the patient, her partner, or other appropriate person(s), the treating oncologist and other team members (e.g. surgeons, obstetricians, pharmacologists and others such as psychologists). The factors to be considered are many but include at least:

- Stage and aggressiveness of the tumour;
- Potential hormonal effects of pregnancy on the tumour;
- Various therapies and their length, efficacy and complications;
- Impact of delaying therapy;
- Expected effects of maternal ill-health on the foetus;
- Stage of pregnancy;
- Foetal assessment and monitoring;
- How and when the baby could be safely delivered;
- Whether the pregnancy should be terminated;
- Legal, ethical and moral issues.

While it is difficult to generalise about the adverse effects of chemotherapy agents administered during the first trimester of pregnancy, with some drugs up to 10% of exposed foetuses exhibit major malformations. After the first trimester, chemotherapy is not usually associated with teratogenesis or adverse developmental outcome. There is some suggestion that in utero exposure to chemotherapeutic agents may cause an increase in the risk of pancytopaenia at birth and possibly subsequent neoplasms in the offspring.

The risks of surgery and anaesthesia during pregnancy are well known and the major problems are associated with hypotension, hypoxia and infection. Maternal well-being should also be considered. Many cancer patients have fever or infections as a result of the tumour or immunosuppression. There may be an association between hyperthermia and teratogenic effects such as neural tube defects and microphthalmia. The other additional maternal problem that can affect the foetus is malnutrition.

2.5.2 During Radiotherapy

Radiotherapy to non-pelvic fields during pregnancy can be performed, but it requires careful estimation of foetal dose and may require additional shielding. A number of cancers occur during pregnancy in locations other than the pelvis or abdomen. Breast cancers complicate about one out of 3,000 pregnancies. This may be treated in a number of ways, including with radiotherapy. Fortunately, the radiotherapy is delivered to sites quite distant from the foetus. Usually during radiotherapy a high-risk obstetrical unit follows such women.

Lymphomas are also relatively common during the reproductive years. Literature in the early 1980s suggested the need for a therapeutic abortion if these diseases appeared early in pregnancy. Now lymphomas can be effectively treated with chemotherapy, and radiotherapy may not be needed at all or may possibly be delayed until late in pregnancy or until after pregnancy.

If radiotherapy is used, it is important to calculate the dose to the foetus before the treatments are given. When external radiotherapy is utilised for treatment of tumours at some distance from the foetus, the most important factor in foetal dose is the distance from the edge of the radiation field. The dose decreases approximately exponentially with distance. Foetal doses below 100 mGy should not be considered a reason for terminating a pregnancy. At foetal doses above this level, informed decisions should be made based upon individual circumstances. Foetal doses for a typical photon treatment regimen for brain cancer are in the range of 30 mGy. For anterior and posterior mantle treatments of the chest for Hodgkin disease, the dose to portions of an unshielded foetus can be 400–500 mGy. With ^{60}Co, at distances greater than 10 cm from the field the dose is higher than with X-ray beams produced by linear accelerators, because of the leakage from the machine head, the side-scattering and the size of the source (1.5–2.5 cm). The dose distribution outside of the primary radiation beam may vary among therapy units, such as linear accelerators, of the same nominal type and energy, as well as with field size. As a result, therapy unit-specific measurements should be made.

Usually, treatment planning software programs are very accurate for estimation of tissue dose in the primary treatment field, but uncertainties are much greater at distances outside the field (for example, at 1 m). In these cases, when dose estimation to peripheral tissues is important, phantom measurements and in vivo dosimetry are usually used.

Additional shielding can reduce the foetal dose by 50%. However, effective shielding often weighs on the order of 200 kg. It can exceed the design limits for many treatment tables and may cause injury to the patient or technician if not properly constructed and handled.

The American Association of Physicists in Medicine (AAPM) has made a series of recommendations (Stovall et al. 1995), which provide points to be considered. Complete all planning as though the patient was not pregnant and as if the foetus is near the treatment beam and do not take portal localisation films with open collimation and blocks removed.

Further recommendations include:

- Medical professionals using radiation should be familiar with the effects of radiation on the embryo and foetus. At most diagnostic levels this would include risk of childhood cancer, while at doses in excess of 100–200 mGy risks related to nervous system abnormalities, malformations, growth retardation and foetal death should be considered. The magnitude of these latter risks differs quite considerably between the various stages of pregnancy.
- All medical practices (both occupational and patient related) involving radiation exposure should be justified (i.e. result in more benefit than risk). Medical exposures should also be justified on an individual basis. This includes considerations balancing medical needs against potential radiation risks. This is done by using judgement rather than numerical calculations. Medical exposure of pregnant women poses a different benefit/risk situation than most other medical exposures. In most medical exposures the benefit and risk are to the same individual. In the situation of in utero medical exposure there are two different entities (the mother and the foetus) who must be considered.
- Before radiation exposure, female patients in the childbearing age group should be evaluated and an attempt should be made to determine who is or could be pregnant.
- Medical radiation applications should be optimised to achieve the clinical purposes with no more radiation than is necessary, given the available resources and technology. If possible, for pregnant patients, the medical procedures should be tailored to reduce foetus dose.
- After medical procedures involving high doses of radiation have been performed on pregnant patients, foetus dose and potential foetus risk should be estimated.
- Pregnant medical radiation workers may work in a radiation environment as long as there is reasonable assurance that the foetal dose can be kept below 100 mGy during the course of pregnancy.
- Radiation research involving pregnant patients should be discouraged.
- Termination of pregnancy at foetal doses of less than 100 mGy is not justified based upon radiation risk. At higher foetal doses, informed decisions should be made based upon individual circumstances.
- Modifications to the treatment plan which would reduce the radiation dose to the foetus by changing field size, angle, radiation energy and field trimmers on the edge nearest the foetus should be considered. If possible use photon energies of less than 25 MV.

- Estimate the dose to the foetus without special shielding, using out-of-beam phantom measurements at the symphysis pubis, fundus and a midpoint.
- If foetal dose is above 50–100 mGy, a shield may be constructed with 4–5 half-value layers of lead. Measure dose to the foetus in a phantom for simulated treatment with the shielding in place, adjusting radiation amount and location.
- Document the treatment plan and discuss it with the staff involved in patient set-up. Document the shielding (perhaps with a photograph).
- Check weight and load-bearing specifications of the treatment couch or other aspects of shielding support. Be present during initial treatment to ensure that shielding is correctly placed. Monitor the foetal size and growth throughout the course of treatment and reassess foetal dose if necessary.
- At completion of treatment, document total dose including range of dose to the foetus during therapy.
- Consider referring the patient to another institution if equipment and personnel are not available for reducing and estimating the foetal dose.

The radiation risk for fatal cancer is conservatively assumed to be 0.6% per 100-mGy foetal dose, corresponding to about 1/17,000 per mGy and a linear dose-response relationship, but many epidemiological studies suggest that the risk may be lower than that assumed here.

Although the exact risk in humans is uncertain, animal data suggest that malformations due to radiation are not likely at doses less than 100–200 mGy. Moreover, these malformations would only be observed if exposure were between the 3rd and 25th weeks of gestation. The risk of malformation is low at 100–200 mGy but will increase with increasing dose. Decreased IQ and possible retardation are only detectable when foetal doses exceed 100 mGy during the 8th to 25th weeks of gestation.

If the foetal absorbed dose is high, for example, in excess of 500 mGy, and it was absorbed during the 3rd to 16th weeks after conception, there is a substantial chance of growth retardation and central nervous system damage. Although it is possible that the foetus may survive doses in this range, the parents should be informed of the high risks involved.

In the intermediate dose range, 100–500 mGy, the situation is less clear-cut, although such circumstances arise relatively infrequently. In this absorbed dose range the risk of a measurable reduction in IQ must be seriously considered if the foetus was exposed between 8 and 15 weeks of gestational age. In such instances, a qualified biomedical or health physicist should calculate the absorbed foetal dose as accurately as possible, and the physician should ascertain the individual and personal situation of the parents. For example, if the dose to the foetus was estimated to be just above 100 mGy and the parents had been trying to have a child for several years, they may not wish to terminate the pregnancy. This should be a personal decision made by the parents after having been appropriately informed.

Regardless of protective measures, radiotherapy involving the pelvis of a pregnant woman almost always results in severe consequences for the foetus, most likely foetal death. Carcinoma of the cervix is the most common malignancy associated with pregnancy. Cervical cancer complicates about one out of 1,250–2,200 pregnancies. This rate, however, varies significantly by country. Cervical cancer is often treated by surgery and/or radiotherapy and the doses required with both forms of radiotherapy will cause termination of pregnancy. If the tumour is infiltrative and is diagnosed late in pregnancy an alternative is to delay treatment until the baby can be safely delivered. Ovarian cancer is quite rare during pregnancy, complicating less than one in 10,000 pregnancies. Exploratory surgery is usually employed to make the diagnosis. Most patients with ovarian carcinoma are treated with chemotherapy. Radiotherapy is rarely used to treat this tumour during pregnancy.

A brachytherapy patient is often kept in the hospital until the sources are removed. While such a patient can occasionally be a source of radiation to a pregnant visiting family member, the potential dose to the family member's foetus is very low, irrespective of the type of brachytherapy. Prostate brachytherapy can be done with permanent implantation of radioactive ^{198}Au or ^{125}I seeds, and the patient is discharged from the hospital with these in place. The short range of the emissions from these radionuclides allows the patient to be discharged since they pose no danger to pregnant family members.

2.5.3 After Radiotherapy

After radiotherapy involving a pregnant patient, careful records of the treatment and of the foetal dose estimation should be maintained. Since there may be foetal consequences, careful counselling and follow-up is recommended.

Since radiotherapy usually involves treatment over several weeks, pregnancy is usually identified before or during treatment. It is extremely rare for a patient to receive a full treatment course of radiotherapy or brachytherapy and then be discovered to be pregnant afterwards. Even with prior counselling and appropriate shielding during treatment, the patient will often want additional information.

The final estimates of the foetal dose should be calculated and registered. This should include details about the technical factors discussed above. An appropriately trained medical physicist should do such calculations and the mother should be informed about the potential risks. Although local regulations vary, it is often necessary to keep these records for many years and usually until the child becomes an adult.

Occasionally, patients who are not pregnant ask when they can become pregnant after radiotherapy. Most radiation oncologists request that their patients not become pregnant for 1–2 years after completion of therapy. This is not primarily related to concerns about potential radiation effects, but rather to considerations about the risk of relapse of the tumour that would require treatment with radiation, surgery or chemotherapy.

2.5.4 Foetal Dose from Radiotherapy

The most common tumours in pregnant women are lymphomas, leukaemias, melanomas and tumours located in the breast, uterine cervix and thyroid. Radiation therapy is often a treatment of choice for these patients. Each pregnant patient presents a unique set of circumstances which the physician must evaluate before deciding whether and how to treat her. Ideally, the chosen treatment should control the tumour and give the foetus the best chance for a normal life. The challenge is to achieve the optimum balance between the risk and the benefit.

The severity and frequency of adverse effects increase with total dose. Therefore, reduction of foetal dose to a level which as is as low as reasonably achievable is of course advisable to reduce the potential risks to the foetus.

The proper treatment of pregnant women with radiation requires advanced consultation between the radiation oncologist, medical oncologist, obstetrician and medical physicist. Special devices to shield the foetus are often only available at large medical institutions, where only a few such patients may be treated annually. As such, technical resources must be allocated to prepare for these patients or they should be referred to those institutions best equipped to manage their treatment. Peripheral dose directly depends upon beam energy, distance from the treatment volume, field size and, to a much lesser extent, depth. Out-of-beam, patient internal and collimator scatter represent the major contribution to the absorbed dose within 10 cm of the field edge. Patient internal scatter dominates from 10 to 20 cm from the field. Head leakage dominates at approximately 30 cm, with patient internal scatter and head leakage approximately equivalent. The use of blocks and wedges may increase the dose near the field edge by a factor of 2–5. It is imperative that the physicist realise that the shielding can only reduce the components of peripheral dose due to collimator scatter and head leakage.

2.5.4.1 Radiation Dose Outside of Treatment Field

A radiation dose outside of a treatment field is the result of photon leakage from the head of the treatment machine, radiation scattered from the collimators and beam modifiers and radiation scattered from within the patient's treatment volume. Collimator scatter accounts for approximately one-third of the dose and predominates near the field edge, while at greater distances treatment unit head leakage predominates. Near the field edge, peripheral dose increases with increasing field size because of internal scatter. The magnitude of this effect is greatest in the first

10 cm from the edge (factor of 10), then decreases with distance (factor of 2). Collimator scatter plus leakage is approximately equal to patient internal scatter. Head leakage can vary by a factor of two, depending upon vendor design, and the peripheral dose can be reduced by placing a lead shield over the critical area. The use of wedges and other beam modifiers can increase the peripheral dose by a factor of 2–4. As with head leakage and collimator scatter, these components can be reduced by shielding the critical area.

Linear accelerators with photon energies greater than 10 MeV produce neutrons in the accelerating guide, the X-ray target, filters, collimators, and the patient. Near the treatment field the neutron dose is less than 5% of the total peripheral dose. The contribution from neutrons may be up to 40% of the total peripheral dose at a distance of 30 cm from the treatment volume. The contribution of neutrons to total dose increases as the megavoltage is increased from 10 to 20 MV and then remains approximately constant. Specific biological data concerning the risk of neutron exposure to the foetus do not exist. The National Council on Radiation Protection (1980) suggests that a negligible biological risk exists from the exposure to incidental neutrons from linear accelerators. The conservative choice is to treat a pregnant patient with photon energies less than 10 MeV, as long as patient care is not compromised.

Electron beam therapy is conceptually similar to photon beam treatment. Because of lower beam currents, head leakage is a smaller fraction of total dose for electron beams; however, other sources of scatter (collimators, blocks, patient) continue to contribute to the overall total dose. The same type of measurements and shields utilised for photon treatments can be used for electron treatments. Use of the photon shielding for electron treatments will reduce foetal dose by more than 50%, partially due to the electron Bremsstrahlung spectrum having a lower mean energy.

2.5.5 Techniques to Estimate and Reduce Foetal Dose

Gestational age is of primary importance to the treating physician, as discussed in Sect. 2.3. Typical anatomical points utilised for foetal dose estimation are the uterine fundus, symphysis pubis and patient umbilicus. The fundus and pubis delineate the limits of the foetal position and the umbilicus represents a generalised mid-foetal position. It should be remembered that foetal orientation changes frequently and no single point can adequately describe the location of the foetal brain, etc. Treatment modification and shielding devices are the primary methods to reduce foetal dose.

Treatment modification usually consists of a combination of many factors, such as change of the field angles, reduction of the field size, choice of a different beam energy and the use of secondary collimators to define the field edge nearest the foetus. The medical physicist must review all treatment parameters to minimise the risk of injury, to the patient or personnel, when using special shielding. Shielding design must allow for treatment with anterior, posterior and lateral fields, above the diaphragm and the extremities. Two types of shielding arrangements described below. Additional details may be found in the scientific literature.

2.5.5.1 Bridge over Patient

A basic shield design consists of a bridge over the patient's abdomen supporting a block of lead or other shielding material with a thickness of five half-value layers (5HVL), allowing the patient to lie in either a supine or prone position. The superior edge of the block must be positioned as near as possible to the inferior edge of the treatment field. This position easily attenuates much of the dose contribution due to head leakage and collimator scatter. For the treatment of a posterior field, the patient may lie prone on a false table top, with the shielding bridge placed over her back.

2.5.5.2 Mobile Shields

Treatment versatility can be increased by coupling the basic bridge over patient design with a frame which supports the lead block such that it does not rest upon the treatment couch. Additionally, a vertical adjustment motor is added to allow for treatment at source-to-skin distance of 80–125 cm and appropriate wheels are attached to allow for easy movement by the treatment staff. The addition of side shielding allows for the treatment of lateral fields. The weight of such a unit may approach 200 kg; it is therefore indispensable to plan appropriate safety procedures both for the patient and the personnel. For posterior fields, a shield fits between the treatment couch and head of the treatment machine. Although the shield is attached to the treatment couch, the contribution of shield and patient weight typically will not exceed the limits defined by the manufacturer.

2.5.5.3 Dosimetry with Shields

The medical physicist is responsible for estimating the dose to the foetus. Dose estimates often require measurements, either in water, solid phantom or anthropomorphic phantom utilising ionisation chambers, diodes or thermoluminescent dosimeters (TLD). The physicist should first estimate/measure the dose to the foetus without special shielding. Additional dose measurement should then be repeated, using special shields as appropriate. Typical measurement points are the fundus, symphysis pubis and umbilicus. The fundus position moves superiorly, with regard to the pubis, as the pregnancy progresses. This position should be carefully monitored during patient treatment and taken into account when determining the total expected foetal radiation dose. Dosimeters may be placed at these three points on the surface of the patient, on a daily basis, as a method of verifying the phantom dose estimates. However, because the daily doses are quite small, statistical variations may result in a wide range of daily dose measurements. The medical physicist should carefully review these results.

2.6 Recommendations

Specific requirements will vary for individual patient treatments. However, the medical physicist in conjunction with the radiation oncologist should carefully review all aspects of the pregnant patient's treatment. The following are minimal requirements to consider before and during the patient's treatment.

- Plan the treatment normally (as if the patient were not pregnant). Modify the treatment plan as appropriate.
- Possible modifications are: changing the field size and angle, selecting a different radiation energy, etc.
- Estimate foetal dose without shielding. Use out-of-beam data measured on the specific treatment unit to be utilised. Typical points of interest are the uterine fundus, the symphysis pubis and a midpoint (umbilicus).
- If dose estimates in item 2 above are not acceptable, design and construct special shielding. Typically five half-value layers of lead or equivalent will be appropriate.
- Final Treatment Plan. Measure out-of-field dose in phantom utilising treatment parameters and shielding (if applicable). Document the results and treatment set-up instructions (including photographs) in the treatment plan. Discuss the set-up with the involved personnel.
- Verify safety, including load-bearing limits of the treatment couch, structural integrity and movement of the shields, etc.
- The physicist should be present at the time of the first session of irradiation and be available for consultation during subsequent sessions.
- Monitor foetal size and location throughout the course of treatment, repeating dose estimates as appropriate. Document the completion of treatment by estimating the total dose to the foetus during the whole course of therapy.
- Refer the patient to another institution for treatment, if appropriate.

References

CT-Expo V. 1.5 Registr. Nr. 3668699175 (2001–2005) Copyright G. Stamm und H.D. Nagel, Hannover-Hamburg

De Maria M, Mazzei F, Tarolo GL (1999) La radioprotezione nelle esposizioni prenatali e neonatali. Rapporto ISTISAN 99/7: 82–98

European Commission(1999) Guidance for protection of unborn children and infants radiated due to parental medical exposures. Radiation Protection 100

Helmrot E, Pettersson H, Sandborg M, Alten JN (2007) Estimation of dose to the unborn child at diagnostic X-ray examinations based on data registered in RIS/PACS. Eur Radiol 17: 205–209

ICRP Publication 60 (1991) 1990 Recommendations of the International Commission on Radiological Protection. Ann ICRP 21: 1–3

IEC EN 60601-2-441/A1 (2004) Particular requirements for the safety of X-ray equipment for computed tomography

Mac Mahon B (1962) Pre-natal X-ray exposure and childhood cancer J Natl Cancer Inst 28: 1173–1191

Naumburg E, Bellocco R, Cnattingius S, Hall P, Boice JD, Eckbom A (2001) Intrauterine exposure to diagnostic X-rays and risk of childhood leukaemia subtypes. Radiat Res 156: 718–723

NCRP Report No. 54 (1977) Medical Radiation Exposure of Pregnant and Potentially Pregnant Women. National Council on Radiation Protection and Measurements, 7910 Woodmont Avenue, Bethesda, MD 20014

Stewart A, Webb K, Giles D (1956) Malignant disease in childhood and diagnostic irradiation in utero. Lancet 2: 447

Stovall M, Blackwell CR, Cundiff J, Novack DH, Palta Jr, Wagner LK, Webster EW, Shalek RJ (1995) Fetal dose from radiotherapy with photon beams: report of AAPM Radiation Therapy Committee Task Group No. 36. Med Phys 22: 1353–1354

Wachsmann F, Drexler G (1976) Graphs and Tables for Use in Radiology, Springer, Berlin

3 Maternal and Fetal Effects of Systemic Therapy in the Pregnant Woman with Cancer

D. Pereg, M. Lishner

Recent Results in Cancer Research, Vol. 178

3.1 Introduction

The diagnosis of cancer and the need to administer chemotherapy during pregnancy pose challenges to the woman, her family, and the medical team. The great challenge is to treat the mother without adversely affecting fetal outcome. The relative rarity of pregnancy-associated cancer precludes conducting large prospective studies to examine the safety of the different chemotherapeutic drugs, and the literature is largely composed of small retrospective studies and case reports. In this chapter we critically review available data, controversies, and unresolved issues regarding the administration of chemotherapy during pregnancy and lactation.

3.2 Pharmacokinetics of Chemotherapeutic Drugs During Pregnancy

When treating pregnant patients with chemotherapy, it is important to consider the normal physiological changes that occur during pregnancy, including an increased plasma volume (by up to 50%) and renal clearance of drugs, the third space created by the amniotic fluid, and a faster hepatic oxidation (Cardonick and Iacobucci 2004; Weisz et al. 2004). These changes may decrease active drug concentrations compared with women who are not pregnant and have the same weight. However, since no pharmacokinetic studies have been conducted in pregnant women receiving chemotherapy, it is still unknown whether pregnant women should be treated with different doses of chemotherapy.

3.3 The Effect of Chemotherapy on the Fetus

Most drugs with a molecular mass of less than 600 kDa are able to cross the placenta (Pacifici and Nottoli 1995). Since the various cytotoxic agents have a molecular mass of between 250 and 400 kDa, virtually all of them can cross the placenta and reach the fetus (Pacifici and Nottoli 1995). However, only few small transplacental studies have been conducted to assess drug concentrations in the amniotic fluid, cord blood, and placental and fetal tissues—with conflicting results.

There are no sufficient data regarding the teratogenicity of most cytotoxic drugs. Almost all chemotherapeutic agents were found to be teratogenic in animals, and for some drugs only experimental data exist (Cardonick and Iacobucci 2004; Koren et al. 2005). However, the chemotherapy doses used in humans are often lower than the minimum teratogenic doses applied in animals. Therefore, it is difficult to extrapolate data from animal models to humans. Furthermore, since cytotoxic drugs are usually not used separately as monotherapy, most human reports arise from exposure to multidrug regimens, making it difficult to estimate the exact effect of each drug. It seems possible that genetic predisposition may explain the differing susceptibility to teratogenicity among patients given the same drugs.

The potential teratogenic effect of any chemotherapeutic agent used during pregnancy depends on the total dose and on the fetal developmental stage at the time of exposure. Chemotherapy during the first trimester may increase the risk of spontaneous abortions, fetal death, and major malformations (Leslie et al. 2005; Zemlickis et al. 1992). Malformations reflect the gestational age at exposure, and the fetus is extremely vulnerable during weeks 2–8, at which organogenesis occurs (Cardonick and Iacobucci 2004; Weisz et al. 2004). During this period, damage to any developing organ may lead to major malformations. After organogenesis, several organs including the eyes, genitalia, the hematopoietic system, and the central nervous system (CNS) remain vulnerable to chemotherapy (Cardonick and Iacobucci 2004, Weisz et al. 2004). Overall, the risk of teratogenesis following cancer treatment appears to be lower than is commonly estimated from animal data. First-trimester exposure to chemotherapy has been associated with 10%–20% risk of major malformations (Weisz et al. 2004). A review of 139 cases of first-trimester exposure to chemotherapy has demonstrated a 17% risk for malformations after single-agent exposure and 25% after exposure to combination chemotherapy (Doll et al. 1998). When folate antagonists were excluded, the incidence of fetal malformations with single-agent chemotherapy during the first trimester declined to 6%. Another study of 210 cases demonstrated 29 fetal abnormalities, of which 27 were associated with first-trimester exposure (Randall 1993). However, these studies included pregnant women who were treated with different chemotherapeutic regimens and covered long periods of time during which the treatment of cancer had changed. Furthermore, these evaluations were based on a collection of case reports, and there may be a reporting bias whereby malformed infants are more likely to be reported after drug exposure than healthy infants. Therefore, it is recommended that when any multidrug chemotherapy is given during the first trimester, pregnancy termination should be strongly recommended.

Besides their direct potential teratogenicity, anticancer chemotherapy agents can adversely affect pregnancy in several other ways and cause spontaneous abortions, intrauterine growth retardation (IUGR), and low birth weight. Chemotherapy is associated with maternal complications such as nausea and vomiting, or cytopenias including neutropenia with an increased susceptibility for infections that can all indirectly affect the fetus. Therefore, proper supportive treatment with antiemetics, growth factors, blood products, and antibiotics is essential and should be administered promptly (the supportive treatment for pregnant patients with cancer is detailed in several chapters in this volume). Furthermore, evidence exists suggesting that anticancer drugs may adversely affect the placenta (Matalon et al. 2004, 2005; DeLoia et al. 1998). For example, the adverse effects of 6-mercaptopurine on the placenta has been documented with inhibition of both migration and proliferation of trophoblast cells in first-trimester human placental explants (Matalon et al. 2005).

Second- and third-trimester exposure are not associated with teratogenic effects but increase the risk for IUGR and low birth weight (Zemlickis et al. 1992). However, the IUGR and low birth weight are not associated with long-term complications, and death rate is relatively low in these circumstances. Therefore, it seems that the advantage of treatment is clear and that multidrug regimens can be administered during this period.

There are several situations that warrant special consideration since the administration of chemotherapy can be more flexible and individualized according to the circumstances. For example, when an early-stage cancer is diagnosed late in the first trimester, it may be possible to consider chemotherapy postponement while keeping the patient under close observation for any sign of disease progression. At the end of the first trimester, proper multidrug chemotherapy should be administered promptly. In rare cases such as in stage I Hodgkin lymphoma restricted to the neck lymph nodes, treatment with local radiotherapy can be considered as a proper yet safe therapy and can replace chemotherapy without adverse fetal outcomes. When pregnancy termination is unacceptable to the patient, a single-agent treatment with anthracycline antibiotics or vinca alkaloids followed by multiagent therapy at the end of the first trimester can be considered. The experience with the different chemotherapeutic drugs is detailed in a subsequent paragraph.

The principles of treatment with anticancer chemotherapy during pregnancy are summarized in Fig. 3.1.

Delivery postponement should be considered for 2–3 weeks after treatment to allow bone marrow recovery. Furthermore, neonates, especially preterm babies, have limited capacity to metabolize and eliminate drugs because of liver and renal immaturity. The delay of delivery after chemotherapy will allow fetal drug excretion via the placenta (Sorosky et al. 1997).

3.4 Long-Term Effects of In Utero Exposure to Chemotherapy

The fact that the CNS continues to develop throughout gestation has raised concerns regarding long-term neurodevelopmental outcome of children exposed to in utero chemotherapy. Other concerns are childhood malignancy and long-term fertility. Information regarding these issues is limited because of the difficulties in long-term follow-up and the relative rarity of such cases. A long-term (up to age 6–29, average 18.7 years) follow-up of 84 children born to mothers with hematological malignancies who were treated with chemotherapy during pregnancy (38 of them during the first trimester) has reported normal physical, neurological, and psychological development (Aviles and Neri 2001). Furthermore, this study has partially addressed the issue of reproduction in that all offspring have shown normal sexual development and 12 of them had become parents to normally developed children. Finally, unlike in utero exposure to radiotherapy, the exposure to chemotherapy during pregnancy was not associated with an increased risk of developing childhood malignancies compared to the general population. This

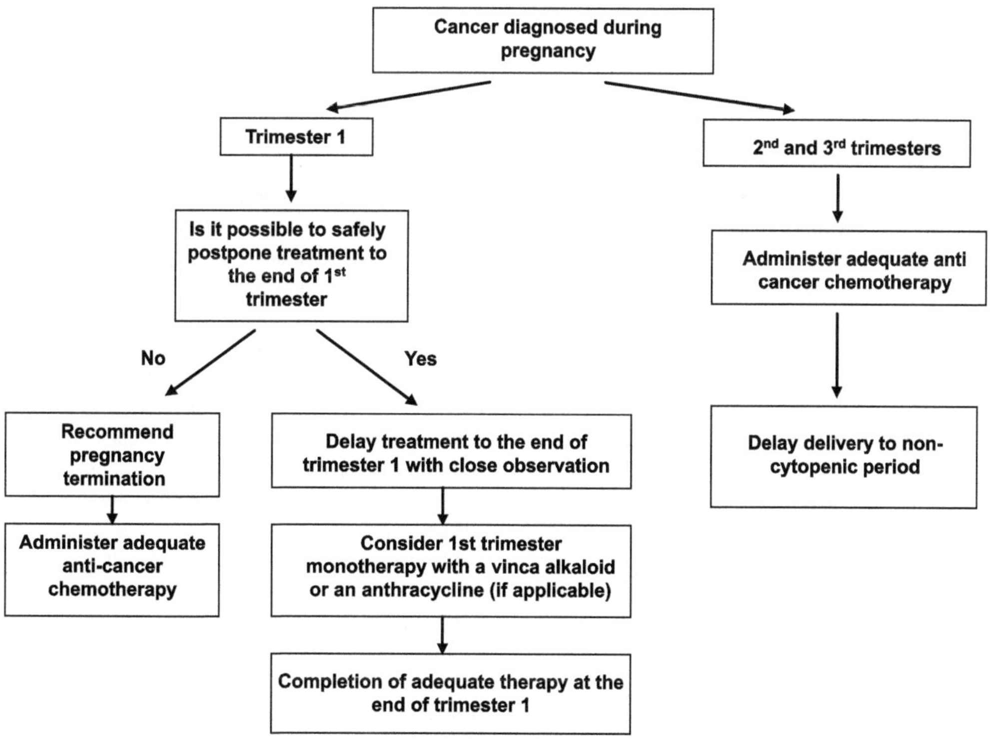

Fig. 3.1 A suggested algorithm for the treatment of pregnant patients with chemotherapy

report was supported by a review summarizing 111 cases of children born to mothers treated with chemotherapy during pregnancy (Nulman et al. 2001). These children, who were followed up for different periods of time (1–19 years) had normal late neurodevelopment based on formal developmental and cognitive tests. In summary, the available data regarding late effect of chemotherapy on children's neurodevelopment are limited, and most reports used a retrospective design in order to recruit a sufficient number of cases. However, the general impression based on the available data suggests that chemotherapy does not have a major impact on later neurodevelopment.

3.5 Breastfeeding and Chemotherapy

The concentration of chemotherapy in breast milk varies among the various agents and is also related to the dose and timing of therapy. Experience regarding chemotherapy during lactation is limited and based only on case reports. While a single case of neonatal neutropenia has been reported after breastfeeding exposure to cyclophosphamide (Durodola 1979), for most chemotherapeutic agents no breastfeeding data are available. However, dose-dependent as well as dose-independent effects of these drugs cannot be ruled out. Although it is unclear how much toxicity can be attributed to these drugs during lactation, most authorities consider breastfeeding as contraindicated while undergoing chemotherapy.

3.6 Chemotherapeutic Agents

We have categorized the different chemotherapeutic drugs according to the classification presented in Harrison's *Principles of Internal Medicine* (16th edition).

3.6.1 Alkylating Agents

Alkylating agents are among the most commonly used chemotherapeutic drugs. The different drugs have antitumor activity against a wide spectrum of malignancies including breast, ovarian, and bladder carcinomas, Hodgkin disease, and non-Hodgkin lymphoma. This chemotherapy group is considered slightly less teratogenic than the antimetabolites. However, first-trimester exposure is associated with an increased risk for malformations, most commonly renal and gastrointestinal, and with limb deformities. Unlike with adult exposure, there are no reports of increased risk for childhood cancer after intrauterine exposure to alkylating agents. The available data regarding treatment with the different alkylating agents during pregnancy are presented in Table 3.1.

3.6.2 Anticancer Antibiotics

3.6.2.1 Anthracyclines

Anthracyclines are an integral part of regimens used for the treatment of different types of cancer including lymphomas, leukemias, and breast, lung, bladder, and gastric carcinomas. The experience with the treatment of anthracyclines during pregnancy is limited mostly to doxorubicin and daunorubicin. Idarubicin, which is more lipophilic compared to other anthracyclines, has an increased placenta transfer and affinity to the DNA, and therefore may be associated with higher rates of adverse fetal outcomes and should be avoided during pregnancy. When doxorubicin is as effective as the other anthracyclines in selected types of cancer, it is the preferred drug during pregnancy. It may also be used as monotherapy during the first trimester, in the rare cases in which postponement of treatment with full multidrug chemotherapy regimens can be considered. Besides their potential teratogenicity, another concern about the administration of anthracyclines during pregnancy is whether they are cardiotoxic to the developing fetus. While most reports have shown no myocardial damage in both gestational and postnatal echocardiogram, a few case reports have demonstrated both transient and permanent cardiomyopathy. The experience with antracyclines during pregnancy is presented in Table 3.2.

3.6.2.2 Other Anticancer Antibiotics

Experience with mitomycin C and actinomycin D and with the topoisomerase inhibitors etoposide and teniposide is extremely limited, and therefore their administration during pregnancy can not be recommended. Most of the experience with bleomycin during pregnancy arises from the treatment of pregnant patients with lymphoma (Table 3.2). Unlike adults, there are no reports of pulmonary damage after intrauterine exposure to bleomycin.

3.6.3 Antimitotic Agents

3.6.3.1 Vinca Alkaloids

This group of chemotherapeutic drugs is commonly used as part of multidrug protocols for treating various malignancies. Vincristine and vinblastine are relatively less teratogenic compared to the other chemotherapeutic drugs, possibly because of their high binding to plasma proteins. Therefore, in the rare cases in which postponement of treatment with full multidrug chemotherapy regimens until the end of the first trimester can be considered, vinca alkaloids may be a safe option for monotherapy. While in adults the treatment with the vinca alkaloids may cause neuropathy, there is no evidence regarding such an effect on fetuses exposed in-utero. Table 3.3 summarizes the main available data regarding the treatment with vinca alkaloids during pregnancy.

3.6.3.2 Taxanes

The experience with paclitaxel during pregnancy is extremely limited, and only a few cases have been reported (Table 3.3). Therefore, taxanes should be avoided throughout pregnancy.

3.6.4 Antimetabolites

Antimetabolites inhibit different biochemical cycles by acting as false substrates, usually as nucleoside analogs that interfere with DNA and RNA synthesis. Among the different anticancer drugs, antimetabolites seem to be associated with a higher risk for adverse fetal outcomes. This was especially true regarding aminopterin, which is an antimetabolite that is no longer in use, and its administration during the first trimester has been associated with high risk for developing the aminopterin syndrome (cranial dysostosis with delayed ossification, hypertelorism, wide nasal bridge micrognatia, and ear anomalies) (Weizz et al. 2004). A very similar pattern of malformation has been described after first-trimester exposure to high-dose methotrexate (>10 mg/week). Furthermore, methotrexate, which is used as an abortifacient in the treatment of ectopic pregnancy, increases the risk for miscarriage when administered early in pregnancy. Table 3.4 summarizes the main available data regarding treatment with antimetabolites during pregnancy.

3.6.5 Miscellaneous Drugs Used for Anticancer Treatment

3.6.5.1 Rituximab

In recent years rituximab has become an integral part of the treatment of intermediate-grade non-Hodgkin lymphomas. Only few cases of rituximab administered during pregnancy have been reported, most of them for the treatment of various autoimmune diseases (Table 3.5). In these reports the administration of rituximab in pregnancy, including during the first trimester, was not associated with an increased risk for adverse fetal outcome.

3.6.5.2 Interferon Alpha

Interferon alpha is used in patients with node-positive malignant melanoma. Most of the experience with interferon arises from its administration to patients with hepatitis and myeloproliferative disorders. To date, there is no evidence regarding any teratogenic effect of interferon (Table 3.5), and it is considered a safe drug to be administered during pregnancy.

Table 3.1 A summary of the main reports regarding treatment with alkylating agents during pregnancy

Drug	Description of study	Outcome of pregnancy	References
Cyclophosphamide	21 patients treated with regimens that include cyclophosphamide. (11 in 1st trimester)	Normal pregnancy outcome	Aviles et al. 1991
	9 mothers treated for acute leukemia. (3 during 1st trimester) with regimens that include cyclophosphamide	No congenital malformations were observed; 1 newborn had pancytopenia and low birth weight	Pizzuto et al. 1980
	57 pregnant patients with breast cancer treated with a combination of cyclophosphamide, doxorubicin and 5-FU (2nd and 3rd trimesters).	1 case of Down syndrome 2 cases of congenital anomalies (clubfoot and congenital bilateral ureteral reflux)	Hahn et al. 2006
	29 breast cancer patients exposed to cyclophosphamide and doxorubicin (all in 2nd and 3rd trimesters)	No congenital malformations were observed 1 case of IUGR	Cardonick and Iacobucci 2004
	5 case reports of treatment with regimens that include cyclophosphamide in 1st trimester	Several malformations were reported including absent big toes in both legs, single left coronary artery, imperforated anus, umbilical hernia, cleft palate, multiple eye defects, esophageal atresia. 1 case was diagnosed with papillary thyroid cancer at 11 years of age and stage III neuroblastoma at 14 years of age	Greenberg and Tanaka 1964; Toledo et al. 1971; Murray et al. 1984; Kirshon et al. 1988; Zemlickis et al. 1993
Busulphan	15 cases (8 during 1st trimester)	2 cases of 2nd-trimester exposure had malformations: pyloric stenosis and unilateral renal agenesis	Cardonick and Iacobucci 2004
Dacarbazine	10 cases treated with ABVD for Hodgkin disease (doxorubicin, bleomycin, vinblastine, and dacarbazine) in all 3 trimesters	Normal pregnancy outcome	Aviles et al. 1991
	4 patients treated with ABVD (2nd and 3rd trimesters)	Normal pregnancy outcome	Lishner et al. 1992
Ifosfamide	2 case reports of 3rd-trimester exposure to ifosfamide and doxorubicin for treating Ewing sarcoma.	Normal pregnancy outcome	Nakajima et al. 2004; Merimsky et al. 1999
Melphalan	1 case report of a patient exposed during 1st trimester	A miscarriage	Zemlickis et al. 1992

Table 3.1 *(continued)* A summary of the main reports regarding treatment with alkylating agents during pregnancy

Drug	Description of study	Outcome of pregnancy	References
Chlorambucil	5 case reports of 1st-trimester exposure	3 cases of normal pregnancy outcome	Nicholson 1968; Jacobs et al. 1981; Ba-Thike and Oo 1990; Shoton and Monie 1953; Steege and Caldwell 1980.
		2 cases of kidney agenesis	
	3 cases of 2nd- and 3rd-trimester exposure	Normal pregnancy outcome	Nicholson 1968
Cisplatin	26 cases of cisplatin exposure during 2nd and 3rd trimesters	1 case of a sensorineural hearing loss with premature delivery at week 26	Cardonick and Iacobucci 2004; Raffles et al. 1989; Elit et al. 1999; Henderson et al 1993; Arango et al. 1994; Bakri and Given 1984; Caluwaerts et al. 2006; Huang et al. 2004; Ferrandina et al. 2005.
		1 case of ventriculomegaly	
		2 cases of fetal death	
		3 cases of premature delivery	
		3 cases of IUGR	
Melphalan	1 case report of a patient exposed during 1st trimester	A miscarriage	Zemlickis et al. 1992

Table 3.2 A summary of the main reports regarding treatment with anticancer antibiotics during pregnancy

Drug	Description of study	Outcome of pregnancy	References
Doxorubicin	Long-term follow-up of 81 children exposed to anthracyclines during all 3 trimesters, among whom 70 were exposed to doxorubicin, 4 to daunorubicin, 4 to idarubicin, and 3 to mitoxantrone	No congenital neurological or psychological abnormalities were observed. Learning and educational performances were normal. There was no myocardial damage in either gestational and postnatal echocardiogram.	Aviles et al. 2006
	57 pregnant patients with breast cancer treated with a combination of cyclophosphamide, doxorubicin, and 5-FU (2nd and 3rd trimesters).	1 case of Down syndrome 2 cases of congenital anomalies (clubfoot and congenital bilateral ureteral reflux)	Hahn et al. 2006
	29 breast cancer patients exposed to cyclophosphamide and doxorubicin (all in 2nd and 3rd trimesters)	No congenital malformations were observed 1 case of IUGR	Cardonick and Iacobucci 2004
	10 cases treated with ABVD for Hodgkin disease (doxorubicin, bleomycin, vinblastine, and dacarbazine) in all 3 trimesters	Normal pregnancy outcome	Aviles et al. 1991
	4 patients treated with ABVD (2nd and 3rd trimesters)	Normal pregnancy outcome	Lishner et al. 1992
Daunorubicin	43 patients who were treated in all 3 trimesters.	One case of malformation:-adherence of the iris (after exposure to daunorubicin and cytarabine during 3rd trimester). 3 cases of intrauterine fetal death (1 exposed in 1st trimester) 5 cases of IUGR (2nd- and 3rd-trimester exposure)	Cardonick and Iacobucci 2004
	9 patients (1 was treated during the 1st trimester)	2 cases of still birth (1 of which had myocardial necrosis)	Gililland and Weinstein 1983
	4 patients treated during 1st trimester	2 cases of spontaneous abortions a few weeks after the initiation of chemotherapy	Alegre et al. 1982; Zuazu et al.1991

Table 3.2 *(continued)* A summary of the main reports regarding treatment with anticancer antibiotics during pregnancy

Drug	Description of study	Outcome of pregnancy	References
Idarubicin	Total of 9 patients treated in 2nd and 3rd trimesters	1 case of transient dilated cardiomyopathy. 2 cases of permanent mild dilated cardiomyopathy, 1 of which had congenital malformations including short limbs and digits and macrognatia)	Aviles et al. 2006; Niedermeier et al. 2005; Siu et al. 2002; Achtari and Hohlfeld 2000; Claahsen et al. 1998; Matsuo et al. 2004
Epirubicin	13 cases of 2nd- and 3rd-trimester exposure	3 fetuses died a few weeks after the initiation of treatment.	Cardonick and Iacobucci 2004
Mitoxantrone	3 cases of 2nd- and 3rd-trimester exposure	Normal pregnancy outcome	Aviles et al. 2006
Bleomycin	23 cases of bleomycin exposure (11 during 1st trimester)	Normal pregnancy outcome	Lishner et al. 1992
	4 patients treated with ABVD (2nd and 3rd trimesters)	Normal pregnancy outcome	Aviles et al. 1991
Etoposide	5 case reports of etoposide exposure (1 case during 1st trimester)	2 premature deliveries with fetal pancytopenia. 1 case of hearing loss.	Arango et al. 1994; Horbelt et al. 1994; Raffles et al. 1989; Brunet et al. 1993; Murray et al. 1994

Table 3.3 A summary of the main reports regarding treatment with antimitotic agents during pregnancy

Drug	Description of study	Outcome of pregnancy	References
Vincristine	28 pregnant patients with hematological malignancies exposed to regimens that contained vincristine during all 3 trimesters	Normal pregnancy outcome	Aviles et al. 1991
	9 patients with acute leukemia exposed to regimens that contained vincristine (5 cases during 1st trimester)	No congenital malformation. 4 cases of IUGR 1 case of severe pancytopenia	Pizzuto et al. 1980
	7 pregnant patients with acute leukemia exposed to regimens that contained vincristine (2nd and 3rd trimesters)	Normal pregnancy outcome	Reynoso et al. 1987
	26 pregnant patients with acute leukemia exposed to regimens that contained vincristine (all 3 trimesters)	1 case of cleft lip and palate, exposed very early in 1st trimester	Mulvihill et al. 1987
	4 patients with hematological malignancies treated with regimens that contained vincristine during the 1stt trimester	1 case of spontaneous abortion 1 case of severe hydrocephalus and death soon after delivery	Zemlickis et al. 1992
Vinblastine	10 cases treated with ABVD for Hodgkin disease (doxorubicin, bleomycin, vinblastine, and dacarbazine) in all 3 trimesters	Normal pregnancy outcome	Aviles et al. 1991
	4 cases treated with ABVD for Hodgkin disease (2nd and 3rd trimesters)	Normal pregnancy outcome	Lishner et al. 1992
	14 cases treated with different multidrug regimens containing vinblastine (2nd and 3rd trimesters)	Normal pregnancy outcome	Doll et al. 1998; Jacobs et al. 1981; Zuazu et al. 1991; Falkson et al. 1980; Ortega 1977.
Paclitaxel	4 case reports of 2nd- and 3rd-trimester exposure	Normal pregnancy outcome	Sood et al. 2001; Mendez et al. 2003; Gonzalez-Angulo et al. 2004; Gadducci et al. 2004.

Table 3.4 A summary of the main reports regarding treatment with antimetabolites during pregnancy

Drug	Description of study	Outcome of pregnancy	References
Methotrexate	20 patients with cancer or rheumatic diseases, with 1st-trimester exposure	7 cases developed a pattern very similar to the aminopterin syndrome (cranial dysostosis with delayed ossification, hypertelorism, wide nasal bridge micrognatia, and ear anomalies). Most of them exposed to high-dose methotrexate (>10 mg/week)	Bawle et al. 1998; Buckleyet al. 1997; Diniz et al. 1978; Milunsky et al. 1968; Powell and Ekert 1971; Dara et al. 1981; Feliu et al. 1988; Addar 2004; Kozlowski et al. 1990.
		1 case of skeletal abnormalities and ambiguous genitalia	
		5 cases of spontaneous abortions	
	18 patients with leukemia (10 treated during 1st trimester)	No congenital malformations	Donnenfeld et al. 1994; Aviles et al. 1991
		4 cases of low birth weight	
		1 case of severe pancytopenia	
5-Fluorouracil	53 cases (5 during 1st trimester)	6 cases of IUGR	Cardonick and Iacobucci 2004
		1 case of fetal death	
		1 case of neonatal death (no obvious cause of death)	
	57 pregnant patients with breast cancer treated with a combination of cyclophosphamide, doxorubicin and 5-FU (2nd and 3rd trimesters).	1 case of Down syndrome	Hahn et al. 2006
		2 cases of congenital anomalies (clubfoot and congenital bilateral ureteral reflux)	

Table 3.4 *(continued)* A summary of the main reports regarding treatment with antimetabolites during pregnancy

Drug	Description of study	Outcome of pregnancy	References
Cytarabine	9 cases of pregnant patients with leukemia treated with regimens including cytarabine (5 treated during 1st trimester)	Normal pregnancy outcome	Aviles et al. 1991
	9 pregnant patients with leukemia (4 exposed during 1st trimester)	No congenital malformations	Taylor et al. 1980
		2 cases of low birth weight	
		1 case of severe pancytopenia	
	4 cases with leukemia treated with cytarabine containing regimens in the 2nd and 3rd trimesters	2 cases of low birth weight	Reynoso et al. 1987
		1 case of severe thrombocytopenia	
	2 case reports of cytarabine exposure during 1st trimester	1 case of severe brachycephaly, hypoplasia of the anterior cranial base and the midface, bilateral four-finger hands and absent radii	Artlich et al. 1994; Maurer et al. 1971
		1 case of group C trisomy mosaicism	
	12 cases of 2nd- and 3rd-trimester exposure	1 case of 46 chromosomes karyotype with gaps and a ring chromosome (the clinical significance is not clear)	Pizzuto et al. 1980; Aviles et al. 2006; Volkenandt et al. 1987; Colbert et al. 1980; O'Donnell et al. 1979
		3 cases of intrauterine death	
		2 cases of severe neonatal pancytopenia	
6-mercaptopurine	49 cases (29 were exposed during 1st trimester)	2 cases of intrauterine death	Cardonick and Iacobucci 2004
		5 cases of IUGR	

Table 3.5 Miscellaneous agents used for anticancer treatment

Drug	Description of study	Outcome of pregnancy	References
Rituximab	4 case reports of rituximab exposure during pregnancy (2 during 1st trimester)	No congenital malformations 1 case of transient complete fetal B-cell depletion However, B-cell recovery was fast, showing a regular immunophenotype without loss of CD20 antigen, no functional deficits, and adequate vaccination IgG titers.	Ojeda-Uribe et al. 2006; Kimby et al. 2004; Scully et al. 2006; Friedrichs et al. 2006
Interferon alpha	14 cases treated for essential thrombocytopenia (2 in 1st trimester)	Normal pregnancy outcome	Vantroyen and Vanstraelen 2002
	27 cases treated for chronic hepatitis or myeloproliferative disorders (6 cases during 1st trimester)	No congenital malformations 4 cases of premature delivery 6 cases of IUGR	Hiratsuka et al. 2000
Imatinib mesylate	21 patients with CML treated in the 1st trimester	4 cases of intrauterine fetal death (1 case with a meningocele) 2 cases of minor malformations (hypospadias in 1 baby and rotation of small intestine in 1 baby)	Ault et al. 2006; Choudhary et al. 2006; Prabhash et al. 2005
Trastuzumab	2 cases of 2nd-trimester exposure	1 case of reversible anhydramnios	Watson 2005; Fanale et al. 2005.
Tamoxifen	2 cases of 2nd-trimester exposure	Normal pregnancy outcome	Andreadis et al. 2004; Isaacs et al. 2001
All-trans retinoic acid	7 cases of 2nd- and 3rd-trimester exposure	Normal pregnancy outcome	Siu et al. 2002; Celo et al. 1994; Delgado-Lamas et al. 2000; Harrison et al. 1994; Incerpi et al. 1997; Stentoft et al. 1994

3.6.5.3 Imatinib Mesylate

This novel tyrosine kinase inhibitor has a major role in the treatment of chronic myeloid leukemia (CML) and of gastrointestinal stromal tumors (GIST). The experience with imatinib during human pregnancy is still limited (Table 3.5). However, animal models suggest that this agent may be teratogenic. Therefore, at this time, imatinib cannot be recommended for treating pregnant patients.

3.6.5.4 Trastuzumab (Herceptin)

This is a monoclonal antibody that blocks the human epidermal growth factor receptor 2 protein and is administered to patients with breast cancer. Currently there are only two reports of treatment with trastuzumab during pregnancy. (Table 3.5)

3.6.5.5 Tamoxifen

Tamoxifen is used to treat patients with hormone receptor-positive breast cancer. The experience with this drug during pregnancy is limited (Table 3.5), and therefore its administration to pregnant patients cannot be recommended.

3.6.5.6 All-*trans* Retinoic Acid

This drug is used for the treatment of patients with promyelocytic leukemia. As with all vitamin A derivatives, its exposure during the first trimester is associated with an extremely high rate (up to 85%) of teratogenicity, including fatal neurological and cardiovascular malformations. Therefore, there is a consensus that any administration of all-*trans* retinoic acid (ATRA) during the first trimester should follow pregnancy termination. Furthermore, it is recommended that women treated with ATRA should be aware of its potential teratogenicity and effective contraception should be used to prevent pregnancy. There are several reports regarding the treatment with ATRA during the second and third trimesters without congenital malformations (Table 3.5)

3.6.6 New Anticancer Agents

The treatment of cancer continues to advance, and new anticancer drugs, many of which are still experimental, are being introduced more rapidly than the accumulation of safety data in pregnancy. Caution is therefore warranted before new agents are administered to pregnant women, even if other drugs from the same class are considered safe. Recently there has been an increasing interest in the development and use of different biological anticancer therapies, the most popular being bevacizumab (Avastin) and cetuximab (Erbitux), which are used most commonly in metastatic colorectal cancer. The fact that bevacizumab is an antiangiogenic factor suggests that it may be associated with severe adverse effects during pregnancy. To our best knowledge, there are no reports regarding treatment with these drugs during pregnancy, and therefore they should not be given to pregnant women.

References

Achtari C, Hohlfeld P (2000) Cardiotoxic transplacental effect of idarubicin administered during the second trimester of pregnancy. Am J Obstet Gynecol 183: 511–512

Addar MH (2004) Methotrexate embryopathy in a surviving intrauterine fetus after presumed diagnosis of ectopic pregnancy: case report. J Obstet Gynaecol Can 26: 1001–1003

Alegre A, Chunchurreta R, Rodriguez-Alarcon J, Cruz E, Prada M (1982) Successful pregnancy in acute promyelocytic leukemia. Cancer 49: 152–153

Andreadis C, Charalampidou M, Diamantopoulos N, Chouchos N, Mouratidou D (2004) Combined chemotherapy and radiotherapy during conception and first two trimesters of gestation in a woman with metastatic breast cancer. Gynecol Oncol 95: 252–255

Arango HA, Kalter CS, Decesare SL, Fiorica JV, Lyman GH, Spellacy WN (1994) Management of chemotherapy in a pregnancy complicated by a large neuroblastoma. Obstet Gynecol 84: 665–668

Artlich A, Moller J, Tschakaloff A, Schwinger E, Kruse K, Gortner L (1994) Teratogenic effects in a case of maternal treatment for acute myelocytic leukaemia--neonatal and infantile course. Eur J Pediatr 153: 488–491

Ault P, Kantarjian H, O'Brien S et al. (2006) Pregnancy among patients with chronic myeloid leukemia treated with imatinib. J Clin Oncol 24: 1204–1208

Aviles A, Diaz-Maqueo JC, Talavera A, Guzman R, Garcia EL (1991) Growth and development of children of mothers treated with chemotherapy during pregnancy: current status of 43 children. Am J Hematol 36: 243–248

Aviles A, Neri N (2001) Hematological malignancies and pregnancy: a final report of 84 children who received chemotherapy in utero. Clin Lymphoma 2: 173–177

Aviles A, Neri N, Nambo MJ (2006) Long-term evaluation of cardiac function in children who received anthracyclines during pregnancy. Ann Oncol 17: 286–288

Ba-Thike K, Oo N (1990) Non-Hodgkin's lymphoma in pregnancy. Asia Oceania J Obstet Gynaecol 16: 229–232

Bawle EV, Conard JV, Weiss L (1998) Adult and two children with fetal methotrexate syndrome. Teratology 7: 51–55

Brunet S, Sureda A, Mateu R, Domingo-Albos A (1993) Full-term pregnancy in a patient diagnosed with acute leukemia treated with a protocol including VP-16. Med Clin (Barc) 100: 757–758

Buckley LM, Bullaboy CA, Leichtman L, Marquez M (1997) Multiple congenital anomalies associated with weekly low-dose methotrexate treatment of the mother. Arthritis Rheum 40: 971–973

Caluwaerts S, VAN Calsteren K, Mertens L et al. (2006) Neoadjuvant chemotherapy followed by radical hysterectomy for invasive cervical cancer diagnosed during pregnancy: report of a case and review of the literature. Int J Gynecol Cancer 16: 905–908

Cardonick E, Iacobucci A (2004) Use of chemotherapy during human pregnancy. Lancet Oncol 5: 283–291

Celo JS, Kim HC, Houlihan C, Canavan BF, Manzullo GP, Saidi P (1994) Acute promyelocytic leukemia in pregnancy: all-*trans* retinoic acid as a newer therapeutic option. Obstet Gynecol 83: 808–811

Choudhary DR, Mishra P, Kumar R, Mahapatra M, Choudhry VP (2006) Pregnancy on imatinib: fatal outcome with meningocele. Ann Oncol 17: 178–179

Claahsen HL, Semmekrot BA, van Dongen PW, Mattijssen V (1998) Successful fetal outcome after exposure to idarubicin and cytosine-arabinoside during the second trimester of pregnancy—a case report. Am J Perinatol 15: 295–297

Colbert N, Najman A, Gorin NC et al. (1980) Acute leukaemia during pregnancy: favourable course of pregnancy in two patients treated with cytosine arabinoside and anthracyclines. Nouv Presse Med 9: 175–178

Dara P, Slater LM, Armentrout SA (1981) Successful pregnancy during chemotherapy for acute leukemia. Cancer 47: 845–846

Delgado-Lamas JL, Garces-Ruiz OM (2000) Acute promyelocytic leukemia in late pregnancy. successful treatment with all-*trans*-retinoic acid (ATRA) and chemotherapy. Hematology 4: 415–418

DeLoia JA, Stewart-Akers AM, Creinin MD (1998) Effects of methotrexate on trophoblast proliferation and local immune responses. Hum Reprod 13: 1063–1069

Diniz EM, Corradini HB, Ramos JL, Brock R (1978) Effect on the fetus of methotrexate (amethopterin) administered to the mother. Presentation of a case. Rev Hosp Clin Fac Med Sao Paulo 33: 286–290

Doll DC, Ringenberg QS, Yarbro JW (1998) Management of cancer during pregnancy. Arch Intern Med 148: 2058–2064

Donnenfeld AE, Pastuszak A, Noah JS, Schick B, Rose NC, Koren G (1994) Methotrexate exposure prior to and during pregnancy. Teratology 49: 79–81

Durodola JI (1979) Administration of cyclophosphamide during late pregnancy and early lactation: a case report. J Natl Med Assoc 71: 165–166

Elit L, Bocking A, Kenyon C, Natale R (1999) An endodermal sinus tumor diagnosed during pregnancy: case report and review of the literature. Gynecol Oncol 72: 123–127

Falkson HC, Simson IW, Falkson G (1980) Non-Hodgkin's lymphoma in pregnancy. Cancer 45: 1679–1682

Fanale MA, Uyei AR, Theriault RL, Adam K (2005) Treatment of metastatic breast cancer with trastuzumab and vinorelbine during pregnancy. Clin Breast Cancer 6: 354–356

Feliu J, Juarez S, Ordonez A, Garcia-Paredes ML, Gonzalez-Baron M, Montero JM (1988) Acute leukemia and pregnancy. Cancer 61: 580–584

Ferrandina G, Distefano M, Testa A, De Vincenzo R, Scambia G (2005) Management of an advanced ovarian cancer at 15 weeks of gestation: case report and literature review. Gynecol Oncol 97: 693–696

Friedrichs B, Tiemann M, Salwender H, Verpoort K, Wenger MK, Schmitz N. (2006) The effects of rituximab treatment during pregnancy on a neonate. Haematologica 91: 1426–1427

Gadducci A, Cosio S, Fanucchi A et al. (2003) Chemotherapy with epirubicin and paclitaxel for breast cancer during pregnancy: case report and review of the literature. Anticancer Res 23: 5225–5229

Gililland J, Weinstein L (1983) The effects of cancer chemotherapeutic agents on the developing fetus. Obstet Gynecol Surv 38: 6–13

Gonzalez-Angulo AM, Walters RS, Carpenter RJ Jr et al. (2004) Paclitaxel chemotherapy in a pregnant patient with bilateral breast cancer. Clin Breast Cancer 5: 317–319.

Greenberg LH, Tanaka KR (1964) Congenital anomalies probably induced by cyclophosphamide. JAMA 188: 423–426

Hahn KM, Johnson PH, Gordon N et al. (2006) Treatment of pregnant breast cancer patients and outcomes of children exposed to chemotherapy in utero. Cancer 107: 1219–1226

Harrison P, Chipping P, Fothergill GA (1994) Successful use of all-*trans* retinoic acid in acute promyelocytic leukaemia presenting during the second trimester of pregnancy. Br J Haematol 86: 681–682

Henderson CH, Elia G, Garfinkel D et al. (1993) Platinum chemotherapy during pregnancy for cystadenocarcinoma of the ovary. Gynecol Oncol 49: 9–94

Hiratsuka M, Minakami H, Koshizuka S, Sato I (2000) Administration of interferon-alpha during pregnancy: effects on fetus. J Perinat Med 28: 372–376

Horbelt D, Delmore J, Meisel R, Cho S, Roberts D, Logan D (1994) Mixed germ cell malignancy of the ovary concurrent with pregnancy. Obstet Gynecol 84: 662–664

Huang HP, Fang CN, Kan YY (2004) Chemotherapy for ovarian mucinous cystadenocarcinoma during pregnancy: a case report. Eur J Gynaecol Oncol 25: 635–636.

Incerpi MH, Miller DA, Posen R, Byrne JD (1997) All-*trans* retinoic acid for the treatment of acute promyelocytic leukemia in pregnancy. Obstet Gynecol 89: 826–828

Isaacs RJ, Hunter W, Clark K (2001) Tamoxifen as systemic treatment of advanced breast cancer during pregnancy—case report and literature review. Gynecol Oncol 80: 405–408

Jacobs C, Donaldson SS, Rosenberg SA, Kaplan HS (1981) Management of the pregnant patient with Hodgkin's disease. Ann Intern Med 95: 669–775

Kimby E, Sverrisdottir A, Elinder G (2004) Safety of rituximab therapy during the first trimester of pregnancy: a case history. Eur J Haematol 72: 292–295

Kirshon B, Wasserstrum N, Willis R, Herman GE, McCabe ER (1988) Teratogenic effects of first-trimester cyclophosphamide therapy. Obstet Gynecol 72: 462–464.

Koren G, Lishner M, Santiago S (2005) The Motherisk guide to cancer in pregnancy and lactation (2nd edition). Motherisk program, Toronto, Canada.

Kozlowski RD, Steinbrunner JV, MacKenzie AH, Clough JD, Wilke WS, Segal AM (1990) Outcome of first-trimester exposure to low-dose methotrexate in eight patients with rheumatic disease. Am J Med 88: 589–592

Leslie KK, Koil C, Rayburn WF (2005) Chemotherapeutic drugs in pregnancy. Obstet Gynecol Clin North Am 32: 627–640

Lishner M, Zemlickis D, Degendorfer P, Panzarella T, Sutcliffe SB, Koren G (1992) Maternal and fetal outcome following Hodgkin's disease in pregnancy. Br J Cancer 65: 114–117

Matalon ST, Ornoy A, Lishner M (2004) Review of the potential effects of three commonly used antineoplastic and immunosuppressive drugs (cyclophosphamide, azathioprine, doxorubicin) on the embryo and placenta. Reprod Toxicol 18: 219–230

Matalon ST, Ornoy A, Lishner M (2005) The effect of 6-mercaptopurine on early human placental explants. Hum Reprod 20: 1390–1397

Matsuo K, Shimoya K, Ueda S, Wada K, Koyama M, Murata Y (2004) Idarubicin administered during pregnancy: its effects on the fetus. Gynecol Obstet Invest 58: 186–188

Maurer LH, Forcier RJ, McIntyre OR, Benirschke K (1971) Fetal group C trisomy after cytosine arabinoside and thioguanine. Ann Intern Med 75: 809–810

Mendez LE, Mueller A, Salom E, Gonzalez-Quintero VH (2003) Paclitaxel and carboplatin chemotherapy administered during pregnancy for advanced epithelial ovarian cancer. Obstet Gynecol 102: 1200–1202

Merimsky O, Le Chevalier T, Missenard G et al. (1999) Management of cancer in pregnancy: a case of Ewing's sarcoma of the pelvis in the third trimester. Ann Oncol 10: 345–350

Milunsky A, Graef JW, Gaynor MF Jr (1968) Methotrexate-induced congenital malformations. J Pediatr 72: 790–795

Mulvihill JJ, McKeen EA, Rosner F, Zarrabi MH (1987) Pregnancy outcome in cancer patients. Experience in a large cooperative group. Cancer 60: 1143–1150

Murray CL, Reichert JA, Anderson J, Twiggs LB (1984) Multimodal cancer therapy for breast cancer in the first trimester of pregnancy. A case report. JAMA 252: 2607–2608

Murray NA, Acolet D, Deane M, Price J, Roberts IA (1994) Fetal marrow suppression after maternal chemotherapy for leukaemia. Arch Dis Child Fetal Neonatal Ed 71: F209–F210

Nakajima W, Ishida A, Takahashi M et al. (2004) Good outcome for infant of mother treated with chemotherapy for ewing sarcoma at 25 to 30 weeks' gestation. J Pediatr Hematol Oncol 26: 308–311

Nicholson HO (1968) Cytotoxic drugs in pregnancy. Review of reported cases. J Obstet Gynaecol Br Commonw 75: 307–312

Niedermeier DM, Frei-Lahr DA, Hall PD (2005) Treatment of acute myeloid leukemia during the second and third trimesters of pregnancy. Pharmacotherapy 25: 1134–1140

Nulman I, Laslo D, Fried S, Uleryk E, Lishner M, Koren G (2001) Neurodevelopment of children exposed in utero to treatment of maternal malignancy. Br J Cancer 85: 1611–1618

O'Donnell R, Costigan C, O'Connell LG (1979) Two cases of acute leukaemia in pregnancy. Acta Haematol 61: 298–300

Ojeda-Uribe M, Gilliot C, Jung G, Drenou B, Brunot A (2006) Administration of rituximab during the first trimester of pregnancy without consequences for the newborn. J Perinatol 26: 252–255

Ortega J (1977) Multiple agent chemotherapy including bleomycin of non-Hodgkin's lymphoma during pregnancy. Cancer 40: 2829–2835

Pacifici GM, Nottoli R (1995) Placental transfer of drugs administered to the mother. Clin Pharmacokinet 28: 235–269

Pizzuto J, Aviles A, Noriega L, Niz J, Morales M, Romero F (1980) Treatment of acute leukemia during pregnancy: presentation of nine cases. Cancer Treat Rep 64: 679–683

Powell HR, Ekert H (1971) Methotrexate-induced congenital malformations. Med J Aust 2: 1076–1077

Prabhash K, Sastry PS, Biswas G et al. (2005) Pregnancy outcome of two patients treated with imatinib. Ann Oncol 16: 1983–1984

Raffles A, Williams J, Costeloe K, Clark P (1989) Transplacental effects of maternal cancer chemotherapy. Case report. Br J Obstet Gynaecol 96: 1099–1100

Randall T (1993) National registry seeks scarce data on pregnancy outcomes during chemotherapy. JAMA 269: 323

Reynoso EE, Shepherd FA, Messner HA, Farquharson HA, Garvey MB, Baker MA (1987) Acute leukemia during pregnancy: the Toronto Leukemia Study Group experience with long-term follow-up of children exposed in utero to chemotherapeutic agents. J Clin Oncol 5: 1098–1106

Scully M, Starke R, Lee R, Mackie I, Machin S, Cohen H (2006) Successful management of pregnancy in women with a history of thrombotic thrombocytopaenic purpura. Blood Coagul Fibrinolysis 17: 459–463

Shoton D, Monie IW (1963) Possible teratogenic effect of chlorambucil on a human fetus. JAMA 186: 180–181

Siu BL, Alonzo MR, Vargo TA, Fenrich AL (2002) Transient dilated cardiomyopathy in a newborn exposed to idarubicin and all-*trans*-retinoic acid (ATRA) early in the second trimester of pregnancy. Int J Gynecol Cancer 12: 399–402

Sood AK, Shahin MS, Sorosky JI (2001) Paclitaxel and platinum chemotherapy for ovarian carcinoma during pregnancy. Gynecol Oncol 83: 599–600

Sorosky JI, Sood AK, Buekers TE (1997) The use of chemotherapeutic agents during pregnancy. Obstet Gynecol Clin North Am 24: 591–599

Steege JF, Caldwell DS (1980) Renal agenesis after first trimester exposure to chlorambucil. South Med J 73: 1414–1415

Stentoft J, Nielsen JL, Hvidman LE (1994) All-*trans* retinoic acid in acute promyelocytic leukemia in late pregnancy. Leukemia 8: 1585–1588

Taylor G, Blom J (1980) Acute leukemia during pregnancy. South Med J 73: 1314–1315

Toledo TM, Harper RC, Moser RH (1971) Fetal effects during cyclophosphamide and irradiation therapy. Ann Intern Med 74: 87–91

Vantroyen B, Vanstraelen D (2002) Management of essential thrombocythemia during pregnancy with aspirin, interferon alpha-2a and no treatment. A comparative analysis of the literature. Acta Haematol 107: 158–169

Volkenandt M, Buchner T, Hiddemann W, Van de Loo J (1987) Acute leukaemia during pregnancy. Lancet 2: 1521–1522

Watson WJ (2005) Herceptin (trastuzumab) therapy during pregnancy: association with reversible anhydramnios. Obstet Gynecol 105: 642–643

Weisz B, Meirow D, Schiff E, Lishner M (2004) Impact and treatment of cancer during pregnancy. Expert Rev Anticancer Ther 4: 889–902

Zemlickis D, Lishner M, Degendorfer P, Panzarella T, Sutcliffe SB, Koren G (1992) Fetal outcome after in utero exposure to cancer chemotherapy. Arch Intern Med 152: 573–576

Zemlickis D, Lishner M, Erlich R, Koren G (1993) Teratogenicity and carcinogenicity in a twin exposed in utero to cyclophosphamide. Teratog Carcinog Mutagen 13: 139–143

Zuazu J, Julia A, Sierra J et al. (1991) Pregnancy outcome in hematologic malignancies. Cancer 67: 703–709.

4 Breast Cancer During Pregnancy: Epidemiology, Surgical Treatment, and Staging

O. Gentilini

Recent Results in Cancer Research, Vol. 178

4.1 Definition and Epidemiology

Historically, pregnancy-associated breast cancer was defined as breast cancer diagnosed during pregnancy and within 1 year of delivery. The present chapter deals with the situation of coincident breast cancer and pregnancy, which represents the real challenge for physicians. In fact, breast cancer diagnosed during lactation does not pose specific therapeutic problems compared to all other breast cancer and therefore is not discussed here. Moreover, the term "pregnancy-associated" somehow implies that cancer might be induced or stimulated by the presence of pregnancy, while it seems more a coincidence rather than an association. From this standpoint, we think that it might be more appropriate to define this clinical scenario simply as breast cancer during pregnancy (BCdP).

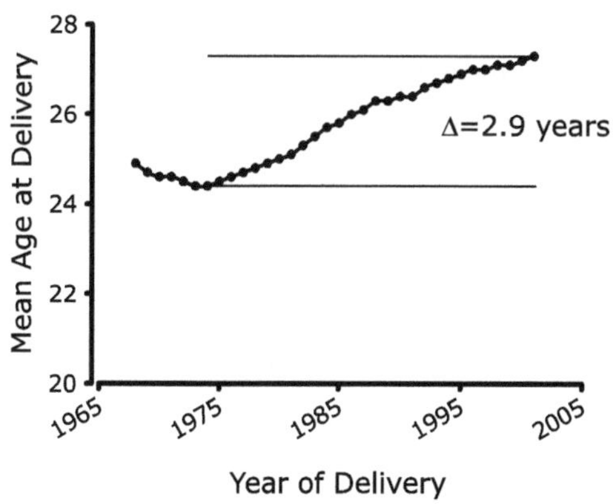

Fig. 4.1 United States of America. The average age of the mothers at delivery increased by 2.9 years between 1974 and 2001

The age of the mother at delivery has been increasing in the last 30 years (Fig. 4.1) and is about 30 years on average in most European countries and a few years younger in the US. Breast cancer is rare in young patients: women below the age of 40 represent less than 10% of patients who develop breast cancer; still, breast cancer is not uncommon in young women. In Western countries, breast cancer is the most common cause of cancer deaths in women aged 30 years and older, and its incidence is much higher than those of Hodgkin disease and other neoplasias commonly associated with young age (Fig. 4.2) (Ries 2006).

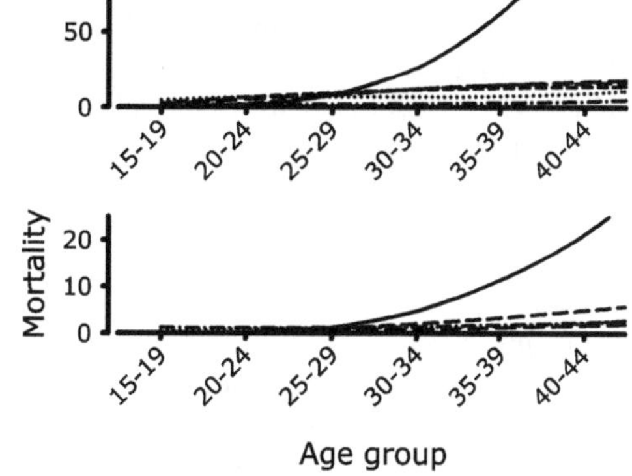

Fig. 4.2 Incidence and mortality of common malignant neoplasias in women of childbearing age

Presently, 1 in 3,000 to 1 in 10,000 pregnancies is complicated by breast cancer (Berry et al. 1999), but with the trend for postponing pregnancy until the thirties and forties it is likely that an increased rate of BCdP will occur.

A Swedish study in women diagnosed with breast cancer before the age of 40 suggested that BRCA1/2 mutation carriers were at increased risk of developing the disease during pregnancy, indicating a role for circulating estrogens in accelerating malignant transformation (Johansson et al. 1998). However, this suggestive hypothesis needs to be confirmed.

4.2 Presentation and Diagnosis

The diagnosis of breast cancer is difficult in pregnancy because of the physiological modifications of the breast in pregnancy. Nevertheless, a painless lump is the most frequent presentation. The diagnostic procedures follow a pattern similar to that in nonpregnant patients, with only slight differences. The diagnosis can often be made with ultrasound alone, which in our opinion should be the first choice as imaging procedure in the presence of a lump. In fact, ultrasound is highly diagnostic in patients with a dense pattern of the breast, as usually happens in young women. Second, the presence of the fetus dictates that the use of ionizing radiation should be limited as much as possible. Therefore, in the presence of a lump, which cannot be diagnosed as certainly benign by ultrasound, histopathologic diagnosis must be performed. Fine-needle aspiration (FNA) or core-needle biopsy can establish the diagnosis. Microhistology is preferable to cytology because FNA has been associated with both false-positive and false-negative results (Mitre et al. 1997; Shannon et al. 2001), the rate of which, however, is very low in expert hands. Microhistology mostly allows diagnosis of invasive cancer and determination of biological features of the tumor that might be important in the decision-making process. It is also important that the pathologist is informed of the presence of pregnancy.

Mammography is possible with proper shielding of the abdomen with minimal exposure of the fetus to ionizing radiation. In fact, with a two-view mammogram the uterine-fetal dose is 4 mGy, well below the threshold for deterministic effects of 100 mGy (Pentheroudakis and Pavlidis 2006). The dense, proliferating mammary glands of young pregnant women may make mammographic diagnosis difficult (sensitivity less than 70%) (Pavlidis and Pentheroudakis 2005; Moore and Foster 2000). Even important masses can be obscured by the normal reaction of the breast to pregnancy, and therefore it is difficult for mammography to be useful to achieve diagnosis in this special setting. However, mammography should be recommended before surgery in order to rule out diffuse microcalcifications in case conservative surgery is planned. From this standpoint, a single projection can be considered to reduce radiation exposure.

The use of MRI to diagnose breast cancer in pregnancy has not been investigated adequately. However, the use of gadolinium contrast media is discouraged, as the contrast media cross the placenta and induce malformations in animal models (Garel et al. 1998). Thus the routine use of breast MRI during pregnancy is discouraged.

4.3 Surgical Treatment of Breast Cancer During Pregnancy

4.3.1 Mastectomy Versus Breast-Conserving Therapy

The occurrence of BCdP poses an acute and dramatic dilemma for the patient, her family, and her physician. The management of BCdP requires a collaborative team effort to provide the best medical options and most effective psychosocial support. Women with BCdP are often influenced by various opinions, which are often radical and difficult to argue against. However, probably more than any other medical condition, BCdP requires a thorough discussion. Obviously, the patient is looking for the physician's recommendation, but it is the physician's role to ensure that the patient is fully aware that she has a variety of treatment options to consider.

Historically, mastectomy was considered to be the standard surgical procedure in pregnant patients with breast cancer (Woo et al. 2003). There are two possible reasons for this: first, patients frequently presented with large tumors as a result of diagnostic delay, and second, there was a concern about the delay before administration of radiotherapy, which is contraindicated during pregnancy.

In our opinion, it is important to inform the patient that mastectomy is not mandatory for the treatment of BCdP (Schwartz et al. 2006). In the experience of the European Institute of Oncology of Milan (Gentilini et al. 2005), tumor size and rate of axillary metastases in patients with BCdP were lower than in previous reports (Berry et al. 1999), probably because of the increased awareness among both patients and physicians. This earlier stage of presentation (median tumor size 2.4 cm) enabled a higher rate of breast-conserving procedures (15 of 21 patients) even though it must be pointed out that all six patients who were diagnosed during the first trimester decided for termination of pregnancy. After a short-term median follow-up (24 months), there were no intrabreast tumor recurrences, and we believe that conservative surgery is a suitable option to discuss with such patients whenever possible. Kuerer et al. reported similar survival rates between patients treated with breast-conserving surgery and those treated with mastectomy (Kuerer et al. 2002). In women diagnosed during the third or the late second trimester, it was suggested that radiotherapy might be postponed until after delivery. Unfortunately, there is limited and retrospective experience published on delayed radiotherapy after breast conservation and its effect on outcome. In a study evaluating 568 patients with T1–T2 N0 breast cancer who underwent lumpectomy and radiotherapy without systemic treatment, a similar rate of recurrence was reported in node-negative patients when radiotherapy started up to 16 weeks after definitive surgery after a median follow-up of 11.2 years (Vujovic et al. 2006). Another retrospective study reported on 13,907 patients aged 65 years or older with stage I–II breast cancer who underwent lumpectomy and radiotherapy taken from the Surveillance, Epidemiology, and End Results (SEER)–Medicare database. The authors concluded that delays of >3 months were associated with poor survival, even though older age, black race, advanced stage, more comorbidities, and unmarried status were associated with longer time intervals between surgery and radiotherapy, and therefore it is not clear whether the association is causal or due to confounding factors (Hershman et al. 2006).

Basically, we suggest that in patients at the second or third trimester, the surgical approach applied to women with BCdP should not significantly differ from that applied to nonpregnant women. The concurrent diagnosis of breast cancer and an unexpected early pregnancy represents the most challenging treatment scenario. It is considered that abortion is not a therapeutic procedure in these cases (Berry et al. 1999), but termination of pregnancy can be considered in order to facilitate completion of treatment. For patients who desire to continue the pregnancy, treatment is possible, but there is a limited number of options during the first weeks of gestation. In fact, chemotherapy is prohibited during the first trimester (Berry et al. 1999; Cardonick and Iacubucci 2004). Surgery is safe at any time (Duncan et al. 1986), but breast conservation performed during the first trimester is probably associated with an excessively long delay in postoperative radiotherapy. Therefore, in a patient at the first trimester who wants to continue the pregnancy and also wishes to conserve the breast all these issues have to be carefully discussed, and the patient has to be informed that a possible increased risk of local recurrence should be considered, even though this is difficult to quantify because of the lack of data.

4.4 Sentinel Node Biopsy

In a review on BCdP, it was stated that axillary dissection is preferred because nodal metastases are commonly found, nodal status affects the choice of adjuvant chemotherapy, and sentinel lymph node biopsy (SLNB) poses an unknown risk to the fetus from the radioisotope (Woo et al. 2003). Patients with BCdP are excluded from the randomized studies on SLNB, and at the Consensus Conference on the role of SLNB in breast carcinoma the panel advised against SLNB in pregnant women until more data are available (Schwartz et al. 2002) More recently, a panel of the American Society of Clinical Oncology concluded that there are insufficient data to recommend the use of SNB in pregnant women with breast cancer (Lyman et al. 2005).

Indeed, when breast cancer is diagnosed during pregnancy, axillary lymph nodes are frequently positive, but when the tumor is diagnosed at an early stage, a considerable proportion of patients have node-negative disease and might therefore benefit from SLNB (Table 4.1).

The decision-making process regarding adjuvant treatment in pregnancy provides limited options. Tamoxifen and other endocrine agents are generally not recommended (Halakivi-Clarke et al. 2000), and other drugs, such as methotrexate (MTX), are strongly contraindicated during pregnancy; in contrast, anthracyclines can be administered during the second and third trimesters (Berry et al. 1999). From this standpoint, axillary staging gives important prognostic information and allows better local control, but should not influence the type of systemic treatment administered during pregnancy.

To evaluate the safety of lymphoscintigraphy and SLNB in pregnant patients, a simulation study was performed in 26 premenopausal nonpregnant women diagnosed with breast cancer. Patients underwent peritumoral injection of approximately 12 MBq of 99m-technetium (^{99m}Tc)-human serum albumin nanocolloids (Gentilini et al. 2004). Static [15 min and 16 h postinjection (p.i.)] and whole body (16 h p.i.) scintigraphic images were acquired. Activity concentration in the urine (0–2 h, 2–4 h, 4–8 h, 8–16 h p.i.) was evaluated by a gamma counter. Activity in the bloodstream was measured at 4 and 16 h p.i. Thermoluminescent dosimeters were placed on the injection site before tracer injection at the epigastrium, umbilicus, and hypogastrum and were removed before surgery.

Scintigraphic imaging showed no diffusion of the radiotracer, except at the injection site and in the sentinel node. Pharmacokinetic data showed that a small amount of the injected radioactivity circulates in the bloodstream and is excreted by the urinary system (<2%). Considering the physical decay of the radiotracer, we can confirm that the level of radioactivity in the body is negligible after each administration of the tracer, posing no significant risk to the fetus. In 23 of 26 patients, all absorbed dose measurements were lower than the sensitivity of the thermoluminescent dosimeters [<10 μgray (μGy)]; in the remaining three patients, the absorbed doses to the epigastrium, umbilicus, and hypogastrium were found to be 100- to 1,000-fold lower than the threshold for deterministic effect. We concluded that, according to our protocol at least, lymphoscintigraphy and SLNB can be safely performed during pregnancy, without any significant risks to the fetus at any phase of pregnancy.

However, there are some practical recommendations that can be followed to further minimize the exposure of the fetus, such as avoiding contact with other patients who might be potential sources of radioactivity (e.g., by scheduling a pregnant patient as the first procedure of the day and keeping the patient in a single-bedded room) and reducing the time interval between lymphoscintigraphy and surgery, with a subsequent possible reduction in the administered radioactivity. Thus, in pregnant patients, SLNB can be performed within 2–3 h after injection of 3–5 MBq of ^{99m}Tc-radiocolloids.

Similar results were reported by Keleher et al. (Keleher et al. 2004). The maximum absorbed dose to the embryo/fetus in pregnant women undergoing breast lymphoscintigraphy

Table 4.1 Rate of node-positive disease in published papers

Author	Accrual	Patients	Tumor size (cm)	Node positive (%)
Berry	1989–1997	26	4.5	67
Middleton	1986–2001	29	4.5	79
Ishida	1978–1988	72	2.8	58
Bonnier	1960–1993	154	2.5	65
Gentilini	1996–2003	21	2.4	48

with 92.5 MBq (2.5 mCi) of ^{99m}Tc-sulfur colloid was found to be 0.0043 Gy under the most adverse conditions in the theoretical model (in which all of the injected radiopharmaceutical travels immediately to the bladder and is eliminated through the process of physical decay). The potentially largest absorbed dose with lymphoscintigraphy remained approximately 12–23 times lower than the threshold associated with reported risk of fetal adverse effects associated with radiation exposure. The authors concluded that the use of ^{99m}Tc-sulfur colloid for pregnant patients with a clinically negative axilla is theoretically safe for the developing embryo/fetus.

4.5 Staging of Patients with Breast Cancer in Pregnancy

The diagnostic work-up of the pregnant woman with cancer should limit exposure to ionizing radiation and be restricted to procedures that do not endanger fetal health. The developing human embryo and fetus are extremely sensitive to ionizing radiation, which might cause pregnancy loss, malformations, growth retardation, and neurobehavioral defects. Most such anomalies appear at fetal doses in excess of 200 mGy, although avoidance of exposure to doses higher than 100 mGy is advised because of the non-deterministic nature of radiobiological events (International Commission on Radiological Protection 2003; Kal and Struikmans 2005).

During the first trimester of pregnancy, only absolutely necessary radiological work-up is justified. When needed, staging of the pregnant woman with cancer should be done by means of chest X-ray and abdominal ultrasound. Chest X-ray seems safe with appropriate radioprotection (lead apron). Radionuclide isotope scans and computerized tomography (CT) scans should be avoided (Nicklas and Baker 2000).

For imaging of the brain, liver, or bones in the context of clinical suspicion for metastases, magnetic resonance imaging (MRI) has been advocated, although the examination was not without drawbacks for the safety of animal embryos. Gadolinium crosses the placenta and causes fetal abnormalities in rats, while the high-energy radio wave-stimulated magnetic fields used carry the risks of fetal heating and cavitation (Garel et al. 1998).

References

Berry DL, Theriault RL, Holmes FA et al. (1999) Management of breast cancer during pregnancy using a standardized protocol. J Clin Oncol 17: 855–861

Bonnier P, Romain S, Dilhuydy JM, Bonichon F, Julien JP, Charpin C, Lejeune C, Martin PM, Piana L (1997) Influence of pregnancy on the outcome of breast cancer: a case-control study. Societe Francaise de Senologie et de Pathologie Mammaire Study Group. Int J Cancer 72(5): 720–727

Cardonick E, Iacubucci A (2004) Use of chemotherapy during pregnancy. Lancet Oncol 5: 283–291

Duncan PG, Pope WDB, Cohen MM et al. (1986) Fetal risk of anesthesia and surgery during pregnancy. Anesthesiology 64: 790–794

Garel C, Brisse H, Sebag G et al. (1998) Magnetic resonance imaging of the foetus. Pediatr Radiol 28: 201–211

Gentilini O, Cremonesi M, Trifirò G et al. (2004) Safety of sentinel node biopsy in pregnant patients with breast cancer. Ann Oncol 15: 1348–1351

Gentilini O, Masullo M, Rotmensz N et al. (2005) Breast cancer diagnosed during pregnancy and lactation: biological features and treatment options. EJSO 31: 232–236

Halakivi-Clarke L, Cho E, Onojafe I, Liao DJ, Clarke R (2000) Maternal exposure to tamoxifen during pregnancy increases carcinogen-induced mammary tumorigenesis among female rat offspring. Clin Cancer Res 6: 305–308.

Hershman DL, Wang X, McBride R, Jacobson JS, Grann VR, Neugut AI (2006) Delay in initiating adjuvant radiotherapy following breast conservation and its impact on survival. Int J Radiat Oncol Biol Phys 65(5): 1353–1360

International Commission on Radiological Protection (2003) Biological effects after prenatal irradiation (embryo and foetus). ICRP publication 90. Ann ICRP 33(1–2): 5–206

Ishida T, Yokoe T, Kasumi F, Sakamoto G, Makita M, Tominaga T, Simozuma K, Enomoto K, Fujiwara K, Nanasawa T et al. (1992) Clinicopathologic characteristics and prognosis of breast cancer patients associated with pregnancy and lactation: analysis of case-control study in Japan. Jpn J Cancer Res 83(11): 1143–1149

Johansson O, Loman N, Borg A et al. (1998) Pregnancy-associated breast cancer in BRCA1 and BRCA2 germ-line mutation carriers. Lancet 352: 1359–1360

Kal HB, Struikmans H (2005) Radiotherapy during pregnancy: fact and fiction. Lancet Oncol6: 328–333

Keleher A, Wendt III R, Delpassand E, Stachowiak AM, Kuerer HM (2004) The safety of lymphatic mapping in pregnant breast cancer patients using Tc-99m sulfur colloid. Breast J 10: 492–495

Kuerer H, Gwyn K, Ames F et al. (2002) Conservative surgery and chemotherapy for breast carcinoma during pregnancy. Surgery 131: 108–110

Lyman GH, Giuliano AE, Somerfield MR et al. (2005) American Society of Clinical Oncology Guideline Recommendations for Sentinel Lymph Node Biopsy in Early-Stage Breast Cancer J Clin Oncol 23: 7703–7720

Middleton LP, Amin M, Gwyn K, Theriault R, Sahin A (2003) Breast carcinoma in pregnant women: assessment of clinicopathologic and immunohistochemical features. Cancer 98(5): 1055–1060

Mitre B, Kaubour A, Mauser N (1997) Fine needle aspiration biopsy of breast carcinoma in pregnancy and lactation. Acta Cytol 41: 1121–1130

Moore HCF, Foster RS (2000) Breast cancer and pregnancy. Semin Oncol 27: 646–653

Nicklas A, Baker M (2000) Imaging strategies in pregnant cancer patients. Semin Oncol;27: 623–632

Pavlidis NA, Pentheroudakis G (2005) The pregnant mother with breast cancer: diagnostic and therapeutic management. Cancer Treat Rev 31(6): 439–447

Pentheroudakis G, Pavlidis N (2006) Cancer and pregnancy: poena magna, not anymore. Eur J Cancer 42: 126–140

Schwartz GF, Giuliano AE, Veronesi U (2002) Consensus Conference Committee. Proceedings of the consensus conference on the role of sentinel lymph node biopsy in carcinoma of the breast, April 19–22, 2001, Philadelphia, Pennsylvania. Cancer 94(10): 2542–2551

Schwartz GF, Veronesi U, Clough K et al. (2006) Proceedings of the Consensus Conference on Breast Conservation, April 28 to May 1, 2005, Milan, Italy Cancer 107(2): 242–250

Shannon J, Douglas-Jones AG, Dallimore NS (2001) Conversion to core-biopsy in preoperative diagnosis of breast lesions: is it justified by results? J Clin Pathol 54: 762–765

Vujovic O, Cherian A, Dar AR, Stitt L, Perera F (2006) Eleven-year follow up results in the delay of breast irradiation after conservative surgery in node-negative breast cancer patients. Int J Radiat Oncol Biol Phys 64(3): 760–764

Woo JC, Yu T, Hurd TC (2003) Breast cancer in pregnancy: a literature review. Arch Surg 138: 91–99

5 Breast Cancer During Pregnancy: Medical Therapy and Prognosis

S. Aebi, S. Loibl

Recent Results in Cancer Research, Vol. 178

5.1 Biological Characteristics of Breast Cancer in Pregnancy

The pathological features of breast cancer diagnosed during pregnancy have been analyzed in numerous studies. Because of the retrospective nature of such studies and the paucity of case-control studies it is impossible to directly compare the biological properties of breast cancer in pregnant and nonpregnant patients of similar age. The vast majority of breast cancers are invasive ductal (Woo et al. 2003). It is likely that, in addition to larger tumor diameters and more frequent involvement of the regional lymph nodes, breast cancers in pregnancy are characterized by poor differentiation and low expression of estrogen and progesterone receptors (Fig. 5.1) (Bonnier et al. 1997; Gentilini et al. 2004; Middleton et al. 2003; Miller et al. 2005; Reed et al. 2003; Ring et al. 2005); a recent review identified 13 studies reporting estrogen receptors in breast cancers diagnosed during pregnancy; estrogen receptors were negative in 138 of 235 patients (59%, 95% confidence interval 52%–65%) (Woo et al. 2003). The proportion of breast cancers with overexpression of HER-2 protein was similar in pregnant and in young nonpregnant patients (Aziz et al. 2003; Colleoni et al. 2002; Middleton et al. 2003).

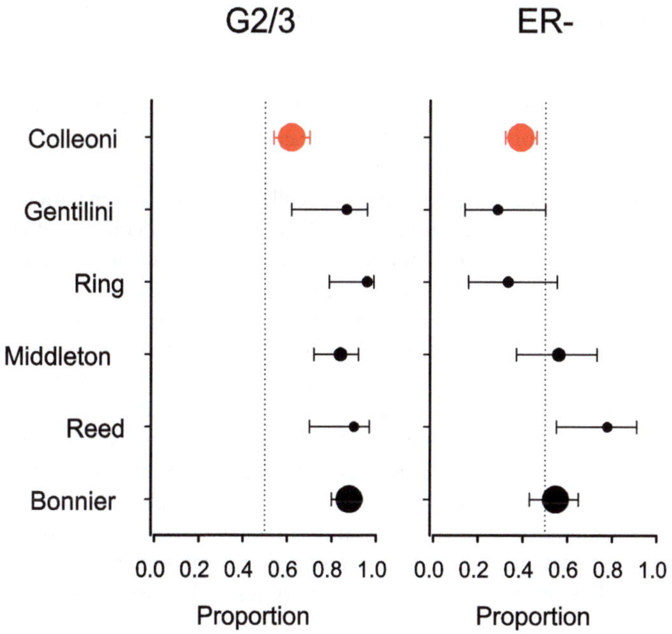

Fig. 5.1 Proportion of patients with intermediate or poorly differentiated and with estrogen receptor-negative tumors in nonpregnant patients aged 35 years (Colleoni et al. 2002) and in pregnant patients (Bonnier et al. 1997; Gentilini et al. 2004; Middleton et al. 2003; Miller et al. 2005; Reed et al. 2003; Ring et al. 2005). Areas represent the sample size, 95% confidence intervals

5.2 Adjuvant Therapies

5.2.1 Indications

The indications for adjuvant chemotherapy in pregnant patients are identical to those in non-pregnant patients. However, adjuvant hormonal therapy and radiation therapy are not indicated in pregnancy, as the initiation of hormonal and radiation therapy is rarely an emergency. Thus preoperative (neoadjuvant) chemotherapy may be indicated for the therapy of locally advanced breast cancer according to recent consensus guidelines (Kaufmann et al. 2006). Recommendations such as those resulting from the St. Gallen consensus conference (Goldhirsch et al. 2005), from national health services, for example, Cancer Care Ontario (Cancer Care Ontario, 2006), or from cancer center networks, for example, the National Comprehensive Cancer Network (Carlson et al. 2006), may be used to determine the appropriateness of postoperative adjuvant chemotherapy.

The timing of chemotherapy is crucial: While it is obviously preferable to postpone chemotherapy until after delivery, this is not always possible. For instance, locally advanced tumors may need to be treated in a neoadjuvant manner. In addition, for patients whose tumors do not express estrogen receptors, a late start of chemotherapy, that is, >3 weeks after surgery, may worsen the prognosis dramatically as compared to an early start of chemotherapy (Colleoni et al. 2000). The efficacy of very late adjuvant chemotherapies, for example, starting later than 8 weeks after surgery, is unknown; thus chemotherapy may need to be started during pregnancy even in patients with estrogen receptor-positive tumors.

5.2.2 Chemotherapy

Chemotherapy is contraindicated in the first trimester of pregnancy as the fetus is undergoing organogenesis and is vulnerable to the teratogenic effects of chemotherapy (Cardonick and Iacobucci, 2004). If chemotherapy cannot be postponed to the second trimester of pregnancy, abortion is indicated. Abortion by itself has never been proven to have a beneficial therapeutic effect in breast cancer (Barthelmes et al. 2005).

In the second and third trimesters chemotherapy is relatively safe, as illustrated by the most recent series of patients reported by investigators from the M.D. Anderson Cancer Center (Hahn et al. 2006) and from the Royal Marsden Hospital (Ring et al. 2005).

The Royal Marsden retrospective series consists of 28 women. The patient and tumor characteristics are summarized in Table 5.1 (Ring et al. 2005). This series is characterized by a nonuniform use of chemotherapy; as in other case series, the use of chemotherapy in the second and third trimesters was safe. Methotrexate is used to induce abortions (Say et al. 2005) and is not of particular importance in the contemporary management of breast cancer. We therefore recommend that methotrexate be avoided during pregnancy.

The largest well-characterized prospective case series of patients with breast cancer in pregnancy was updated recently by investigators from the M.D. Anderson Cancer Center (Hahn et al. 2006). This series is characterized by a standardized approach to the management of breast cancer in pregnancy; the patient and tumor characteristics are summarized in Table 5.1. All patients were treated with FAC during the second and third trimesters of pregnancy. In this series, some patients received postpartum adjuvant therapy consisting of taxanes and tamoxifen.

Both case series report favorable fetal outcomes with no reason to suspect an increased risk of malformations. Similar results have been reported in a case collection of Canadian patients reported by the Toronto group (Zemlickis et al. 1996) and in a systematic review of the literature (Woo et al. 2003).

In recent years taxanes (paclitaxel and docetaxel) have become important components of adjuvant therapy (Henderson et al. 2003; Mamounas et al. 2005; Martin et al. 2005). Their use in pregnancy has been reported in a small number of patients with breast (De Santis et al. 2000; Gadducci et al. 2003; Nieto et al. 2006; Potluri et al. 2006) and other neoplasias. So far, there is no evidence of a detrimental effect of taxane use after the first trimester. However, given the proven efficacy of the sequential use of taxanes (Henderson et al. 2003; Mamounas et al. 2005; Roché et al. 2004), taxanes may be candidate drugs for use after delivery.

In summary, doxorubicin, cyclophosphamide, and fluorouracil have been used in a reasonably large number of patients and may be considered safe for use after the first trimester of pregnancy. To date, while no definite and consistent adverse fetal effects have been observed with taxanes, their safety record is very limited.

Table 5.1 Recent studies of chemotherapy for early breast cancer during pregnancy

	MD Anderson Cancer Center [Hahn et al. 2006]	Royal Marsden and London Hospitals [Ring et al. 2005]
Number of patients	57	24 [+ 4 stage IV]
Age at diagnosis	33.5 (24–45)	33 (28–42)
Median gestational age at diagnosis	17.4 (2–33)	17 weeks (4–33)
Stage at diagnosis		
I	3	2
II	28	11
III	26	11
[IV]	0	[4]
Histology		
Invasive ductal	45	19
Other	8	5
Unknown	4	0
Histologic grade		
1	1	0
2	9	6
3	45	17
Unknown	2	1
Estrogen receptor		
Positive	11	11
Negative	25	8
Unknown	21	5
HER-2		
Positive	10	5
Negative	25	7
Unknown	22	12

AC: doxorubicin (50–60 mg/m^2), cyclophosphamide (600 mg/m^2), q 3 weeks

EC: epirubicin (60–100 mg/m^2), cyclophosphamide (600 mg/m^2), q 3 weeks

CMF: cyclophosphamide 100–150 mg orally days 1–14, methotrexate 40 mg/m^2 days 1 and 8, fluorouracil 600 mg/m^2 days 1 and 8, q 4 weeks

FAC, fluorouracil 500 mg/m^2, doxorubicin 50 mg/m^2, fluorouracil 500 mg/m^2, q 3 weeks

Table 5.1 *(continued)* Recent studies of chemotherapy for early breast cancer during pregnancy

	MD Anderson Cancer Center [Hahn et al. 2006]	Royal Marsden and London Hospitals [Ring et al. 2005]
Local therapy		
Mastectomy	42	17
Breast-conserving surgery	15	10
Postpartum radiation therapy	Not reported	17
Gestational age at start of chemotherapy	23 weeks (11–34)	20 weeks (15–33)
Chemotherapy		
Neoadjuvant	25	7
Adjuvant	32	17
[Palliative]		[4]
AC		11
EC		5
CMF		12
FAC	57	
Gestational age at delivery	37 weeks (29–42)	37 weeks (30–40)
Cesarean section	21	6
Birth weight	2.89 kg (1.4–4.0)	3.0 kg (1.4–3.5)
		None <10th percentile for gestational age
Fetal/infant follow-up	2–157 months	Not reported
Fetal outcomes	4 required neonatal ventilation	1 abortion after inadvertent first-trimester chemotherapy with CMF
	1 subarachnoid hemorrhage	2 neonatal respiratory distress
	1 Down syndome	1 hemangioma on the abdomen.
	18 school-age children; 2 special attention schooling	
Median maternal follow-up	38.5 months	40.5 months
Maternal outcomes (stages I–III)		
OS	77%	67%
DFS	70%	63%

AC: doxorubicin (50–60 mg/m^2), cyclophosphamide (600 mg/m^2), q 3 weeks

EC: epirubicin (60–100 mg/m^2), cyclophosphamide (600 mg/m^2), q 3 weeks

CMF: cyclophosphamide 100–150 mg orally days 1–14, methotrexate 40 mg/m^2 days 1 and 8, fluorouracil 600 mg/m^2 days 1 and 8, q 4 weeks

FAC, fluorouracil 500 mg/m^2, doxorubicin 50 mg/m^2, fluorouracil 500 mg/m^2, q 3 weeks

5.2.3 Supportive Care

Antiemetics such as short-term glucocorticosteroids and most serotonin receptor III antagonists are considered safe in pregnancy. Ondansetron has the longest safety record, and no increased frequency of untoward effects has been reported in connection with treating pregnant patients (Einarson et al. 2004). Currently, ondansetron is considered a pregnancy class B drug in the United States. Tropisetron, an antiemetic in frequent use in Europe, has been classified as a class C drug based on malformations observed following in utero exposure in laboratory rodents; in our view, there is no indication for tropisetron in pregnancy. Granisetron and palonosetron have rarely been used in pregnancy. To date, therefore, the serotonin receptor III antagonist of choice is ondansetron.

Granulocyte colony-stimulating factor (GCSF, e.g., filgrastim) is known to cross the placenta and has been used occasionally in pregnant patients; as of December 3, 2006, Medline contains fewer than five reports about the use of filgrastim in pregnancy. Filgrastim and pegfilgrastim are category C drugs because of the induction of abortion and malformations in rodents.

Erythropoietin and darbepoietin have been used in a small number of pregnant patients undergoing dialysis treatment for renal failure; so far, no malformations could be attributed to the use of erythropoietins. Both drugs belong to pregnancy category C. In the context of cancer chemotherapy, dose adaptations and transfusions may be preferable to the use of G-CSFs and erythropoietins.

5.2.4 Trastuzumab

Trastuzumab is effective adjuvant therapy in patients with HER-2-amplified breast cancer. It has been investigated in randomized trials in parallel to sequential taxanes (Romond et al. 2005; Slamon et al. 2005) and after the completion of chemotherapy (Piccart-Gebhart et al. 2005) with similar efficacy at 1–2 years of follow-up. Trastuzumab is known to cross the placenta in primate models; it is labeled as a category B drug in the United States, because no harm has been observed in monkeys. It has been used in very few pregnant patients to treat early (Waterston and Graham, 2006) and metastatic (Fanale et al. 2005; Watson 2005) breast cancer. Whereas no malformations or fetal deaths were described, one fetus developed reversible oligohydramnios (Watson 2005); whether or not this was the consequence of intrauterine heart failure is not known.

At the present time, it seems prudent to consider the efficacy of the sequential use of chemotherapy and trastuzumab and to defer the adjuvant therapy with trastuzumab to the postpartum period.

5.2.5 Hormonal Therapy

Tamoxifen has been reported to cause malformations of the genital tract and of the skeleton in rodents; in addition, the development of the uterus was impaired after exposure to tamoxifen, resembling the changes induced by diethylstilbestrol, a known carcinogen (Barthelmes and Gateley 2004). The effect of tamoxifen on the human fetus is less well known: Whereas cases with malformations have been reported (Cullins et al. 1994; Tewari et al. 1997), others had favorable outcomes of pregnancy (Isaacs et al. 2001; Oksuzoglu and Guler 2002), and a recent review of tamoxifen during pregnancy revealed that at least 100 women became pregnant while on tamoxifen or used tamoxifen during pregnancy. Only one case of ambiguous genitalia was observed; other congenital defects were observed, with no typical pattern appearing (Barthelmes and Gateley 2004). At present, therefore, adjuvant therapy with tamoxifen should be started after pregnancy. Adjuvant aromatase inhibitors have been used during early pregnancy in at least one patient without any manifest adverse fetal effects (Smith et al. 2006). Aromatase inhibitors such as letrozole are being used for the induction of ovulation in survivors of breast cancer without any evidence of harm to the fetus (Oktay et al. 2005). Nevertheless, the efficacy of aromatase inhibitors in premenopausal women is unproven, and the use of such agents during pregnancy is discouraged.

5.2.6 Radiation Therapy

Adjuvant radiation therapy exposes the fetus to ionizing radiation. The absorbed dose depends on the gestational age and the position of the fetus (Bradley et al. 2006). Whether or not detrimental effects of adjuvant radiation therapy are to be anticipated is still a matter of debate (Kal and Struikmans 2005; Mazonakis et al. 2003). However, the start of adjuvant radiation therapy is never urgent; delays of radiation therapy of up to 3–4 months result in outcomes similar to those with earlier initiation (Hebert-Croteau et al. 2004; Hershman et al. 2006; Vujovic et al. 2006). In most cases, therefore, the initiation of radiation therapy can be safely delayed until after delivery.

5.2.7 Systemic Palliative Therapy

For patients with metastatic breast cancer, the same principles apply as for patients with early breast cancer. Generally speaking, chemotherapy is possible in the second and third trimesters, and radiation therapy and hormonal therapies should preferably be deferred until after delivery. The choice of chemotherapy is identical to the adjuvant situation. The use of cytotoxic drugs during pregnancy has been reported, for example vinorelbine (Cuvier et al. 1997; Fanale et al. 2005) or docetaxel (De Santis et al. 2000; Nieto et al. 2006; Potluri et al. 2006). Although no adverse outcomes of pregnancy have been reported, the low number of patients precludes any useful conclusion.

Lapatinib, an inhibitor of EGF receptor and HER-2 kinase activity, was used inadvertently in one pregnant patient: No adverse outcome was observed (Kelly et al. 2006). For trastuzumab the same considerations apply in advanced and early breast cancer. We are not aware of any report of bevacizumab during pregnancy; based on the experience of thalidomide, however, it is obvious that antiangiogenic agents may have catastrophic consequences when used during early pregnancy.

5.2.8 Bisphosphonates

At present, bisphosphonates are effective and licensed for the treatment of hypercalcemia, prevention of fractures, and skeletal pain due to metastatic involvement of bones (Pavlakis et al. 2005). They have not been approved for the adjuvant treatment of breast cancer, although randomized studies have shown them to reduce the occurrence of bone metastases (Diel et al. 1998; Powles et al. 2006). Bisphosphonates have been used in a small number of patients during pregnancy without any reported negative fetal effects. However, one must be aware of potential undesired effects of bisphosphonates. First, they can induce hypocalcemia, which in turn can reduce the contractility of the uterus; this was associated with neonatal deaths, and hypocalcemia should be treated with intravenous calcium supplementation (Culbert and Schfirin 2006). Second, bisphosphonates cross the placenta; the fetal osteoclast activity could be inhibited, giving rise to skeletal abnormalities. So far, none have been reported, however. Given the small numbers of patients who have been treated during pregnancy, adverse effects cannot be excluded (Illidge et al. 1996). Therefore, the use of bisphosphonates is not recommended during pregnancy.

5.3 Maternal Prognosis and Fetal Outcomes

5.3.1 Maternal Prognosis

The prognosis of breast cancer depends on the involvement of axillary lymph nodes, tumor size, and differentiation; sex hormone receptors are important predictors of the response to adjuvant therapy. Whether or not the maternal prognosis for breast cancer during pregnancy is worse has been a matter of debate. Given the known unfavorable biological characteristics, breast cancer in pregnancy has been regarded as particularly aggressive. However, in the majority of retrospective case-control studies with multivariate statistical analysis of prognostic and predictive factors, the prognosis of women with breast cancer during pregnancy did not appear to differ from that of nonpregnant patients of the same age and stage of disease (Table 5.2). Thus the conventional belief of an inferior prognosis is probably based on a higher proportion of patients with adverse prognostic factors such as more advanced stage at diagnosis; nonstandardized and suboptimal therapies may have contributed to this clinical impression. At present, therefore, standard prognostic and predictive factors should be used to estimate the risk of recurrence and death from breast cancer as well as the likely effectiveness of medical therapies.

Table 5.2 Selected studies comparing the prognosis of patients with pregnancy-associated breast cancer and nonpregnant controls [modified from Loibl et al. 2006]

Author	Number of patients	Survival type	Subgroup	Survival rate PABC %	Survival rate non-PABC %	P value
Nugent and O'Connell 1985	19 PABC 157 controls	5 y OAS	All	56	56	n.s.
Petrek et al. 1991	63 PABC	5 y OAS	All	61	73	n.s.
			N0	82	82	n.s.
			N+	47	59	n.s.
		10 y OAS	all	45	62	n.s.
			N0	77	75	n.s.
			N+	25	41	n.s.
Ishida et al. 1992	192 PABC 191 controls	10 y OAS	All	55	79	0.001
			N0	85	93	0.05
			N+	37	62	0.01
Zemlickis et al. 1992	118/102 PABC 269 controls	10 y OAS	All	40	48	0.6
Chang et al. 1994	21 PABC 199 controls	5 y OAS	All	57	70	n.s.
Guinee et al. 1994	26 pregnant (66 PABC)	5 y OAS	All	40	70	<0.0001
Anderson et al. 1996	22 PABC 205 controls	10 y OAS	I-IIA	73	74	n.s.
			IIB-IIIA	17	47	
Bonnier et al. 1997	154 PABC (62 pregnant) 308 controls	5 y RFS	All	69	81	0.01
		5 y MFS	all	45	68	0.0009
			N0	63	77	n.s.
			N+	31	63	0.0001
		5 y OAS	all	61	75	0.001
Ibrahim et al. 2000	72 PABC 216 controls	5 y OAS	All	55*	51*	n.s.
Zhang et al. 2003	88 PABC (33 pregnant) 176 controls	5 y OAS	All	40%	57%	0.05
		10 y OAS		36%	55%	

PABC, pregnancy associated breast cancer; *OAS*, overall survival; *RFS*, recurrent free survival; *MFS*, metastasis-free survival; *N0*: nodal negative; *N+*: nodal positive; *estimate from published figure

5.3.2 Children with In Utero Exposure to Chemotherapy

Early toxicities of cytotoxic treatment on the fetus include anemia, neutropenia, and alopecia depending on the timing of the therapy in relation to delivery (Giacalone et al. 1999). Usually, newborns will recover from these side effects. However, the neonatologist should be aware of these possible complications and monitor the newborn adequately.

Little is known about the possible delayed effects of exposure to antineoplastic agents in utero. Major concerns include physical and mental development, heart function, secondary malignancies, and infertility. A large study with a median follow-up of 18.7 years on 84 children who were born to mothers who received chemotherapy during pregnancy for hematologic malignancies, did not reveal any congenital neurological and psychological abnormalities and, indeed, showed normal learning and educational behavior (Aviles and Neri 2001).

Some data can be extrapolated from children who have received chemotherapy for acute leukemia. However, the amount of drugs given in children is comparatively high, the type of drugs used differs between leukemia and breast cancer, and in the pregnant breast cancer patient only a percentage of the delivered drug will reach the fetus. A study by Kremer et al. (Kremer et al. 2001) reported a 5% cumulative rate of anthracycline-induced clinical heart failure 15 years after therapy in a cohort of 607 children. The incidence increased with the cumulative dose of anthracyclines and with the time of follow-up. In two reviews by the same authors the incidence of subclinical cardiotoxicity and heart failure after anthracycline-containing chemotherapy ranged from 0% to 57% and 0%–16%, respectively (Kremer et al. 2002a, 2002b). However, most of the trials had limitations and the authors recommended new studies with well-defined patient groups. A case report of fetal echocardiography sequences during maternal anthracycline-containing chemotherapy revealed no changes of the shortening fraction as well as the biometry of the ventricular cavities (Meyer-Wittkopf et al. 2001).

5.3.3 In Utero Exposure to Hormonal Therapy

Neonatal defects produced by tamoxifen have been described in the genital tract in female mice (Cunha et al. 1987). Although tamoxifen has been given safely in patients with metastatic breast cancer without damage to the child (Isaacs et al. 2001; Oksuzoglu and Guler 2002), there are other reports of birth defects such as Goldenhar syndrome (Cullins et al. 1994) and ambiguous genitalia (Tewari et al. 1997) in human embryos (Woo et al. 2003). Hormone treatment, if indicated, should start after delivery and after completion of chemotherapy.

5.3.4 In Utero Exposure to Trastuzumab

A small number of case reports have been published describing the use of trastuzumab in pregnant patients. In one of those cases a reversible anhydramnios was reported (Watson 2005). In two cases there was no detrimental effect on the pregnancy (Fanale et al. 2005; Waterston and Graham 2006). The United States Food and Drug Administration has labeled trastuzumab as a pregnancy category B drug. Studies in monkeys showed placental transfer, but no harm to the fetuses was observed. Nevertheless, at present, we discourage the use of trastuzumab in pregnant patients.

5.4 Role of Cancer Registries in the Improvement of Care for Patients with Breast Cancer in Pregnancy

In the treatment of the pregnant breast cancer patient, the evidence upon which we base decisions has been largely limited to case reports, case-control studies, and retrospective cohorts. The German Breast Group has launched a prospective registry for women with breast cancer during pregnancy. So far, data on 72 patients have been collected. All women with a diagnosis of breast cancer during pregnancy can be registered independently of the therapy used. The primary end point of the registry is the outcome of the baby 4 weeks after delivery. Secondary end points are the outcome of the mother, the pregnancy, the outcome of the child after 5 years, the biological and histologic properties of the cancer, the stage at the time of diagnosis, the therapies used, and the methods used during pregnancy to diagnose cancer. Randomized controlled studies are unlikely to succeed because of the rarity of the condition. Thus it is critical that collection of prospective data such as those collected in the database of the German Breast Group/Breast International Group be continued.

References

Anderson BO, Petrek JA, Byrd DR et al. (1996) Pregnancy influences breast cancer stage at diagnosis in women 30 years of age and younger. Ann Surg Oncol 3: 204–211

Aviles A and Neri N (2001) Hematological malignancies and pregnancy: a final report of 84 children who received chemotherapy in utero. Clin Lymphoma 2: 173–177

Aziz S, Pervez S, Khan S et al. (2003) Case control study of novel prognostic markers and disease outcome in pregnancy/lactation-associated breast carcinoma. Pathol Res Pract 199: 15–21

Barthelmes L and Gateley CA (2004) Tamoxifen and pregnancy. Breast 13: 446–451

Barthelmes L, Davidson LA, Gaffney C et al. (2005) Pregnancy and breast cancer. BMJ 330: 1375–1378

Bonnier P, Romain S, Dilhuydy JM et al. (1997) Influence of pregnancy on the outcome of breast cancer: a case-control study. Societe Francaise de Senologie et de Pathologie Mammaire Study Group. Int J Cancer 72: 720–727

Bradley B, Fleck A, Osei EK (2006) Normalized data for the estimation of fetal radiation dose from radiotherapy of the breast. Br J Radiol 79: 818–827

Cancer Care Ontario (2006) Breast Cancer Evidence-based Series and Practice Guidelines, Vol. 2006, Cancer Care Ontario

Cardonick E and Iacobucci A (2004) Use of chemotherapy during human pregnancy. Lancet Oncol 5: 283–291

Carlson RW, Anderson BO, Burstein HJ et al. (2006) NCCN Clinical Practice Guidelines in Oncology. Breast Cancer

Chang YT, Loong CC, Wang HC et al. (1994) Breast cancer and pregnancy. Zhonghua Yi Xue Za Zhi (Taipei) 54: 223–229

Colleoni M, Bonetti M, Coates AS et al. (2000) Early start of adjuvant chemotherapy may improve treatment outcome for premenopausal breast cancer patients with tumors not expressing estrogen receptors. The International Breast Cancer Study Group. J Clin Oncol 18: 584–590

Colleoni M, Rotmensz N, Robertson C et al. (2002) Very young women (<35 years) with operable breast cancer: features of disease at presentation. Ann Oncol 13: 273–279

Culbert EC and Schfirin BS (2006) Malignant hypercalcemia in pregnancy: effect of pamidronate on uterine contractions. Obstet Gynecol 108: 789–791

Cullins SL, Pridjian G, Sutherland CM (1994) Goldenhar's syndrome associated with tamoxifen given to the mother during gestation. JAMA 271: 1905–1906

Cunha GR, Taguchi O, Namikawa R et al. (1987) Teratogenic effects of clomiphene, tamoxifen, and diethylstilbestrol on the developing human female genital tract. Hum Pathol 18: 1132–1143

Cuvier C, Espie M, Extra JM et al. (1997) Vinorelbine in pregnancy. Eur J Cancer 33: 168–169

De Santis M, Lucchese A, De Carolis S et al. (2000) Metastatic breast cancer in pregnancy: first case of chemotherapy with docetaxel. Eur J Cancer Care (Engl) 9: 235–237

Diel IJ, Solomayer EF, Costa SD et al. (1998) Reduction in new metastases in breast cancer with adjuvant clodronate treatment. N Engl J Med 339: 357–363

Einarson A, Maltepe C, Navioz Y et al. (2004) The safety of ondansetron for nausea and vomiting of pregnancy: a prospective comparative study. BJOG 111: 940–943

Fanale MA, Uyei AR, Theriault RL et al. (2005) Treatment of metastatic breast cancer with trastuzumab and vinorelbine during pregnancy. Clin Breast Cancer 6: 354–356

Gadducci A, Cosio S, Fanucchi A et al. (2003) Chemotherapy with epirubicin and paclitaxel for breast cancer during pregnancy: case report and review of the literature. Anticancer Res 23: 5225–5229

Gentilini O, Cremonesi M, Trifiro G et al. (2004) Safety of sentinel node biopsy in pregnant patients with breast cancer. Ann Oncol 15: 1348–1351

Giacalone PL, Laffargue F, Benos P (1999) Chemotherapy for breast carcinoma during pregnancy: A French national survey. Cancer 86: 2266–2272

Goldhirsch A, Glick JH, Gelber RD et al. (2005) Meeting highlights: international expert consensus on the primary therapy of early breast cancer 2005. Ann Oncol 16: 1569–1583

Guinee VF, Olsson H, Moller T et al. (1994) Effect of pregnancy on prognosis for young women with breast cancer. Lancet 343: 1587–1589

Hahn KM, Johnson PH, Gordon N et al. (2006) Treatment of pregnant breast cancer patients and outcomes of children exposed to chemotherapy in utero. Cancer 107: 1219–1226

Hebert-Croteau N, Freeman CR, Latreille J et al. (2004) A population-based study of the impact of delaying radiotherapy after conservative surgery for breast cancer. Breast Cancer Res Treat 88: 187–196

Henderson IC, Berry DA, Demetri GD et al. (2003) Improved outcomes from adding sequential Paclitaxel but not from escalating Doxorubicin dose in an adjuvant chemotherapy regimen for patients with node-positive primary breast cancer. J Clin Oncol 21: 976–983

Hershman DL, Wang X, McBride R et al. (2006) Delay in initiating adjuvant radiotherapy following breast conservation surgery and its impact on survival. Int J Radiat Oncol Biol Phys 65: 1353–1360

Ibrahim EM, Ezzat AA, Baloush A et al. (2000) Pregnancy-associated breast cancer: a case-control study in a young population with a high-fertility rate. Med Oncol 17: 293–300

Illidge TM, Hussey M, Godden CW (1996) Malignant hypercalcaemia in pregnancy and antenatal administration of intravenous pamidronate. Clin Oncol (R Coll Radiol) 8: 257–258

Isaacs RJ, Hunter W, Clark K (2001) Tamoxifen as systemic treatment of advanced breast cancer during pregnancy—case report and literature review. Gynecol Oncol 80: 405–408

Ishida T, Yokoe T, Kasumi F et al. (1992) Clinicopathologic characteristics and prognosis of breast cancer patients associated with pregnancy and lactation: analysis of case-control study in Japan. Jpn J Cancer Res 83: 1143–1149

Kal HB and Struikmans H (2005) Radiotherapy during pregnancy: fact and fiction. Lancet Oncol 6: 328–333

Kaufmann M, Hortobagyi GN, Goldhirsch A et al. (2006) Recommendations from an international expert panel on the use of neoadjuvant (primary) systemic treatment of operable breast cancer: an update. J Clin Oncol 24: 1940–1949

Kelly H, Graham M, Humes E et al. (2006) Delivery of a healthy baby after first-trimester maternal exposure to lapatinib. Clin Breast Cancer 7: 339–341

Kremer LC, van Dalen EC, Offringa M et al. (2001) Anthracycline-induced clinical heart failure in a cohort of 607 children: long-term follow-up study. J Clin Oncol 19: 191–196

Kremer LC, van der Pal HJ, Offringa M et al. (2002a) Frequency and risk factors of subclinical cardiotoxicity after anthracycline therapy in children: a systematic review. Ann Oncol 13: 819–829

Kremer LCM, van Dalen EC, Offringa M et al. (2002b) Frequency and risk factors of anthracycline-induced clinical heart failure in children: a systematic review. Ann Oncol 13: 503–512.

Loibl S, von Minckwitz G, Gwyn K et al. (2006). Breast carcinoma during pregnancy. International recommendations from an expert meeting. Cancer 106: 237–246

Mamounas EP, Bryant J, Lembersky B et al. (2005) Paclitaxel after doxorubicin plus cyclophosphamide as adjuvant chemotherapy for node-positive breast cancer: results from NSABP B-28. J Clin Oncol 23: 3686–3696

Martin M, Pienkowski T, Mackey J et al. (2005) Adjuvant docetaxel for node-positive breast cancer. N Engl J Med 352: 2302–2313

Mazonakis M, Varveris H, Damilakis J et al. (2003) Radiation dose to conceptus resulting from tangential breast irradiation. Int J Radiat Oncol Biol Phys 55: 386–391

Meyer-Wittkopf M, Barth H, Emons G et al. (2001) Fetal cardiac effects of doxorubicin therapy for carcinoma of the breast during pregnancy: case report and review of the literature. Ultrasound Obstet Gynecol 18: 62–66

Middleton LP, Amin M, Gwyn K et al. (2003) Breast carcinoma in pregnant women: assessment of clinicopathologic and immunohistochemical features. Cancer 98: 1055–1060

Miller KD, Chap LI, Holmes FA et al. (2005) Randomized Phase III trial of capecitabine compared with bevacizumab plus capecitabine in patients with previously treated metastatic breast cancer. J Clin Oncol 23: 792–799

Nieto Y, Santisteban M, Aramendia JM et al. (2006) Docetaxel administered during pregnancy for inflammatory breast carcinoma. Clin Breast Cancer 6: 533–534

Nugent P and O'Connell TX (1985) Breast cancer and pregnancy. Arch Surg 120: 1221–1224

Oksuzoglu B and Guler N (2002) An infertile patient with breast cancer who delivered a healthy child under adjuvant tamoxifen therapy. Eur J Obstet Gynecol Reprod Biol 104: 79

Oktay K, Buyuk E, Libertella N et al. (2005) Fertility preservation in breast cancer patients: a prospective controlled comparison of ovarian stimulation with tamoxifen and letrozole for embryo cryopreservation. J Clin Oncol 23: 4347–4353

Pavlakis N, Schmidt R, Stockler M (2005) Bisphosphonates for breast cancer. Cochrane Database Syst Rev: CD003474

Petrek JA, Dukoff R, Rogatko A (1991) Prognosis of pregnancy-associated breast cancer. Cancer 67: 869–872

Piccart-Gebhart MJ, Procter M, Leyland-Jones B et al. (2005) Trastuzumab after adjuvant chemotherapy in HER2-positive breast cancer. N Engl J Med 353: 1659–1672

Potluri V, Lewis D, Burton GV (2006) Chemotherapy with taxanes in breast cancer during pregnancy: case report and review of the literature. Clin Breast Cancer 7: 167–170

Powles T, Paterson A, McCloskey E et al. (2006) Reduction in bone relapse and improved survival with oral clodronate for adjuvant treatment of operable breast cancer [ISRCTN83688026]. Breast Cancer Res 8: R13

Reed W, Hannisdal E, Skovlund E et al. (2003). Pregnancy and breast cancer: a population-based study. Virchows Arch 443: 44–50

Ring AE, Smith IE, Jones A et al. (2005) Chemotherapy for breast cancer during pregnancy: an 18-year experience from five London teaching hospitals. J Clin Oncol 23: 4192–4197

Roché H, Fumoleau P, Spielmann M et al. (2004) Five-year analysis of the PACS 01 trial: 6 cycles of FEC100 cs. 3 cycles of FEC100 followed by 3 cycles of docetaxel (D) for the adjuvant treatment of node positive breast cancer. Breast Cancer Res Treat 88 Suppl 1: S16

Romond EH, Perez EA, Bryant J et al. (2005) Trastuzumab plus adjuvant chemotherapy for operable HER2-positive breast cancer. N Engl J Med 353: 1673–1684

Say L, Kulier R, Gulmezoglu M et al. (2005) Medical versus surgical methods for first trimester termination of pregnancy. Cochrane Database Syst Rev: CD003037

Slamon D, Eiermann W, Robert N et al. (2005) Phase III trial comparing AC-T with AC-TH and with TCH in the adjuvant treatment of HER2 positive early breast cancer patients: first interim efficacy analysis. Breast Cancer Res Treat 89, Suppl. 1: S5 (Abstract #1)

Smith IE, Dowsett M, Yap YS et al. (2006) Adjuvant aromatase inhibitors for early breast cancer after chemotherapy-induced amenorrhoea: caution and suggested guidelines. J Clin Oncol 24: 2444–2447

Tewari K, Bonebrake RG, Asrat T et al. (1997) Ambiguous genitalia in infant exposed to tamoxifen in utero. Lancet 350 :183

Vujovic O, Yu E, Cherian A et al. (2006) Eleven-year follow-up results in the delay of breast irradiation after conservative breast surgery in node-negative breast cancer patients. Int J Radiat Oncol Biol Phys 64: 760–764

Waterston AM and Graham J (2006) Effect of adjuvant trastuzumab on pregnancy. J Clin Oncol 24: 321–322.

Watson WJ (2005) Herceptin (trastuzumab) therapy during pregnancy: association with reversible anhydramnios. Obstet Gynecol 105: 642–643

Woo JC, Yu T, Hurd TC (2003) Breast cancer in pregnancy: a literature review. Arch Surg 138: 91–98; discussion 99

Zemlickis D, Lishner M, Degendorfer P et al. (1996) Maternal and fetal outcome following breast cancer in pregnancy. In Cancer in pregnancy. Maternal and fetal risks., Koren, G., Lishner, M. & Farine, D. (eds) pp. 95–115. Cambridge University Press: New York

Zemlickis D, Lishner M, Degendorfer P et al. (1992) Maternal and fetal outcome after breast cancer in pregnancy. Am J Obstet Gynecol 166: 781–787

Zhang J, Liu G, Wu J et al. (2003) Pregnancy-associated breast cancer: a case control and long-term follow-up study in China. J Exp Clin Cancer Res 22: 23–27

6 Subsequent Pregnancy After Breast Cancer

F. Peccatori, S. Cinieri, L. Orlando, G. Bellettini

Recent Results in Cancer Research, Vol. 178

6.1 Introduction

Approximately 213,000 new cases of breast cancer were diagnosed in the US during 2006. Of these, 25% and 10% occurred in women younger than 50 and 40 years, respectively (Howe et al. 2006).

As women are delaying childbearing for personal reasons, including cultural, educational, and professional reasons (Ventura 1989), there has been an increasing number of patients in whom breast cancer occurs before the completion of their reproductive project.

Breast cancer is a potentially curable disease when diagnosed early and if appropriate local and systemic treatment is delivered.

Even very young women with breast cancer, who have a notably worse prognosis than older patients (Aebi et al. 2006), can now live longer and healthier: More effective and tailored therapies have become available as adjuvant treatment for early breast cancer, including dose-dense chemotherapy and trastuzumab (Smith et al. 2007). Moreover, the role of endocrine responsiveness in very young patients has been elucidated (Colleoni et al. 2006), and innovative trials exploring the combination of LH-RH analogs and aromatase inhibitors versus LH-RH analogs and tamoxifen are ongoing (Goldhirsch et al. 2006). As a result of earlier diagnosis and better care, in the US and in most European countries, breast cancer mortality has been decreasing in all age cohorts since the beginning of the 1980s (Levi et al. 2007).

Estrogens are causally linked to the development of breast cancer: Age at menarche, age at first full-term pregnancy, parity, breast feeding, and oral contraceptive use are some of the recognized factors that influence breast cancer incidence in young women (Russo and Russo 2006). Moreover, endocrine manipulation has been used as an effective treatment for advanced and early breast cancer, as recently confirmed by the EBCTG meta-analysis (Clarke 2006).

For these reasons, the possible promotional effect of gestational estrogens on micrometastases has raised concern about the safety of a subsequent pregnancy in breast cancer patients.

In this chapter the different aspects of pregnancies subsequent to breast cancer diagnosis and treatment are elucidated and illustrated.

6.2 Breast Changes During Pregnancy and Lactation

During intrauterine life the mammary ducts develop in cellular sheets arising from the nipple epithelium. Around puberty in the female adolescent, the gradual rise of ovarian estrogens and insulin-like growth factor-1 (IGF-1) induces ductal proliferation and lobular formation. During the fertile years, the process of cellular proliferation, differentiation, and apoptosis is related to the different phases of the ovarian cycle, reflecting the different hormonal levels of the follicular and the luteinic phase. Estrogens prevail during the follicular-proliferative phase, peaking during ovulation, while progesterone is the main hormone secreted by the corpus luteum during the luteinic-secretory phase. However, it is only during pregnancy and lactation that the mammary gland fully develops (Russo and Russo 2004).

During pregnancy the mammary gland is exposed to very high levels of ovarian estrogens and progestins, pituitary prolactin, and placental lactogens. Early pregnancy is typically characterized by steady estrogen and human chorionic gonadotrophin increase and by placental estrone and human placental lactogen production during the second and third trimesters (Numan 1994). These increased levels of hormones induce ductal proliferation and alveolar formation, with typical histopathologic changes.

During lactation the mammary glands undergo terminal differentiation of the lobuloalveolar structures (Fig 6.1) and produce a lactescent fluid rich in water, proteins, carbohydrates, and lipids: the milk.

Milk production can exceed 800 ml per day and is finely regulated by the pituitary hormones prolactin and oxitocin, which induce milk production and ejection, respectively. The lactating breast is also capable of downregulating milk production by FIL (factor inhibiting lactation) when the amount of milk exceeds the baby's needs (Riordan 2005).

After the weaning of the baby, the differentiated lobuloalveolar structures undergo apoptosis with an active role of extracellular matrix-degrading proteinases and inflammatory cytokines of the TNF family. This leads to basement membrane degradation, epithelial cell detachment, and subsequent apoptosis of the unwanted secretory mammary epithelium (Schedin 2006).

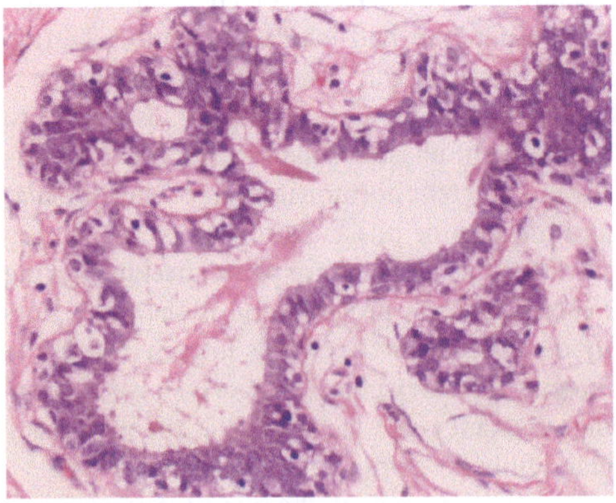

Fig. 6.1 Human lactating breast. (H&E, ×200)

6.3 Effects of Pregnancy After Breast Cancer on Survival and Risk of Recurrence

6.3.1 Published Clinical Data on Subsequent Pregnancies: Survival

Most of the published evidence about the effect on survival of subsequent pregnancy in breast cancer patients comes from case series or case-control studies, and thorough reviews and commentaries have been published (Upponi et al. 2003; Surbone 2002; Surbone and Petrek 1997, 1998). Cases are defined as patients affected by breast cancer who eventually became pregnant, while controls are defined as patients with breast cancer who did not became pregnant. There is also a number of population-based studies, some of which report results as relative risk of death compared to controls.

Overall, the large majority of the published studies report that subsequent pregnancy is not detrimental for survival. On the contrary, survival of women who had given birth or had a pregnancy after breast cancer was better than controls in most studies. In population-based studies, where the matching is usually more precise and includes age, stage of disease, and year of breast cancer diagnosis, relative risk of death was always inferior for cases than for controls. In three of seven studies, results were statistically significant (Ives et al. 2004, Mueller et al. 2003; Sankila et al. 1994). The study by Kroman (Kroman et al. 1997) and that by Mueller (Mueller et al. 2003), which are the ones with the higher number of cases, are analyzed here in more detail. Kroman et al. reported results obtained from the Danish registry, which retained data about diagnosis and follow-up of 5,725 women with breast cancer aged 45 or younger at the time of diagnosis. Of these, 173 women (3%) became pregnant after breast cancer. Women with full-term pregnancy had a nonsignificant reduction of the risk of dying (RR 0.55, 95% CI 0.28–1.06) compared to controls. The control choice was very meticulous, including age at diagnosis, disease stage, and reproductive history before diagnosis. Results were not influenced by age, tumor characteristics at diagnosis (including tumor size, nodal status, or grade), or pregnancy outcome. In the study by Mueller et al., the authors conducted a cohort study using data from three population-based cancer registries in United States, linked to birth certificate data in each state (Seattle, Washington; Detroit, Michigan; Los Angeles, California). Four hundred thirty-eight women were identified as having births after breast cancer and matched with 2,775 women without births. After adjustment for stage, age, year of diagnosis, and race, women with birth after 10 months or more after diagnosis had a statistically significant decrease in the risk of dying (RR 0.54, 95% CI 0.41–0.71). In subgroup analysis, cases with local disease or regional disease at diagnosis had a decreased risk (RR 0.59 and 0.54, respectively) compared to controls. The same holds true for cases with node-positive (RR 0.65), tumors smaller or larger than 2 cm (RR 0.70 and 0.52, respectively), or among women who had received chemotherapy or other treatments including hormone manipulation or radiation therapy (RR 0.54, 0.36, and 0.44, respectively). Also in case-control studies and case series, 5-year and in some instances 10-year overall survival of cases was consistently better than controls, regardless of node involvement, when assessed. Tables 6.1, 6.2, and 6.3 summarize the results of case series, case-control studies, and population-based studies.

In conclusion, women treated for breast cancer who wish to become pregnant should be informed that pregnancy is possible and does not seem to be associated with a worse prognosis for their breast cancer. However, they should be made aware that the evidence remains rather scanty and that the issue is still controversial (see also Sect. 6.4).

Table 6.1 Case series studies: survival data

Author	Publication year	No. of cases	% 10y OS (n–/n+)
Aerial	1989	46	77/56
Clark	1989	136	76/63
Ribeiro	1986	57	64/26
Harvey	1981	41	80/79
Cheek	1973	10	50*/NS
Rissanen	1969	53	70°
Holleb	1962	52	64/38*
White	1955	269	51/34.6
White	1954	208	49/16.8*

10y OS, 10-years overall survival; *n*–, node negative; n+, node positive; *5-year survival; ° *n*– and *n*+; *NS*, not stated

Table 6.2 Case-control studies: survival data

Author	Publication year	No. of cases	% 5y OS cases	% 5y OS controls
Gelber	2001	94	92	85
Lethaby	1996	14	100	80
Sankila	1994	91	87.5	63
Cooper	1970	32	94	71

5y OS, 5-years overall survival

Table 6.3 Population-based studies: survival data

Author	Publication year	No. of cases	RR of death (95% CI)
Ives	2006	123	0.59 (0.37–0.95)
Blakely	2004	47	0.71 (0.25–1.95)
Mueller	2003	438	0.54 (0.41–0.71)
Velentgas	1999	53	0.80 (0.30–2.30)
Kroman	1997	173	0.55 (0.28–1.06)
Von Schoulz	1995	50	0.48 (0.18–1.29)
Sankila	1994	91	0.20 (0.10–0.50)

RR, risk ratio, *CI*, confidence interval

6.3.2 Published Clinical Data on Subsequent Pregnancies: Local Recurrences and Distant Metastases

In some published studies, survival is not the only outcome measure. Recurrence and distant metastases are analyzed, too. For example, Malamos (Malamos et al. 1996) reported that patients with subsequent pregnancies have a local recurrence rate of 14% compared to 39% for the nonpregnant group. Sutton (Sutton et al. 1990) reported similar results, with 28% recurrence rate in the pregnant group compared to 46% in the nonpregnant group. On the other hand, in the study from von Shoultz (von Schoultz et al. 1995) the relapse rate was 24% in the pregnant group compared to 8% in the nonpregnant group.

Even if data are not conclusive, pregnancy after breast cancer does not seem to increase the rate of local recurrence or of distant metastases.

6.3.3 Interval Between Diagnosis and Pregnancy

There has been debate about how long a woman should wait after breast cancer diagnosis or treatment to plan a pregnancy. Few studies have investigated the subject. In three series no differences in survival were found, according to time from diagnosis to pregnancy (Harvey et al. 1981; Mignot et al. 1986; Sankila et al. 1994). In another report (Clark and Chua 1989), 5-year survival was worse for patients becoming pregnant within 6 months of diagnosis (53.8%), compared to those who became pregnant after 6 months but before 2 years (78%) and those who became pregnant after 5 years (100%). A recent population-based study (Mueller et al. 2003) reported an increased risk of mortality if pregnancy occurred within 3 months of diagnosis (RR 1.7; 95% CI 1.2–2.6), while no differences were found in the other cohorts (Table 6.4).

In another population study (Ives et al. 2006), outcome was analyzed with a Cox's proportional hazard model with time-dependent variables stratified by time from diagnosis. Authors reported a non-statistically significant better outcome for women who waited at least 6 months after diagnosis (RR 0.45, 95% CI 0.16–1.28), while subsequent pregnancy after 2 years from diagnosis significantly improved survival (RR 0.48, 95% CI 0.27–0.83, $p=0.009$). The authors concluded that in women with localized disease, conception after 6 months from diagnosis is unlikely to affect survival (Ives et al. 2006).

In common clinical practice, though, it is still suggested to wait at least 2 years from diagnosis

Table 6.4 Risk of mortality according to the time interval from diagnosis to pregnancy (modified from Mueller et al. 2003)

Time to pregnancy (years)	RR (95% CI)
2–2.9	0.49 (0.27–0.86)
3–3.9	0.30 (0.12–0.71)
4–4.9	0.19 (0.05–0.81)

before attempting conception, to allow early recurrences to manifest.

Other factors like risk at diagnosis, adjuvant treatment length, residual fertility, and age at conception should be taken into consideration when counseling young patients about interval time between diagnosis and pregnancy.

6.4 Concerns About Published Data: Methodological Issues

One of the major concerns about the published studies is that they might not be representative of the entire population who became pregnant after breast cancer diagnosis and treatment. In the different studies the percentage of pregnancies varies from 3% to 8%, so that some of the studies could be biased or underpowered to really describe the reported events (Gemignani and Petrek 1999). Only a dedicated register that thoroughly analyzes reproductive events after breast cancer could help in having meaningful figures. The second concern is the so-called "healthy mother effect" (Sankila 1994). Women who became pregnant after breast cancer could have more favorable characteristics than women who did not become pregnant. Those who feel well have children, while women who have had a recurrence after diagnosis do not. This could represent a bias even if cases and controls were well matched at diagnosis. In some studies the healthy mother effect has been taken into consideration for the control choice. For example, in the study by Gelber (Gelber et al. 2001) cases who had a pregnancy after breast cancer were matched with controls who had at least a disease-free interval equal to or longer than the time from diagnosis to pregnancy completion. In this study survival was more favorable in the pregnancy group (RR 0.44, 95% CI 0.21–0.96). Another issue is the difficulty in controlling for biological factors and risk determinants in the statistical model used, as data are often incomplete in retrospective studies and also in population-based studies. For example, the effects of pregnancy according to estrogen receptor status at diagnosis is still an unresolved issue, and no study so far has had the statistical power to assess any difference in survival for women with endocrine-responsive tumors versus endocrine-nonresponsive tumors. Another major concern is the methodology of many studies. In case series or retrospective case-control studies, the denominator of the population is often unknown. Also, the definition of pregnancy varies in many studies: Some consider only "full-term pregnancies," others "any pregnancy," including those that end in miscarriage or induced abortion. Again, only a prospective registry would help in making this issue unequivocal.

6.5 Is Pregnancy Protective? Possible Immunologic and Endocrine Explanations

Regardless of the concerns about methodology that have been raised in the previous paragraph, if we assume that the reported data are true and that pregnancy after breast cancer improves survival, we should try to find a plausible biological explanation. Unfortunately, we do not have an experimental model that helps us in testing the different hypotheses that have been made, and we have to rely on speculation alone.

The first hypothesis postulates that in pregnancies subsequent to breast cancer diagnosis, an alloimmunization against breast cancer occurs (Janerich 2001). According to this hypothesis, breast cancer and fetal cells share common antigens. During pregnancy, the mother's immunity is boosted against breast cancer cells by circulating fetal cells, whose presence has been recently confirmed (Mavrou et al. 2006). The activated immune system would then eliminate quiescent tumor cells, thus accounting for the better survival of patients with subsequent pregnancies (Botelho and Clark 1998).

The second hypothesis is endocrine. As already described, pregnancy is characterized by conspicuous changes in the endocrinologic milieu of the pregnant mother. If the combination of high estrogen levels, progesterone, and HCG has the capability to induce apoptosis in endocrine-responsive breast tumor cells (Guzman et al. 1999), then pregnancy could act as another endocrine treatment, whose mechanism of action is not fully understood. Clearly, further research is needed to clarify this issue.

6.6 Birth Outcome After Chemo-Endocrine Treatment for Breast Cancer

One of the major concerns of patients who receive adjuvant chemotherapy or hormonal therapy after surgery for breast cancer is the potential delayed teratogenicity of such treatments. Even if many years have elapsed since the administration of cytotoxic agents or hormones, the concern that permanent damage of the oocyte has occurred is not unfounded. Some cytotoxic agents bind to the DNA of resting cells, others interfere with specific metabolic pathways; hormones can have a long half-life and remain in tissues for years. Cytotoxic chemotherapy can indeed permanently damage the primordial oocytes, reducing their amount and inducing amenorrhea or early premature menopause (Warne et al. 1973). A comprehensive review of amenorrhea after adjuvant chemotherapy for breast cancer has been recently published (Walshe et al. 2006). The process of oocyte maturation and selection is very well regulated, and only a very few primordial oocytes reach the stage of mature oocytes; damaged oocytes are usually eliminated. Taking into account the time of oocyte maturation, the practical advice is to wait at least 6 months from the end of chemotherapy, to be sure that any damaged oocyte will be replaced by a normal one.

For hormonal therapy, data are less conclusive. Tamoxifen is the drug that has been studied in the most detail. The half-life of long-term tamoxifen is highly variable and ranges from 3 to 21 days. However, tamoxifen and its metabolites have been detected in various concentrations in several tissues more than 1 year following withdrawal after chronic use (Lien et al. 1991). Even if tamoxifen is known to increase the incidence of endometrial cancer in long-term users, no data are available regarding a direct gonadotoxicity or genotoxicity of this drug. On the contrary, tamoxifen has been used to improve oocyte pickup during assisted reproduction and is licensed in UK for this purpose. Therefore, the practical advice is to wait 3–6 months after tamoxifen withdrawal before attempting conception.

Aromatase inhibitors have a definite role in the adjuvant treatment of postmenopausal breast cancer patients. Trials to address the role of the combination of LHRH analog and aromatase inhibitors in premenopausal breast cancer patients are ongoing. Also, aromatase inhibitors, and in particular letrozole, have been used to induce ovulation (Oktay et al. 2005). A warning about the risk of congenital cardiac and bone malformation after letrozole use for infertility has been recently denied. In a survey of 911 newborns prenatally exposed to letrozole, malformations were not increased in the treated group (Tulandi et al. 2006).

Few papers have analyzed birth outcome after breast cancer. In all papers the induced abortion rate is quite high, ranging from 20% to 44% (Kroman et al. 1997; Velentgas et al. 1999; Gelber et al. 2001; Blakely et al. 2004). This high rate of induced abortion probably reflects the uncertainties of patients and physicians about the safety of pregnancy after breast cancer. In one paper (Gelber et al. 2001), 23 of 33 "therapeutic" abortions (69%) were recorded as recommended by the doctors. The miscarriage rate in the different reports varies from 9% to 28% (Kroman et al. 1997; Velentgas et al. 1999; Gelber et al. 2001; Blakely et al. 2004) and is influenced by the proportion of induced abortions. In one report (Velentgas et al. 1999) patients with previous breast cancer diagnosis had a miscarriage rate of 24% compared to 18% in age-matched women without cancer. No differences were found among women who received adjuvant chemotherapy or radiation compared to women who did not receive any adjuvant treatment.

In another well-conducted population-based cohort study (Langagergaard et al. 2005), among 216 births occurring after breast cancer diagnosis, the offspring sex ratio was 50% male and 50% female, with a gestational age at birth of 39.2 weeks (± 2.4 weeks). These data were similar to those of the comparison cohort of 10,453 births occurring in women without previous breast cancer. Moreover, the crude and adjusted prevalence of preterm birth, low birth weight, stillbirth, and abnormalities were not different from the comparison cohort. The authors suggest that a previous breast cancer diagnosis does not influence periconceptional life events, as demonstrated by the equal proportion of male and females in the offspring. A higher miscarriage rate would have resulted in a lower proportion of males, partly because male embryos have a higher abortion rate (Hansen et al. 1999). In conclusion, birth outcome after breast cancer is not different from that of the normal population. A careful monitoring of pregnancy is needed to ensure proper care in the first weeks of gestation.

6.7 Breast-Feeding in Women with Pregnancies After Breast Cancer

Breast-feeding is considered by many women an integral part of pregnancy.

While there is no doubt that breast-feeding is valuable for the newborn, reducing neonatal infections, autoimmune diseases, allergies, and subsequent risk of childhood obesity (Zembo 2002), the safety and feasibility of breast-feeding after breast cancer remains an open issue.

No reports specifically address the safety of breast-feeding in women who become pregnant after breast cancer. No prospective or retrospective case-control studies have been reported, with relative risks or matching and comparison of women who nursed and women who bottle-fed their babies. The numbers are simply too low, and in some cohort-studies the information is missing. However, in some series lactation has been described in approximately 30% of cases (Gelber et al. 2001), and overall survival of the cases, including women who nursed, was better compared to that of women who did not have a child (RR 0.44, 95% CI 0.21–0.96). In the general population, breast-feeding can effectively reduce breast cancer incidence. Each year of breast-feeding is associated with a 4.3% reduction (Collaborative Group on Hormonal Factors in Breast Cancer 2002). Moreover, lactation delays ovulation, reduces intramammary estrogens and carcinogens, and induces a protective lobuloalveolar differentiation of the mammary gland, as already described (Riordan 2005).

The concern that long-term lactation could delay breast examination or radiological evaluation is unrealistic. Ultrasound can be safely and effectively performed during lactation, and mammogram or breast magnetic resonance can be done after having drained the lactating breasts (Obenauer and Dammert 2007).

There have been reports of women who have had a unilateral mastectomy and breast-fed their babies after a subsequent pregnancy (Gelber et al. 2001). The notion that one breast is enough is reinforced by the historical practice of wet nurses, who could breast-feed more than three babies at the same time, and by the common experience of twin lactation and of babies whose choice is to nurse from one breast only (Riordan 2005). The mother should be also reassured about the adequacy of milk production by a single breast and encouraged to seek early advice if latching problems occur. If pain and nipple abrasion occur, the mother should improve the baby's latch-on, trying to cover the entire nipple-areola complex with the baby's mouth. She should also try to alter the baby's position frequently, to provide optimal drainage to all portions of the breast and optimal breast stimulation.

Some common features are reported in women who underwent conservative surgery and breast irradiation for breast cancer and subsequently tried to nurse (Higgins and Haffty 1994; Tralins 1995; Moran et al. 2005):

- There is little or no enlargement of the treated breast during pregnancy in more than 80% of patients. This observation was also made by our group and is probably related to radiotherapy-induced fibrosis (Fig. 6.2).
- The treated breast has less likelihood of having a full milk supply; lactation can be absent in approximately 40% of cases.
- Difficulty with latch-on sometimes occurs because the nipple on the breast may not extend as completely as might be expected.
- The ability to lactate and breast-feed from the untreated breast is normal.

In a report of 53 patients who became pregnant and delivered after radiation, 18 (34%) were able to lactate. Although all 18 patients were able to exhibit some level of lactation, only 13 women chose to breast-feed. Of the five who did not breast-feed, three reported insufficient milk as a reason (Tralins 1995). In the SOGC clinical practice guidelines on breast cancer, pregnancy, and breast-feeding (Helewa et al. 2002) is stated: "There is no evidence that breast feeding increases the risk of breast cancer recurring or of a second breast cancer developing, nor that

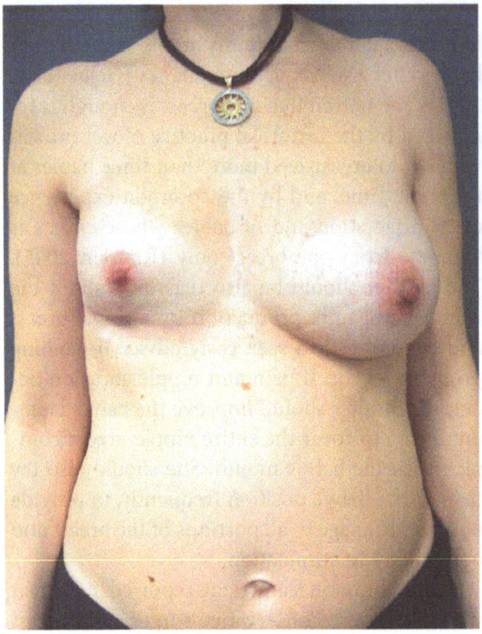

Fig. 6.2 Pregnant breasts after right breast quadrantectomy and axillary clearance+ radiotherapy (45 Gy + 10 Gy boost) 6 years earlier. Note right breast hypotrophia compared to the normal left breast. Twenty weeks of pregnancy

it carries any health risk for the child. Women previously treated for breast cancer who do not show any evidence of residual tumor should be encouraged to breast-feed their children."

6.8 Pregnancy After Breast Cancer in Women with BRCA1 and BRCA2 Mutations

There are no data that specifically address the issue of pregnancy after breast cancer occurring in women with BRCA1 or BRCA2 mutation. BRCA1 and -2 genes are located on chromosome 17 q12–21 and 13 q12–13, respectively, and their mutation is genetically transmitted, with an autosomal dominant pattern at variable penetrance. Families with BRCA1 mutation have an increased risk of breast and ovarian cancer, which can be estimated around 65% (95% CI 51–75%) and 39% (95% CI 22–51%), respectively, by age 70 (Antoniou et al. 2003). In families with BRCA2 mutation, breast cancer risk at age 70 was 45% (95% CI 33–54%) and ovarian cancer risk 11% (95% CI 4.1–18%), and there was also a higher colon and pancreatic cancer incidence (Antoniou et al. 2003). Typically, breast cancer occurs at a younger age (mean age at diagnosis 34.1) (Jernstrom et al. 2004) and in BRCA1 carriers tends to be endocrine nonresponsive, with non-overexpressed or amplified HER-2 (Turner and Reis-Filho 2006).

Reproductive factors have been studied in BRCA1 and -2 carriers, with controversial results. An early report suggested that parity could increase breast cancer risk in BRCA1 carriers (Narod 2002), but a larger retrospective study of 1,260 carriers did not confirm this finding and even observed decreased breast cancer risk in BRCA1 carriers with more than four children (OR = 0.62, 95% CI 0.41–0.94,) versus nulliparous carriers (Cullinane et al. 2005). In BRCA2 carriers, parity caused a borderline increase in risk for breast cancer before age 50 years (OR = 1.17 for each pregnancy, 95% CI 1.01–1.36) (Cullinane et al. 2005). In a case-only study, young age at first pregnancy delayed onset of breast cancer in carriers (King et al. 2003), and a retrospective study of 1,601 carriers found that in women over 40 years of age each full-term pregnancy reduced breast cancer risk by 14% (95% CI 6–22%).

In a case-control study of 965 BRCA1 and 280 BRCA2 carriers, BRCA1 carriers who breast-fed for over 1 year were less likely to have had breast cancer than those who never breast-fed (OR = 0.55, 95% CI 0.38–0.80). No effect was observed in BRCA2 carriers (Jernstrom et al. 2004). In another cohort study of 1.601 carriers, though, the effect was less striking (HR = 0.89, 95% CI 0.62–1.27) (Andrieu et al. 2006).

In conclusion, pregnancy after breast cancer in BRCA1 or BRCA2 carriers should not be discouraged because of the concern that it may increase breast cancer incidence. Breast-feeding could be protective in BRCA1 carriers and should be encouraged. A comprehensive genetic counseling, inclusive of risk reduction strategies, prenatal diagnosis options, and psychological support is warranted (Friedman and Kramer 2005).

References

Aebi S, Castiglione M (2006) The enigma of young age. Ann Oncol 17(10): 1475–1477

Aerial IM, Kempner R (1989) The prognosis of patients who become pregnant after mastectomy for breast cancer. Int Surg 74: 185–187

Andrieu N, Goldgar DE, Easton DF, Rookus M, Brohet R, Antoniou AC, Peock S, Evans G, Eccles D, Douglas F, Nogues C, Gauthier-Villars M, Chompret A, Van Leeuwen FE, Kluijt I, Benitez J, Arver B, Olah E, Chang-Claude J (2006) Pregnancies, breast-feeding, and breast cancer risk in the International BRCA1 and BRCA2 Carrier Cohort Study (IBCCS). J Natl Cancer Inst 98: 535–544

Antoniou A, Pharoah PD, Narod S, Risch HA, Eyfjord JE, Hopper JL, Loman N, Olsson H, Johannsson O, Borg A, Pasini B, Radice P, Manoukian S, Eccles DM, Tang N, Olah E, Anton-Culver H, Warner E, Lubinski J, Gronwald J, Gorski B, Tulinius H, Thorlacius S, Eerola H, Nevanlinna H, Syrjakoski K, Kallioniemi OP, Thompson D, Evans C, Peto J, Lalloo F, Evans DG, Easton DF (2003) Average risks of breast and ovarian cancer associated with BRCA1 or BRCA2 mutations detected in case series unselected for family history: a combined analysis of 22 studies. Am J Hum Genet 72: 1117–1130

Blakely LJ, Buzdar AU, Lozada JA, Shullaih SA, Hoy E, Smith TL, Hortobagyi GN (2004) Effects of pregnancy after treatment for breast carcinoma on survival and risk of recurrence. Cancer 100(3): 465–469

Botelho F, Clark DA (1998) How might pregnancy immunize against breast cancer? Am J Reprod Immunol 39: 279–283

Cheek JH (1973) Cancer of the breast in pregnancy and lactation. Am J Surg 126: 729–731

Clark RM, Chua T (1989) Breast cancer and pregnancy: the ultimate challenge. Clin Oncol 1: 11–18

Clarke M (2006) Meta-analyses of adjuvant therapies for women with early breast cancer: the Early Breast Cancer Trialists' Collaborative Group overview. Ann Oncol 17 Suppl 10: x59–x62

Collaborative Group on Hormonal Factors in Breast Cancer (2002) Breast cancer and breastfeeding: collaborative reanalysis of individual data from 47 epidemiological studies in 30 countries, including 50302 women with breast cancer and 96973 women without the disease. Lancet 360(9328): 187–195

Colleoni M, Rotmensz N, Peruzzotti G, Maisonneuve P, Orlando L, Ghisini R, Viale G, Pruneri G, Veronesi P, Luini A, Intra M, Cardillo A, Torrisi R, Rocca A, Goldhirsch A (2006) Role of endocrine responsiveness and adjuvant therapy in very young women (below 35 years) with operable breast cancer and node negative disease. Ann Oncol 17(10): 1497–1503

Cooper DR, Butterfield J (1970) Pregnancy subsequent to mastectomy for cancer of the breast. Ann Surg 17: 429–433

Cullinane CA, Lubinski J, Neuhausen SL, Ghadirian P, Lynch HT (2005) Effect of pregnancy as a risk factor for breast cancer in BRCA1/BRCA2 mutation carriers. Int J Cancer 117: 988–991

Friedman LC, Kramer RM (2005) Reproductive issues in women with BRCA mutations J Natl Cancer Inst Monogr 34: 83–86

Gelber S, Coates AS, Goldhirsch A et al. (2001) Effect of pregnancy on overall survival after the diagnosis of early stage breast cancer. J Clin Oncol 19: 1671–1675

Gemignani ML, Petrek JA (1999) Pregnancy after breast cancer. Cancer Control 6(3): 272–276

Goldhirsch A, Coates A, Gelber R, Glick J, Thurlimann B, Senn HJ (2006) First—select the target: better choice of adjuvant treatments for breast cancer patients. Ann Oncol 17(12): 1772–1776

Guzman RC, Yang J, Rajkumar L, Thordarson G, Chen X, Nandi S (1999) Hormonal prevention of breast cancer: mimicking the protective effect of pregnancy. Proc Natl Acad Sci USA 96(5): 2520–2525

Hansen D, Moller H, Olsen J (1999) Severe periconceptional life events and the sex ratio in offspring: follow up study based on five national registers. BMJ 319(7209): 548–549

Harvey JC, Rosen PP, Ashikari R, Robbins GF, Kinne DW (1981) The effect of pregnancy on the prognosis of carcinoma of the breast following radical mastectomy. Surg Gynecol Obstet 153: 723–725

Helewa M, Levesque P, Provencher D, Lea RH, Rosolowich V, Shapiro HM; Breast Disease Committee and Executive Committee and Council, Society of Obstetricians and Gynaecologists of Canada (2002) Breast cancer, pregnancy, and breastfeeding. J Obstet Gynaecol Can 24(2): 164–180

Higgins S, Haffty BG (1994) Pregnancy and lactation after breast-conserving therapy for early stage breast cancer. Cancer 73(8): 2175–2180

Holleb AI, Farrow JH (1962) The relation of carcinoma of the breast and pregnancy in 283 patients. Surg Gynecol Obstet 115: 65–71

Howe HL, Wu X, Ries LA, Cokkinides V, Ahmed F, Jemal A, Miller B, Williams M, Ward E, Wingo PA, Ramirez A, Edwards BK (2006) Annual Report to the Nation on the Status of Cancer, 1975–2003, Featuring Cancer among U.S. Hispanic/Latino Populations. Cancer 107: 1711–1742

Ives A, Saunders C, Bulsara M, Semmens J (2006) Pregnancy after breast cancer: population based study. BMJ; doi 10.1136/bmj.39035.667176.55

Janerich DT (2001) The fetal antigen hypothesis: cancers and beyond. Med Hypotheses 56(1): 101–103

Jernstrom H, Lubinski J, Lynch HT, Ghadirian P, Neuhausen S, Isaacs C, Weber BL, Horsman D, Rosen B, Foulkes WD, Friedman E, Gershoni-Baruch R, Ainsworth P, Daly M, Garber J, Olsson H, Sun P, Narod SA (2004) Breast-feeding and the risk of breast cancer in BRCA1 and BRCA2 mutation carriers. J Natl Cancer Inst 96: 1094–1098

King MC, Marks JH, Mandell JB (2003) Breast and ovarian cancer risks due to inherited mutations in BRCA1 and BRCA2. Science 302: 643–646

Kroman N, Jensen MB, Melbye M et al. (1997) Should women be advised against pregnancy after breast cancer treatment? Lancet 350: 319–322

Langagergaard V, Gislum M, Skriver MV, Norgard B, Lash TL, Rothman KJ, Sorensen HT (2006) Birth outcome in women with breast cancer. Br J Cancer 94(1): 142–146

Lethaby AE, O'Neill MA, Mason BH, Holdaway IM, Harvey VJ (1996) Overall survival from breast cancer in women pregnant or lactating at or after diagnosis. Int J Cancer 67: 751–755

Levi F, Lucchini F, Negri E, La Vecchia C (2007) Continuing declines in cancer mortality in the European Union. Ann Oncol 18: 593–595

Lien EA, Solheim E, Ueland PM (1991) Distribution of tamoxifen and its metabolites in rat and human tissues during steady-state treatment. Cancer Res 51(18): 4837–4844

Malamos NA, Stathopoulos GP, Keramopoulos A, Papadiamantis J, Vassilaros S (1996) Pregnancy and offspring after the appearance of breast cancer. Oncology 53: 471–475

Mavrou A, Kouvidi E, Antsaklis A, Souka A, Kitsiou Tzeli S, Kolialexi A (2007) Identification of nucleated red blood cells in maternal circulation: A second step in screening for fetal aneuploidies and pregnancy complications. Prenat Diagn 27: 150–153

Mignot L, Morvan F, Berdah J, Querleu D, Laurent JC, Verhaeghe M, Fontaine F, Marin JL, Gorins A, Marty M (1986) Pregnancy after treated breast cancer. Results of a case-control study Presse Med 15(39): 1961–1964

Moran MS, Colasanto JM, Haffty BG, Wilson LD, Lund MW, Higgins SA (2005) Effects of breast-conserving therapy on lactation after pregnancy. Cancer J 11(5): 399–403

Mueller BA, Simon MS, Deapen D, Kamineni A, Malone KE, Daling JR (2003) Childbearing and survival after breast carcinoma in young women. Cancer 98(6): 1131–1140

Narod SA (2002) Modifiers of risk of hereditary breast and ovarian cancer. Nat Rev Cancer 2: 113–123

Numan M (2004) In Physiology of Reproduction, eds. Knobil E, Neill JD. Raven, New York, 221–302

Obenauer S, Dammert S (2007) Palpable masses in breast during lactation. Clin Imaging 31(1): 1–5

Oktay K, Buyuk E, Libertella N, Akar M, Rosenwaks Z (2005) Fertility preservation in breast cancer patients: a prospective controlled comparison of ovarian stimulation with tamoxifen and letrozole for embryo cryopreservation. J Clin Oncol 23(19): 4347–4353

Ribeiro G, Jones DA, Jones M (1986) Carcinoma of the breast associated with pregnancy. Br J Surg 73: 607–609

Riordan J (ed) (2005) Breastfeeding and human lactation (3rd ed). Jones and Bartlett Publishers

Rissanen PM (1969) Pregnancy following treatment of mammary carcinoma. Acta Radiol Ther Phys Biol 8: 415–422

Russo J, Russo IH (2004) Development of the human breast. Maturitas 49(1): 2–15

Russo J, Russo IH (2006) The role of estrogen in the initiation of breast cancer. J Steroid Biochem Mol Biol 102(1–5): 89–96

Sankila R, Heinavaara S, Hakulinen T (1994) Survival of breast cancer patients after subsequent term pregnancy: "Healthy mother effect". Am J Obstet Gynecol 170: 818–823

Schedin P (2006) Pregnancy associated breast cancer and metastases. Nat Rev Cancer 6: 281–291

Smith I, Procter M, Gelber RD, Guillaume S, Feyereislova A, Dowsett M, Goldhirsch A, Untch M, Mariani G, Baselga J, Kaufmann M, Cameron D, Bell R, Bergh J, Coleman R, Wardley A, Harbeck N, Lopez RI, Mallmann P, Gelmon K, Wilcken N, Wist E, Sanchez Rovira P, Piccart-Gebhart MJ; HERA study team (2007) 2-year follow-up of trastuzumab after adjuvant chemotherapy in HER2-positive breast cancer: a randomised controlled trial. Lancet 369(9555): 29–36

Surbone A, Petrek JA (1997) Childbearing issues in breast carcinoma survivors. Cancer 79: 1271–1278

Surbone A, Petrek JA (1998) Pregnancy after breast cancer. The relationship of pregnancy to breast cancer development and progression. Critical Rev Oncol Hematol 27: 169–178

Surbone A (2002) The complex relationship between pregnancy and breast cancer. Expert Opin Pharmacother 3(4): 429–431

Tralins AH (1994) Lactation after conservative breast surgery combined with radiation therapy. Am J Clin Oncol 18(1): 40–43

Tulandi T, Martin J, Al-Fadhli R, Kabli N, Forman R, Hitkari J, Librach C, Greenblatt E, Casper RF (2006) Congenital malformations among 911 newborns conceived after infertility treatment with letrozole or clomiphene citrate. Fertil Steril 85(6): 1761-1765

Turner NC and Reis-Filho JS (2006) Basal like breast cancer and the BRCA1 phenotype. Oncogene 25: 5846–5853

Upponi SS, Ahmad F, Whitaker IS, Purushotham AD (2003) Pregnancy after breast cancer (Review). Eur J Cancer 39(6): 736–741

Velentgas P, Daling JR, Malone KE et al. (1999) Pregnancy after breast carcinoma- outcomes and influence on mortality. Cancer 85: 2424–2432

Ventura SJ (1989) First births to older mothers, 1970–86. Am J Public Health 79: 1675

von Schoultz E, Johansson H, Wilking N, Rutqvist L-E (1995) Influence of prior and subsequent pregnancy on breast cancer prognosis. J Clin Oncol 13: 430–434

Walshe JM, Denduluri N, Swain SM (2006) Amenorrhea in premenopausal women after adjuvant chemotherapy for breast cancer. J Clin Oncol 24(36): 5769–5779

Warne GL, Fairley KF, Hobbs JB, Martin FI (1973) Cyclophosphamide-induced ovarian failure. N Engl J Med 289(22): 1159–1162

White TT (1954) Carcinoma of the breast and pregnancy. Ann Surg 139: 9–18

White TT (1955) Prognosis of breast cancer for pregnant and nursing women. Surg Gynecol Obstet 100: 661–666

Zembo CT (2002) Breastfeeding. Obstet Gynecol Clin North Am 29(1): 51–76

7 Cervical and Endometrial Cancer During Pregnancy

S. Kehoe

Recent Results in Cancer Research, Vol. 178

7.1 Introduction

Though cancer is a rare event during pregnancy, of those which are recorded, cervical cancer is one of the commonest encountered. As the age group who embark on starting a family correlates with a higher incidence of cervical cancer, the coincidental finding of this association is understandable. This contrasts with endometrial cancer—a disease primarily developing after the menopause, when of course, pregnancy is not feasible. Therefore, in pregnancy-related cancers, these two form either end of the spectrum of diseases. As with all such situations, care is complicated because of the desire (or not) to continue with a pregnancy and the endeavour to balance the probabilities of achieving a live baby without compromising the mother's survival prospects.

7.2 Cervical Carcinoma

The incidence of cervical cancer detected during pregnancy or in the early post-partum period is similar to the expected incidence in that age population, which is not surprising considering that sexual intercourse and parity are recognised risk factors (Munoz et al. 2002). Equally, the immunosuppressive impact of pregnancy should, if anything, encourage an increased incidence of cervical cancer.

7.2.1 HPV in Pregnancy

HPV 16 and 18 are two of the human papillomavirus family most commonly found in cervical cancer and are known risk factors for developing this malignancy (Khan et al. 2005). It is estimated that up to 80% of women will have been carriers of this virus at sometime during their sexually active life (www.cdc.gov/std/HPV/STDFact 2006). There are conflicting reports as to the impact of pregnancy on the viral presence or load. Smith et al. (1991) were one of the first to examine the prevalence of HPV in pregnancy, comparing 69 pregnant women with a control population. HPV 16/18/31/33 and 35 were found equally in both groups, though HPV6/11 were not detected in the pregnant women. However, the researchers did note an increased detection rate of HPV from 8% in the first trimester to 23% in the third trimester, an increase presumed due to activation of latent HPV. A more recent study, again using a control population, found HPV prevalence in pregnancy at 10.1% and 11.4% in the control group, which was a non-significant difference, and the prevalence did not alter according to gestational age (Chan et al. 2002). Another study agreed with this when examining women with ASCUS smears in pregnancy, whereby the prevalence of HPV infection and their subtypes were the same as in the non-pregnant population (Lu et al. 2003).

The actual viral load could be more pertinent. A small series involving 25 pregnant women, 24 controls and 40 women with cervical cancer noted a high viral load in cervical cancer patients, a low load in non-pregnant women and a mid-range load in pregnant women (Bandyopadhyay and Chatterjee 2006). In the same study the incidence of HPV prevalence was 68% in pregnant and only 25% in non-pregnant women.

Therefore, regarding HPV in pregnancy, it seems at least as prevalent compared to the non-pregnant population, and might be increased. Another important fact to note is that in HPV-positive women, increased parity is recognised as an independent increase risk factor for cervical squamous carcinomas (Munoz 2002)

7.2.2 Incidence of Cervical Cancer

The reported incidence of cervical cancer in pregnancy ranges from 1/1,200 to 1/10,000 pregnancies, though the latter rate seems most representational (Nguyen et al. 2000). Of all the types of cancers reported in pregnancy, cervical cancer is one of the commonest and accounts for up to 50% of pregnancy-related cancers.

7.2.3 Clinical Presentation

The clinical presentation of cervical cancer can be confusing because of the other pregnancy-related symptoms, such as occasional bleeding—be it a threatened miscarriage or ante-partum haemorrhage. In such cases the cervix does require an examination at some stage, but because of rarity of this disease, often the physician will omit to perform such an examination, and on some occasions the disease is detected during vaginal examination in labour. The potential ways in cases can be encountered in pregnancy are shown in Table 7.1. As compared with cervical cancer outside pregnancy, the disease stage tends to be earlier, with a three-fold increased chance of having stage I disease (Zemlickis et al. 1991), as compared to non-pregnant women. There is no evidence that histopathologies differ greatly from those outside pregnancy, with the vast majority having squamous cell carcinomas. The timing of presentation seems mainly to be in the first trimester of pregnancy, though notably in the studies reported by Sood et al. (2000) and van der Vange (1995) a large cohort of patients were diagnosed during the post-partum period (up to 6 months after delivery) (Table 7.2).

Table 7.1 Presentation of cervical cancer in pregnancy

Abnormal smear
Post-coital bleeding
Frank malignancy noted on examination
Abnormal vaginal bleeding during pregnancy
Detection at examination in labour
Abnormal post-partum bleeding

Histological proof of cancer is mandatory before embarking on any form of therapy. This can be obtained by with punch biopsy, loop cone biopsy or knife wedge biopsy. In all cases, the enhanced vasculature of the pregnant cervix will increase the possibility of significant haemorrhage after a biopsy. The timing of the biopsy may also be relevant to the mother. For example, a punch biopsy alone would probably not incur an increased risk of spontaneous miscarriage, but there may be a case to wait until after 8 weeks so that the majority of naturally spontaneous miscarriages have already occurred. Such matters require careful discussion with the patient.

Table 7.2 Presentation, stage and survival in cervical cancer

Reference	Cases	Presentation			Disease Stage		5-Year survival
		Trimester		PP	I	II/III/IV	
		Ist	Other				
Germann	21	13	7	1	15	6	82%
Tarushim	28	20	5	3	22	6	72%
Van der Vange	44	23*	21	32	12		80%
Sood	93	13	43	27	69	24	—
Jones	161	50	111		118	43	82%

PP = Post-partum

7.2.4 Management

Besides the disease stage influencing care, the patient's views need to be respected. Her choice with regarding to continuation of the pregnancy requires careful counselling, and indeed the care of the patient in some cases will require a multidisciplinary team, which includes obstetrical and neo-natal experts. A frame of potential care is shown in Fig. 7.1.

7.2.4.1 Staging

The decision as to the optimum therapy for a women with cervical carcinoma requires appropriate staging procedures. These are determined by the FIGO criteria and include the use of imaging, clinical examination, cystoscopy and sigmoidoscopy. Naturally, not all of these procedures may be deemed safe or wise in pregnancy—particularly if the women wishes her pregnancy to continue. Nevertheless, MRI scanning, though not for general use, would seem to be safe (Hand et al. 2006), with the fetus having reduced absorption rates of 50% that of the mother. Also, it is possible to reduce the exposure of the fetus by using various radiation protective methods. On balance, the possible risk of imaging exposure, whilst to be avoided before 12 weeks of gestation, is less than the risk of not ensuring, as much as possible, accurate information regarding the disease stage. Most, therefore, would deem an MRI of the pelvis and a clinical examination a minimal requirement in this situation.

There is also the possibility—in particular if the pregnancy has been prolonged to consider laparoscopic evaluation of the pelvic nodes—to ensure they are negative for disease (Stan 2005).

There are certain clinical situations in which the decisions are clear. In stage Ia1 completely excised at conisation, the pregnancy can continue. Also, when the pregnancy is at a stage where fetal maturity is sufficient, prolongation of the pregnancy is unnecessary. Delivery should be expedited and appropriate therapy commenced, which in many cases will be a Caesarean section combined with a Wertheim hysterectomy.

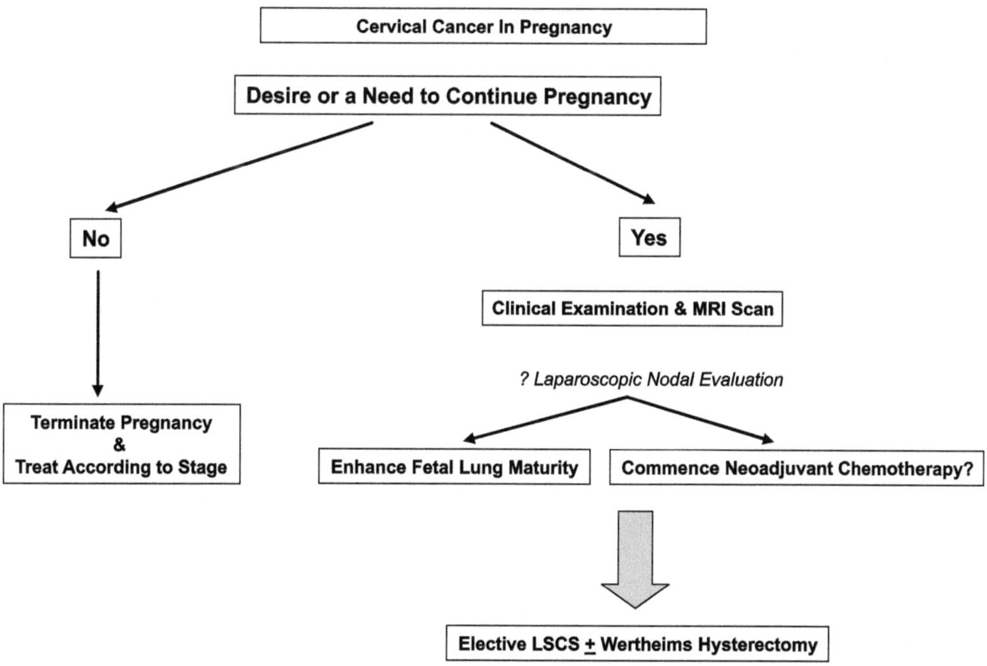

Fig. 7.1 Cervical cancer in pregnancy

In the first trimester, when the mother expresses a desire for treatment, a termination of pregnancy can be undertaken and appropriate care administered. The difficult area is when the pregnancy is going to be prolonged and what effect this may have on the mother's survival. There are no specific or correct recommendations in the latter situation, except careful counselling and respecting the individual's views.

7.2.5 Mode of Delivery

The mode of delivery may be important. It would be difficult to justify proceeding with a vaginal delivery considering the implications of cervical tears and haemorrhage. There is some evidence that vaginal delivery impacts on survival. A retrospective study examined 57 women who had cervical cancer diagnosed during pregnancy, with 27 diagnosed post-partum. (Sood et al. 2000). A matched control population (no pregnancy within the preceding 5 years of cervical cancer diagnosis) was used as the comparator. In 7 women who had caesarean section 1 developed a recurrence, compared with 10 of 17 who had vaginal deliveries ($p=0.04$). Multivariate analysis revealed vaginal delivery to be the most important prognosticator for recurrence (OR 6.9, 95% CI 1.45–32.8). The wide confidence intervals reflect the small numbers in this series, and are contrary to those reported in a smaller study of 44 women (van der Vange et al. 1995) but they do support intuition, in that presumably the forces on the cervix during vaginal delivery increase the probabilities of disseminating tumour cells, or altering local growth or other factors rendering tumour growth more likely.

7.2.6 Survival

The survival for women with cervical cancer in pregnancy is excellent overall, due to the fact that the disease is mainly early at presentation (Table 7.3). Therapeutic interventions can be introduced quickly in many cases, and even chemotherapy can by utilised whilst permitting the pregnancy to proceed (Caluwaerts 2006). Prognosis for women with cervical cancer I pregnancy seems equal to non-pregnant women with similar-stage disease (Jones et al. 1996; Zemlickis et al. 1991).

7.3 Endometrial Cancer

As pregnancy itself is dependent on a suitable endometrial environment to be successful, and with endometrial cancer a disease predominantly of the post-menopausal woman, co-existence of endometrial cancer and pregnancy is a very rare event.

The vast majority of reports on this condition are case reports only; a selection of cases over the recent years is given in Table 7.3. The largest series reported consists of five cases (Schammel et al. 1998) and only those cases with de novo endometrial carcinoma and diagnosed within 6 months post-partum are included. There is a supposed larger group in the California Cancer Study (Smith et al. 2003), with 22 cases diagnosed pre-pregnancy, 11 during pregnancy and 44 post-partum. The post partum period was longer, and importantly, the registry linked "other"/unknown gynaecological cancers with

Table 7.3 Cases reporting endometrial cancer and pregnancy (up to 6 months PP)

Ref	Cases	Detection
Itoh [2004]	1	6 months PP
Vaccarello [1999]	3	1–D/C, 2 PP (4 months)
Kovacs [1996]	1	D/C 7 weeks
Ichikawa [2001]	1	6 months PP
Schammel [1998]	5	4–D/C, I at LSCS
Foersterling [1999]	1	PP
Ayhun [1999]	1	D/C
Ojomo [1993]	1	PP (with ovarian cancer)
Schneller [1994]	1	D/C (elective TOP)
Leunen [2003]	1	PP
Stead [1997]	1	With ectopic
Victoriano [1998]	1	D/C

uterine cancers. Further work would be required to elicit more definitive outcomes on this group.

7.3.1 Clinical Presentation

From the 18 cases in Table 7.2, 50% of cases were diagnosed in the post-partum period.

This was primarily due to persisting irregular and abnormal bleeding, and hence in such clinical situations it can be recommended that some sampling of the endometrium be considered when found.

The second commonest clinical scenario was evacuation of the uterus for miscarriage, persistent bleeding or elective termination of pregnancy during the first trimester. In all these cases, endometrial carcinoma cannot have been anticipated. The only pertinent point would be that consideration be given to histological evaluation of all specimens, appreciating that this would have to be judged against the cost efficacy of introducing such a recommendation.

In two cases, the disease was detected in conjunction with ovarian malignancy. This is a high rate, 2 of 18 cases, but the synchronous occurrence of these malignancies is well known.

7.3.2 Management

In all cases, the management of endometrial cancer is comparable with that of the non-pregnant women. Unlike cervical cancer, the issue of prolonging pregnancy does not exist, because of the time at which these cancers are detected. Staging according to FIGO (www.figo.org/content/PDF/staging-booklet) should be undertaken, and surgery considered as the optimum therapy where feasible.

7.3.3 Survival

As the reported cases are so few, there is little to discuss regarding outcomes, though there would not seemingly be any indication that the outcomes differ greatly.

References

Ayhan A, Gunalp S, Karaer C, Gokoz A, Oz U (1999) Endometrial adenocarcinoma in pregnancy. Gynecol Oncol 75(2): 298–299

Bandyopadhyay S, Chatterjee R(2006) HPV viral load determination during pregnancy as a possible cervical cancer risk. J Exp Clin Cancer Res 25(1): 29–38

Caluwaerts S, van Calsteren K, Mertens L, Lagae L, Moerman P, Hanssens M, Wuyts K, Vergote I, Amant F (2006) Neoadjuvant chemotherapy followed by radical hysterectomy for invasive cervical cancer diagnosed during pregnancy: report of a case and review of the literature. Int J Gynecol Cancer 16(2): 905–908

CDC. Genital HPV infection. Genital HPV infection (web site). Available at: http://www.cdc.gov/std/HPV/STDFact-HPV.htm

Chan PK, Chang AR, Tam WH, Cheung JL, Cheng AF (2002) Prevalence and genotype distribution of human cervical human papilloma virus infection: comparison between pregnant women and non-pregnant controls. J Med Virol 67(4): 583–588

Charkviani L, Charkviani T, Natenadze N, Tsitsishvili Z (2003) Cervical carcinoma and pregnancy. Clin Exp Obstet Gynecol 30(1): 19–22

Foersterling DL, Blythe JG (1999) Ovarian carcinoma, endometrial carcinoma and pregnancy. Gynecol Oncol 72(3): 425–426

Germann N, Haie-Meder C, Morice P, Lhomme C, Duvillard P, Hacene K, Gerbaulet A (2005) Management and clinical outcomes of pregnant patients with invasive cervical cancer. Ann Oncol 16(3): 397–402

Hand JW, Li Y, Thomas EL, Rutherford MA, Hajnal JV (2006) Prediction of specific absorption rate in mother and fetus associated with MRI examinations during pregnancy. Magn Reson Med 55(4): 883–893

Ichikawa Y, Takano K, Higa S, Tanabe M, Wada A, Sugita M, Tsunoda H, Nishida M (2001) Endometrial carcinoma coexisting with pregnancy, presumed to derive from adenomyosis: a case report. Int J Gynecol Cancer 11(6): 488–490

Itoh K, Shiozawa T, Shiohara S, Ashida T, Konishi I (2004) Endometrial carcinoma in a septate uterus detected 6 months after full-term delivery: case report and review of the literature Gynecol Oncol 93(1): 242–247

Jones WB, Shingleton HM, Russell A, Fremgen AM, Clive RE, Winchester DP, Chmiel JS (1996) Cervical carcinoma and pregnancy. A national patterns of care study of the American College of Surgeons. Cancer 77(8): 1479–1488

Khan MJ, Castle PE, Lorincz AT, Wacholder S, Sherman M, Scott DR, Rush BB, Glass AG, Schiffman M (2005) The elevated 10-year risk of cervical precancer and cancer in women with human papilloma (HPV) virus type 16 or 18 and the possibility of utility of type-specific HPV testing in clinical practice. J Natl Cancer Inst 97(14): 1072–1079

Kovacs AG, Cserni G (1996) Endometrial cancer in early pregnancy. Gynecol Obstet Invest 41(1): 70–72

Leunen K, Amant F, Debiec-Rychter M, Croes R, Hagemeijer A, Schoenmakers EF, Vergote I (2003) Endometrial stromal sarcoma presenting as postpartum haemorrhage: report of a case with sole t(10;17)(q22;p13) translocation. Gynecol Oncol 91(1): 265–271

Lu DW, Pirog EC, Zhu X, Wang HL, Pinto KR (2003) Prevalence and typing of HPV DNA in atypical squamous cells in pregnant women. Acta Cytol 47(6): 1008–1016

McPherson CP, Sellers TA, Potter JD, Bostick RM, Folsom AR (1996) Reproductive factors and risk of endometrial cancer: the Iowa Women's Health study. Am J Epidemiol 143(12): 1195–1202

Munoz N, Franceschi S, Bosetti C, Moreno V, Herrero R, Smith JS, Shah KV, Meijer CJ, Bosch FX (2002). The role of parity and human papillomavirus in cervical cancer: the IARC multicentric case-control study. Lancet 359(9312): 1093–1101

Nguyen C, Montz FJ, Bristow RE (2000) Management of stage 1 cervical cancer in pregnancy. Obstet Gynecol Surv 55(10): 633–643

Ojomo EO, Ezimokhai M, Reale FR, Nwabineli NJ (1993). Recurrent post-partum haemorrhage caused by endometrial carcinoma co-existing with endometrioid carcinoma of the ovary in a full term pregnancy. Br J Obstet Gynaecol 100(5): 489–491

Schammel DP, Mittal KR, Kaplan K, Deligdisch L, Tavassoli FA (1998) Endometrial adenocarcinoma associated with intrauterine pregnancy. A report of five cases and a review of the literature. Int J Gynecol Pathol 17(4): 327–335

Schneller JA, Nicastri AD (1994) Intrauterine pregnancy coincident with endometrial cancer: a case study and review of the literature. Gynecol Oncol 54(1): 87–90

Smith EM, Johnson SR, Jiang D, Zaleski S, Lynch CF, Brundage S, Anderson RD, Turek LP (1991) The association between pregnancy and human papilloma virus prevalence. Cancer Detect Prev 15(5): 397–402

Smith LH, Danielsen B, Allen ME, Cress R (2003) Cancer associated with obstetric delivery: results of linkage with the California cancer registry Am J Obstet Gynecol 189(4): 1128–1135

Sood AK, Sorosky JI, Mayr N, Anderson B, Buller RE, Niebyl J (2000) Cervical cancer diagnosed shortly after pregnancy: prognostic variables and delivery routes. Obstet Gynecol 95(6 Pt 1): 832–838

Stan C, Megevand E, Irion O, Wang C, Bruchim I, Petignat P (2005) Cervical cancer in pregnant women: Laparoscopic evaluation before delaying treatment. Eur J Gynaecol Oncol 26(6): 649–650

Stead JA, Behnam KM (1997) Co-existing endometrial adenocarcinoma and tubal ectopic pregnancy: a case report. W V Med J 93(3): 133–135

Takushi M, Moromizato H, Sakumoto K, Kanazawa K (2002) Management of invasive carcinoma of the uterine cervix associated with pregnancy: outcome of intentional delay in treatment. Gynecol Oncol 87(2): 185–189

Vaccarello L, Apte SM, Copeland LJ, Boutselis JG, Rubin SC (1999) Endometrial carcinoma associated with pregnancy: report of three cases and review of the literature. Gynecol Oncol 74(1): 118–122

Van der Vange N, Weverling GJ, Ketting BW, Ankum WM, Samlal R, Lammes FB (1995). The prognosis of cervical cancer associated with pregnancy: a matched cohort study. Obstet Gynecol 85: 1022–1026

Victoriano MJ (1998) Endometrial carcinoma co-existing with an intrauterine pregnancy: a case report. Philipp J Obstet Gynecol 22(4): 135–146

Zemlickis D, Lishner M, Degendorfer P, Panzarella T, Sutcliffe S, Koren G. (1991) Maternal and fetal outcome after invasive cervical cancer in pregnancy. J Clin Oncol 9(11): 1956–1961

8 Ovarian Cancers in Pregnancy

C. Sessa, M. Maur

Recent Results in Cancer Research, Vol. 178

8.1 Introduction

Pregnancy and its associated hormonal changes are inversely related to the risk of developing ovarian adenocarcinoma. Ovarian cancer is, however, the second most frequent gynecologic cancer in pregnancy. The incidence of ovarian masses in pregnancy is between 1% and 4% (Goff et al. 2000; Bernhard et al. 1999; Marino and Craigo 2000).

The majority of these masses are corpus luteum or other functional cysts that usually resolve by 16 weeks of gestation. Some adnexal masses, however, persist, and 1–8% of these masses are of malignant origin. The average estimated incidence of ovarian tumors in pregnancy is approximately 1 in 1,000 deliveries. (Creasman et al. 1971; Whitecar et al. 1999; Sherard et al. 2003; Schmeler et al. 2005).

Adnexal masses are usually asymptomatic and are found during routine ultrasound or at the time of cesarean section. The first symptoms occur at about 16 weeks, when the uterus is enlarged; the most frequent symptoms are torsion (15%), pelvic pain, hemorrhage, rupture, and infection.

Ultrasound examination is the ideal method for detection and surveillance since it is sensitive enough to detect adnexal masses; it can also evaluate their structural characteristics and distinguish between simple cysts and complex masses with characteristics of either low malignant potential (LMP) tumors or ovarian cancers (Boulay and Podczaski 1998). It is best used in combination with a high-frequency transvaginal transducer applied transabdominally (Sherer et al. 1999). In addition, the use of color Doppler imaging has been shown to significantly improve the ability to distinguish between benign and malignant disease (Cohen and Fishman 2002).

There is general agreement that observation and repeated ultrasound between 14 and 16 weeks of pregnancy are appropriate for those masses less than 6 cm, unilateral, unilocular, mobile, and asymptomatic. For an adnexal mass exceeding 6 cm, with complex structure or ascites or persisting after 16 weeks of gestation, surgical intervention is important to obtain a final histologic diagnosis and rule out malignancy. Laparotomy or laparoscopy is warranted and should not be delayed (Dudkiewicz et al. 2002). The incidence of spontaneous abortus after surgery in the first trimester was reported as 10%, and elective surgery for lesions with low suspicion of malignancy should be delayed until the second trimester (16–18 weeks of gestation) to decrease the risk of fetal complications. A mass that is first diagnosed in the third trimester is best managed by awaiting fetal maturity only if the clinical suspicion of malignancy is low (Zanotti et al. 2000).

Staging is primarily surgical, and laparoscopy may be an initial approach to assess adnexal masses in patients who do not have evidence of extraovarian pathology (Parulaker 2005).

At diagnosis the majority of adnexal masses are benign and confined to the ovaries. Among malignant ovarian tumors in pregnancy, epithelial tumor is the most frequent histotype (35%), followed by germ cell/sex cord stromal tumors (mostly dysgerminomas; 35%) and borderline malignant tumors (30%). The metastatic involvement of the ovary by another primary site (Krukenberg tumor) has rarely been reported.

Ovarian germ cell and borderline malignant tumors are most often diagnosed at an early stage (80% FIGO stage I–II). Granulosa, Sertoli-Leydig, and „unclassified" sex cord stromal tumor types have been reported as well. Other benign conditions of sex cord stromal tissues can mimic malignancy like luteoma of pregnancy, luteinized follicular cysts, granulosa cell proliferations, hilus cell hyperplasia, and ectopic deciduas.

Several authors have recently published retrospective analyses on clinicopathological characterization of ovarian cancer in pregnancy. Leiserowitz (Leiserowitz et al. 2006) reported a population-based study of 4,846,505 obstetrical patients; 9,375 women had a hospital diagnosis of an ovarian mass associated with pregnancy, of whom 87 had ovarian cancers and 115 LMP tumors. The occurrence rate was 0.93% ovarian cancers over the total number of ovarian masses diagnosed during pregnancy. In summary, ovarian cancers and LMP tumors were: FIGO stages IA–IB in 65% and 81%, respectively, of cases, FIGO stage IC in 6.9% and 7.8%, FIGO stages III and IV in 23%, and 4.4%, 4.6%, and 6.1% cases were of unknown stages.

Zhao and co-workers (Zhao et al. 2006) have summarized their experience on ovarian cancer in pregnancy, analyzing data on treatment, follow-up, and outcome. The incidence of ovarian carcinoma in pregnancy in their series was 0.073 of 1,000 pregnancies; 41% were germ cell tumors, 27.3% LMP tumors, 23% invasive epithelial tumors, and 9% sex cord stromal tumors. More than 70% of patients were diagnosed at stage I. The presence of ascites at diagnosis seemed to be a negative prognostic factor.

CA125 levels are elevated with wide spontaneous fluctuations in pregnancy, mainly during the first trimester and immediately after delivery because of chorionic invasion (Aslam et al. 2000; Schmeler et al. 2005). CA125 peaks at about the 10th week of gestation and then at delivery. In the second and third trimesters CA125 levels are low in maternal serum (Kobayashi et al. 1989) but high in the amniotic fluid. High maternal CA125 levels are caused by chorionic invasion or placental separation (Moore et al. 1992). In addition, CA125 can be elevated in many of the benign conditions frequent in this population, particularly in endometriosis.

For all the above-mentioned reasons, CA125 is not a "good" biomarker for diagnosis and follow-up of ovarian cancer during pregnancy.

Table 8.1 Management of ovarian cancer in pregnancy

Diagnostic laparotomy mandatory if adnexal masses
Symptomatic
>5 cm by 16 weeks
Increasing size and/or complex structure
Frozen section analysis
Intraoperative decision-making based on
Histology
Extent of disease
Gestational age
Patient desires

8.2 Treatment

The clinical characteristics and prognosis of ovarian cancer in pregnant women are similar to those of nonpregnant women. Management of these cases depends on tumor histology, stage of disease, and term of pregnancy (Table 8.1).

8.3 Surgery

Surgery is the cornerstone of treatment (Table 8.2). Laparotomy with midline incision at 16–18 weeks of gestation is recommended, with unilateral oophorectomy or adnexectomy together with careful examination of the contralateral ovary to complete the staging.

The subsequent surgical treatment depends on the results of frozen sections. For advanced disease, an adequate staging with debulking surgery must be pursued, similarly to what is recommended in nonpregnant women. This may include omental biopsy/sampling, peritoneal biopsies, and pelvic washing for cytology. In case of ovarian dysgerminoma, pelvic/paraaortic node biopsy is mandatory to reduce the risk of understaging. Biopsy of the contralateral ovary is warranted only if it is macroscopically involved. Pregnancy can be continued after a conservative surgery.

The majority of malignant ovarian germ cell tumors could be treated by conservative surgery without compromising survival because of their

Table 8.2 Surgery in the management of ovarian cancer in pregnancy

Main features
Laparotomy with midline incision
Pelvic washing, peritoneal biopsies
Omentectomy, nodal sampling
Delivery by cesarean section
Germ cell tumors
Unilateral salpingo-oophorectomy
Routine biopsy of "normal" contralateral ovary no longer recommended
Systematic lymphadenectomy only for dysgerminoma
Debulking if advanced stage
Epithelial tumors
LMP, invasive early stage
Conservative surgery
Invasive advanced stage
Debulking according to
Extent of disease
Gestational age
Hysterectomy not mandatory

sensitivity to the standard combination regimen (cisplatin, bleomycin, etoposide/vinblastine) (Tewari et al. 2000; Zhao et al. 2006).

The same conservative management (monolateral salpingo-oophorectomy) could be used for stage IA, low-grade epithelial ovarian cancer. All higher-stage tumors should undergo more aggressive surgery with TAHBSO, omentectomy, nodal sampling, biopsies of the liver and diaphragm, and peritoneal cytology visualization.

In patients with advanced disease, the decision for such an aggressive surgical approach should take into account fetal viability and patient health and preference. If a patient wishes to continue pregnancy, hysterectomy is not done, unless it might contribute significantly to tumor debulking (Zanotti et al. 2000; Boulay and Podczaski 1998; Zhao et al. 2006); after the 7th week of gestation bilateral salpingo-oophorectomy is compatible with continuation of pregnancy since the hormonal production is taken up by the trophoblast. During the third trimester a long delay is not justified; in case of delivery of a viable fetus, cesarean section and radical surgical hysterectomy should be performed.

Jackisch and co-workers (Jackisch et al. 2003) reported a vertical transmission of malignant cells to the placenta or fetus. For this reason macroscopic and histopathologic examination of the placenta, with study of the intravillous spaces and villi and cytological examination of umbilical cord blood should be routinely done in every case of malignancy in pregnancy. Fetal metastases occur in no less than 25% of cases.

8.4 Chemotherapy

Chemotherapy is contraindicated during the first trimester of pregnancy because of the high rate of abortion and abnormal fetus development (10% for single agent, 25% for combination regimens), whereas it is compatible in the second or third trimester when the risk of congenital malformation for fetuses is no greater than in the general population. Some oncologists have recently employed neoadjuvant chemotherapy during the last two trimesters to postpone radical surgery after delivery by cesarean section.

However, the nonteratogenic effects of chemotherapy such as intrauterine growth restriction (low birth weight) or effects on the central nervous system should also be taken into account. At time of delivery, the expected bone marrow depression and potential complications such as bleeding or infections should be taken into account. Self-limiting fetal hematopoietic depression has also been described, and the neonate should be monitored for that. No studies so far have evaluated the long-term consequences for children exposed to intrauterine chemotherapy for gynecologic malignancies; there are, however, limited data suggesting that, in patients with hematologic or other solid tumors, long-term consequences might be absent. Different regimens have been used such as vinca alkaloids, actinomycin-D, cyclophosphamide, bleomycin, cisplatin, and etoposide, and more recently carboplatin, anthracycline, and paclitaxel with good fetal outcome and significant tumor response (Mendez et al. 2003; Sood et al. 2001).

8.5 Conclusions

Some preliminary conclusions can be drawn on the clinical management of ovarian neoplasia in pregnancy.

The first main decision to be taken refers to time of treatment, immediate or delayed up to postpartum; in this process of decision making, stage of disease, histologic type, and gestational age should be the driving key factors.

Open questions, still a matter of discussion and evaluation, are the maximum acceptable delay of treatment, the long-term effects of chemotherapies, and the safety and increasing role of conservative surgery.

References

Aslam N, Ong C, Woelfer B, Nicolaides K, Jurkovic D (2000) Serum CA125 at 11–14 weeks of gestation in women with morphologically normal ovaries. BJOG 107: 689–690

Bernhard LM, Klebba PK, Gray DL, Mutch DG (1999) Predictors of persistence of adnexal masses in pregnancy. Obstet Gynecol 93(4): 585–569

Boulay R, Podczaski E (1998) Ovarian cancer complicating pregnancy. Obstet Gynecol Clin N Am 25: 385–399

Cohen L, Fishman DA (2002) Ultrasound and ovarian cancer. Cancer Treat Res 107: 119–132

Creasman WT, Rutledge F, Smith JP (1971) Carcinoma of the ovary associated with pregnancy. Obstet Gynecol 38: 111–116

Dudkiewicz J, Kowalski T, Grzonka D, Czarnecki M (2002) Ovarian tumors in pregnancy. Ginekol Pol 73: 342–345

Goff BA, Paley PJ, Koh W-J, Petersdorf SH, Douglas JG, Greer BE (2000) Cancer in the pregnant patient. In: Hoskins WJ, Perez CA, Young RC, editors. Principles and practice of gynecologic oncology, third ed. Philadelphia, Lippincott Williams and Wilkins, p. 501–528

Jackisch C, Louwen F, Schwenkagen A et al. (2003) Lung cancer during pregnancy involving the products of conception and a review of the literature. Arch Gynecol Obstet 268: 69–77

Kobayashi F, Sagawa N, Nakamura K et al. (1989) Mechanism and clinical significance of elevated CA 125 levels in the sera of pregnant women. Am J Obstet Gynecol 160: 563–566

Leiserowitz GS, Xing G, Cress R, Brahmbhatt B, Dalrymple JL, Smith LH (2006) Adnexal masses in pregnancy: how often are they malignant?. Gynecol Oncol 101: 315–321

Marino T, Craigo SD (2000) Managing adnexal masses in pregnancy. Contemp Ob/Gyn 45(5): 130–143

Mendez LE, Mueller A, Salom E, Gonzalez-Quintero VH (2003) Paclitaxel and carboplatin chemotherapy administered during pregnancy for advanced epithelial ovarian cancer. Obstet Gynecol 102: 1200–1202

Moore JL, Martin JN (1992) Cancer and pregnancy. Obstet Gynecol Clin North Am 19: 815–827

Parulaker W (2005) Ovarian tumors and pregnancy. In Cancer in Pregnancy and Lactation, second ed. By G. Koren, M.Lishner, S. Santiago, Mother Risk Program, Toronto, Canada

Schmeler KM, Mayo-Smith WW, Peipert J, Weitzen S, Manuel MD, Gorinier M (2005) Adnexal masses in pregnancy: surgery compared with observation. Obstet Gynecol 105(5): 1098–1103

Sherard GB, Hodson CA, Williams HJ, Semer DA, Hadi HA, Tait DL (2003) Adnexal masses and pregnancy: a 12-year experience. Am J Obstet Gynecol 189: 358–363

Sherer DM, Eisenberg C, Abulafia O (1999) Transabdominal application of transvaginal tranducer enhancing depiction of mature cystic teratoma at 34 weeks' gestation. Am J Perinatol 16(7): 361–363

Sood AK, Shahin MS, Sorosky JI (2001) Paclitaxel and platinum chemotherapy for ovarian carcinoma during pregnancy. Gynecol Oncol 83(3): 599–600

Tewari K, Cappuccini F, Disaia PJ, Berman ML, Manetta A, Kohler MF (2000) Malignant germ cell tumors of the ovary. Obstet Gynecol 95: 128–133

Whitecar MP, Turner S, Higby MK (1999) Adnexal masses in pregnancy: a review of 130 cases undergoing surgical management. Am J Obstet Gynecol 181: 19–24

Zanotti KS, Belinson JL, Kennedy AW (2000) Treatment of gynaecologic cancers in pregnancy. Semin Oncol 27: 686–698

Zhao XY, Huang HF, Lian LJ, Lang JH (2006) Ovarian cancer in pregnancy: a clinicopathological analysis of 22 cases and review of the literature. Int J Gynecol Cancer 16: 8–15

9 Fertility After the Treatment of Gynecologic Tumors

V. Kesic

Recent Results in Cancer Research, Vol. 178

Gynecologic cancer is a particularly distressing type of cancer because it affects women not only in terms of physical ability and social life, but also in sexual responsiveness, body image, and, particularly important, future reproductive capabilities. The majority of these cancers are diagnosed at postmenopausal age. This is why preservation of fertility has not been a common problem in gynecologic oncology. However, 21% of patients are women in the reproductive age group, yet to complete or commence a family [Makar and Trope 2001]. For a young women, the fact that she will not be able to have children is often more disastrous than having a malignant disease. Women with a history of gynecologic cancer, who have lost their fertility as a result of their cancer treatment, experience pronounced feelings of depression, grief, stress, and sexual dysfunction [Carter et al. 2005].

From 1970 to 2000, the mean age of women giving birth for the first time increased by 3.5 years (from 21.4 to 24.9 years) [Mathews and Hamilton 2002]. In the US, between 1990 and 2002, the birth rate increased by 31% in women aged 35–39 and by 51% in women in the age group of 40–45 [Seli and Tangir 2005]. The incidence of cervical, ovarian, and even endometrial cancer in these age groups should not be disregarded (Table 9.1).

Because of both increasing survival rates and delayed childbearing, especially in Western countries, preservation of fertility in female patients diagnosed with cancer has become an important health issue.

Recent advances in staging and understanding of the natural history of gynecologic cancers have led to new approaches to treatment. More conservative methods have emerged as the alternative treatment modalities for these women, as they may allow for future fertility without compromising long-term survival. The treatment can now often be tailored to the extent of the disease.

Table 9.1 Surveillance, epidemiology, and end results data: age-specific incidence of gynecologic cancers, 1997–2001

Age (years)	Uterine corpus [a]	Ovarian [a]	Cervical [a]
<20	0	0.7–1.4	0
20–24	0	1.6	1.5
25–29	1.2	1.9	6.6
30–34	2.9	2.9	11.3
35–39	6.4	5.4	12.7
40–44	12.9	9.2	14.6
45–49	24.0	16.6	14.9

[a] Rates per 100,000 people

From Reis et al. [2004]

Today, in a young patient with gynecologic cancer preservation of fertility is possible and depends primarily on the stage of the disease and the type of cancer.

9.1 Cervical Cancer

9.1.1 Epidemiology

Cervical cancer is the second most common cancer among women worldwide, with almost half a million new cases each year, comprising about 12% of all cancers in women. There are great variations in cervical cancer incidence rates throughout the world, with the average age-standardized rate for the world population being 15.0 per 100,000 women. The majority of these cases (75%) occur in less developed regions, where the average age-standardized rate per 100,000 is 19.1 compared to 10.3 in more developed countries [Ferlay 2004].

The age distribution of cervical cancer shows a typical increase from the age of 30, with a peak in incidence in women aged 45–49 and 70–74. Although cervical screening has reduced the incidence of cervical cancer, overall the incidence is increasing in younger women. Forty-three percent of women diagnosed with cervical cancer are younger than 45 [Seli and Tangir 2005].

9.1.2 Risk Factors

Cervical squamous carcinoma and its precursor cervical intraepithelial neoplasia (CIN) have multifactorial etiology. Nowadays, human papillomavirus (HPV) infection, easily transmitted during sexual intercourse, is considered the most important risk factor for cervical cancer [Bosch et al. 2002]. HPV infection alone is necessary, but not sufficient, to induce carcinoma in an immunocompetent host. Factors that determine which HPV infections will develop into squamous intraepithelial lesions have been poorly identified. Cigarette smoking, infection by other microbial agents, specific vitamin deficiency, hormonal influences, and, most of all, a compromised immune system are believed to be cofactors in cervical carcinogenesis [Schiffman and Brinton 1995].

The natural history of cervical cancer is still not completely understood. It has been looked upon as a sequential multistep process: from a normal cervical epithelium through HPV infection to CIN to invasive cancer. The duration of the progress from precancerous stage to invasive cancer is supposed to exceed 10 years. CIN can be detected easily and treated effectively by local excision.

9.1.3 Staging and Treatment

Treatment of invasive cervical cancer is affected by the stage of the disease. The currently used International Federation of Gynecology and Obstetrics system of staging (FIGO staging) is based on anatomical extent of the disease and on clinical evaluation. Surgery is the mainstay of treatment for early-stage disease, while radiotherapy is used for more advanced stages.

However, certain early phases of invasive carcinoma have limited metastatic potential and therefore are most likely curable by nonradical treatment. Interest in defining this substage of cervical cancer is motivated by the desire to preserve fertility and prevent the potential complications of radical treatment. The concept of conservative treatment for early cervical cancer is not new. In 1951, Franz Novak from Ljubljana proposed trachelectomy as a reliable treatment approach for carcinoma in situ of the cervix and published the first paper on this subject in *Acta Cytologica Yugoslavica*. The first conservative surgical approach to early invasive cancer was proposed by Aburel in 1954 as subfundic radical hysterectomy, but until the introduction of laparoscopy this technique did not become widely accepted [Aburel 1981].

Today, the options for conservative (fertility preserving) surgical treatment of early cervical cancer include:

- Excisional cone biopsy (conization)
- Radical vaginal trachelectomy
- Radical abdominal trachelectomy

Excisional cone biopsy (conization) is the standard treatment for almost all CIN lesions and for carefully selected cases of microinvasive cervical cancer. Cone-shaped local excision, if the lesion is removed in its entirety, is sufficient treatment for these cases.

Radical vaginal trachelectomy (RVT) involves a two-step procedure consisting of laparoscopic pelvic (with or without paraaortic) lymphadenectomy and, if node negative, radical vaginal trachelectomy (removal of the entire cervix and paracervical tissues). This operation was introduced by Daniel Dargent, who published the results of the first successful conservative approach for invasive cervical cancer in 1994 [Dargent et al. 1994]. Since Dargent's first reports on RTV the technique has not changed much, and today it is known as Dargent's operation.

Abdominal radical trachelectomy is another surgical technique for conservative management of cervical carcinoma [Smith et al. 1997]. The technique is similar to a standard radical hysterectomy and lymphadenectomy. The ovarian vessels are not ligated and after the lymphadenectomy and skeletonization of the uterine arteries, only the cervix, parametrium, and vaginal cuff are excised. Recently, this procedure has been performed even during pregnancy [Ungar et al. 2006].

It should be emphasized that all these options can only be used in a highly selected group of patients. The choice of each option is based on the stage of the disease and histological prognostic factors. If distant spread is very unlikely, simple but complete excision of the lesion suffices. If it is likely that the cancer has spread, then an extended operation should be performed.

9.1.4 Stage Ia—Microinvasive Disease

The category of microinvasive carcinoma of the cervix (FIGO stage Ia) applies to a tumor less than 5 mm in depth and less than 7 mm in width. Generally, this stage has limited metastatic potential. Unfavorable prognostic criteria are based on histological findings of:

- Deeper stromal invasion
- Capillary-like space involvement
- Poor differentiation
- Confluent growth pattern

The diagnosis of Stage Ia cervical squamous cell carcinoma should be based on cone biopsy, preferably using a technique that does not result in cauterized margins. Ideally, each patient with microinvasive cancer should be evaluated individually and management should be planned in cooperation with an experienced pathologist.

The choice of operation in microinvasive disease depends on the risk for nodal involvement, which is generally low. The patients most at risk of nodal metastases or central pelvic recurrence are those with definitive evidence of tumor emboli in lymph-vascular spaces.

9.1.4.1 Stage Ia1 Cervical Cancer

Several studies have suggested that FIGO stage Ia1 disease, defined as minimal microscopic invasion (depth <3 mm, width <7 mm), can be managed conservatively [Nam et al. 2002]. The treatment options for stage Ia1 cervical cancer, in the absence of lymphovascular invasion, are:

- Conization, in women wishing to retain their reproductive potential, assuming complete excision of the lesion is possible, or
- Simple hysterectomy, in women who do not wish to retain fertility

Lymph node metastases are extremely rare in this group of patients, and lymphadenectomy is not necessary.

In the largest series published, no recurrence was reported all 200 patients with stage Ia1 cervical cancer and no lymphovascular space involvement (LVSI) treated by laser conization and followed for a median time of 117 months (range 72–240 months) [Ueki et al. 2004].

Although lymphovascular invasion is generally considered a poor prognostic factor in cervical cancer, the prognostic significance of lymphovascular space involvement in stage Ia1 is not clearly defined. Therefore, some authors think that in the presence of lymphovascular space involvement, even stage Ia1 requires radical treatment [Lu and Burke 2000].

Treatment options for stage Ia1 with lymphovascular invasion include

- Modified radical hysterectomy with pelvic node dissection
- Radical trachelectomy with laparoscopic pelvic node dissection if fertility is desired

9.1.4.2 Stage Ia2 Cervical Cancer

The incidence of lymphovascular space invasion and the risk of pelvic node metastases increase with depth of invasion.

Patients with stage Ia2 (depth 3–5 mm, width <7 mm) have a risk of nodal disease of approximately 8% [Benedet and Anderson 1996]. Accordingly, unless there are strong reasons for conservative treatment, the patient can be treated by primary radical hysterectomy, modified radical hysterectomy with pelvic lymphadenectomy, or primary radiotherapy. Radical vaginal trachelectomy and laparoscopic pelvic lymphadenectomy may be an option where preservation of fertility is desired.

More recent studies have suggested that the rate of lymph node involvement in this group of patients (Ia2) who do not have lymphovascular invasion may be much lower and have questioned whether conservative therapy might be adequate for patients believed to have no residual disease following conization [Creasman et al. 1998]. Stage Ia2 with no lymphovascular invasion can be treated effectively by complete excision (conization or extrafascial hysterectomy), although radical trachelectomy/hysterectomy may be warranted. Pelvic node dissection is of questionable value in this group of patients.

Recommended treatment for Stage Ia2 cases with unfavorable pathological characteristics (lymphovascular invasion) is:

- Radical hysterectomy with pelvic node dissection
- Radical trachelectomy with laparoscopic pelvic node dissection, in young women if pregnancy is desired

9.1.5 Stage Ib (Invasive) Disease

Most patients with early-stage cervical cancer are treated by either radical surgery or radical radiotherapy. Both treatment modalities have proven to be equally effective, and there is no high level of evidence to support the choice of either radical surgery or radiation therapy in the treatment of early-stage invasive cervical cancer.

The standard surgical procedure in an early-stage cervical cancer (FIGO stage Ib) is radical hysterectomy (RH) with pelvic lymphadenectomy. The operation involves removal of the uterus and the paracervical tissues surrounding cervix and the upper vagina. With radical surgery ovarian function can be preserved and vaginal stenosis avoided, which is of great advantage over irradiation, especially for younger patients. Both modalities, however, permanently destroy fertility. It was estimated that nearly half of all patients younger than 40 years of age who might otherwise undergo a radical hysterectomy may be candidates for a fertility-sparing procedure [Sonoda et al. 2004]

Radical vaginal trachelectomy and laparoscopic pelvic lymphadenectomy may be an option in small (<2 cm) cervical cancer where preservation of fertility is desired. Before the option of RVT is considered, a thorough gynecologic and colposcopic examination should be performed. Any specimen for histological examination (biopsy or cone) must be extensively reviewed and all histological prognostic factors must be assessed (tumor size, depth of invasion, histology type, differentiation, and presence of lymphovascular invasion/LVSI)

Over the more than 10 years since this operation was introduced into the practice, the requirements for performing trachelectomy have been well defined. The eligibility criteria for radical trachelectomy include:

- Strong desire to preserve fertility
- Patient <40
- Stage Ia1 with positive LVSI
- Ia2, Ib1; tumor <2 cm, or <3 cm if exophytic
- No evidence of lymph node and/or distant metastases
- Limited endocervical involvement on colposcopy
- Exclusion of unfavorable histology
- Adequate cervical length (>2 cm)

Treatment of bulky stage Ib tumors (primary tumor >4 cm, FIGO stage Ib2) is difficult, and whatever primary treatment is chosen, the recurrence rate is higher compared to stage Ib1 disease. Neoadjuvant chemotherapy followed by radical surgery, instead of conventional chemoradiation, has been suggested as an option that may improve survival in patients with stage Ib2 disease [Benedetti-Panici et al. 2002]. It offers the advantages of surgery, and the neoadjuvant chemotherapy will keep to a minimum the risk of extracervical spread of the tumor without combining surgery and radiotherapy. Similarly, neoadjuvant chemotherapy followed by fertility-sparing surgery has emerged as a possible alternative to conventional treatment in locally advanced cervical cancer [Plante and Roy 2006].

9.1.6 Oncological Outcome

Patient selection is the most critical part of the decision to perform conservative surgical treatment for early cervical cancer. Based on the published studies, in carefully selected cases oncological outcome does not differ between standard treatment (RH) and RVH. The summarized data from the literature on 319 RTV confirm an overall recurrence rate of 4.1% and a death rate of 2.5% [Plante et al. 2004]. The most significant predictor of tumor recurrence is tumor size. In six of eight patients from Leitao's analysis of previously published studies, the tumor size was >2 cm [Leitao and Chi 2005]. Adenocarcinoma histology and lymphovascular space involvement are relative contraindications for RVT. Despite the favorable oncological outcome reported in studies published up to now, the long-term results of this procedure are still to be evaluated. Therefore, patients should always be fully informed and aware of the possible risks of choosing the conservative treatment option.

9.1.7 Obstetrical Outcome

Pregnancies have been documented after RVT. Recently, Plante and colleagues reported on pregnancy outcomes for 72 patients who had undergone a vaginal radical trachelectomy. Thirty-one women (43%) had a total of 50 pregnancies. There were eight (16%) first-trimester miscarriages and two (4%) second-trimester miscarriages, and two women (4%) had therapeutic abortions. Thirty-six of these pregnancies (72%) resulted in third-trimester deliveries. Twenty-eight of them were term deliveries. Two patients were pregnant at the time of publication [Plante et al., 2005].

The most recent review of 16 published studies (1998–2005) identified 355 cases of RVT in total [Boss et al. 2005]: 153 (43%) of these patients attempted to conceive, and 70% of those who attempted actually become pregnant. These 107 women had 161 pregnancies resulting in first-trimester abortion in 22%, second-trimester abortion in 8%, and premature delivery in 21% patients. The rate of early abortion is similar to that in the general population. However, the rates of late pregnancy losses (>14 weeks) and premature deliveries are higher. Possible explanations include loss of cervical substance and strength to hold pregnancy, loss of the natural cervical barrier to infection, and subclinical infection due to the presence of cerclage. The total 161 pregnancies resulted in term delivery (>36 gestational weeks) in 49% of patients.

Successful pregnancies and deliveries have also been reported after abdominal trachelectomies [Palfalvi et al. 2003; Rodriguez et al. 2001].

9.2 Endometrial Cancer

9.2.1 Epidemiology

Endometrial cancer is the most common gynecologic malignancy in the developed world. One to three percent of postmenopausal women will develop endometrial cancer by the age of 75. Worldwide, endometrial cancer is uncommon before the age of 40. It is primarily a postmenopausal disease. However, 25% of cases occur in premenopausal patients, with 3%–14% occurring in patients younger than 40.

9.2.2 Risk Factors

The etiology of endometrial cancer is not fully understood. Most cases appear sporadically, whereas about 10% are hereditary. Hereditary endometrial cancers are developed in women carrying the autosomally dominant inheritance for nonpolyposis colorectal cancer (HNPCC). These women have 10 times higher risk for endometrial cancer compared to the general population [Munstedt et al. 2004]. For the majority of endometrial cancers that are nonhereditary, the risk is increased by any factor that increases exposure to unopposed estrogen (e.g., hormone replacement therapy, obesity, anovulatory cycles, estrogen-secreting tumors). Young patients who develop endometrial cancer often have some degree of hyperestrogenism, anovulation, obesity, and lipid and carbohydrate imbalance. Nearly half of these patients are nulliparous [Leitao and Chi 2005].

9.2.3 Staging and Treatment

Stage of disease is the most important prognostic factor for endometrial cancer. Other prognostic factors within the same stage correlating with survival have been identified:
- Tumor grade
- Tumor size (depth of myometrial invasion)
- Lymphovascular space involvement
- Histotype (papillary-serous, clear cell)

Staging and standard treatment of endometrial cancer include:
- Adequate incision
- Peritoneal washings
- Careful inspection with excision of all suspicious lesions
- TAH + BSO
- Immediate resection of the uterus
- Pelvic and para-aortic lymph node sampling

Approximately 90% of endometrial cancers in very young women (<30 years of age) are well-differentiated lesions limited to the endometrium [Farhi et al. 1986]. After surgery alone in this stage (FIGO stage Ia) 5-year survival has been shown to be nearly 100%. Thus hormonal therapy emerged as an alternative for young patients with an early-stage endometrial cancer wishing to retain their fertility. High remission rates are seen in well-selected stage 1, grade 1 endometrial cancer of young women using hormone therapy as fertility-preserving treatment.

If conservative treatment of early endometrial cancer is considered, pretreatment evaluation must be done thoroughly and should include:
- Comprehensive gynecologic and family history
- Complete physical evaluation
- Routine blood and urine studies
- Serum levels of Ca 125
- D&C
- Radiologic imaging (preferably contrast-enhanced MRI)

Imaging methods are of particular importance, since in the absence of surgical staging it is difficult to assess the depth of myometrial invasion. Comparison of transvaginal ultrasound (TVS), computed tomography (CT), and MRI demonstrated no statistical difference among the three modalities in overall performance, but assessment of myometrial invasion was best achieved with contrast-enhanced MRI [Kinkel et al. 1999].

Currently used conservative hormonal treatment for early endometrial cancer is progestin therapy (200–500 mg/day MPA or 160–320 mg/day megestrol acetate orally). Many other hormones such as gonadotropin releasing hormone analogs (GnRHa), selective receptor modulators, and others were investigated as alternative options for conservative treatment of endometrial hyperplasia and endometrial cancer. Tamoxifen may be a valuable adjunct to progestin therapy. GnRHa have been used adjunctively to tamoxifen as second-line hormone therapy for fertility sparing after progestin failed. Aromatase inhibitors have shown their potential in treating endometrial cancer and endometrial hyperplasia as a single agent or in combination with progestins. Intrauterine progestins seem efficacious in treating endometrial hyperplasia; their application to endometrial cancer patients, however, have been limited to postmenopausal women with poor surgical risk [Lai and Huang 2006].

During follow-up, patients treated conservatively for endometrial cancer should be closely monitored, including D&C (or at least endometrial office sampling) every 3–6 months or sooner if necessary. If the disease is persisting the options would be to continue therapy, to increase the therapy, or to advise hysterectomy. Hysterectomy should be offered if patient complies poorly with medication or follow-up, if there is evidence of progressive disease, if the patient is unable or no longer desires to continue with medical therapy, or if childbearing is complete [Leitao and Chi 2005].

9.2.4 Oncological Outcome

The first report on conservative treatment for endometrial carcinoma dates from 1985. Bokhman and colleagues reported on 19 patients under the age of 37 with localized well or moderately differentiated endometrial carcinoma treated by curettage and progestin alone. Fifteen patients were without evidence of disease at 3–9 years of follow-up [Bokhman et al. 1985]. Gotlieb has the same concept of conservative treatment of endometrial cancer. In 2003, he published reports on conservative management and follow-up of 13 patients over a period of 30 years. The mean follow-up was 82 months. All patients responded to conservative treatment within a mean period of 3.5 months. Six patients (46%) recurred within a median of 40 months (range 19–358 months). During the median duration of treatment of 9–29 months, response rates of 58%–75% have been achieved.

The largest published review paper to date on conservative treatment for endometrial cancer, based on a MEDLINE 1966–2003 search, found among 79 papers 27 articles that included 81 patients suitable for the study. Hormonal treatment induced response in 62 patients (76%) with a median time to response of 12 weeks (range 4–60 weeks). The disease recurred in 15 (24%) of these patients with a median time to recurrence of 19 months (range 6–44 months). Retreatment with progestagens resulted in second response in five (71%) patients. In total, 52 (4%) of 81 patients responded to at least one course of hormonal therapy and were disease free. Nineteen (24%) patients did not respond to therapy at all [Ramirez et al. 2004].

Investigating the prediction of response to the therapy, Amant [Amant et al. 2006] recently concluded that conservative hormonal treatment for endometrial cancer may be acceptable for:

- Young women
- Well-differentiated endometrioid adenocarcinoma
- No myometrial invasion
- No evidence of LVSI or extrauterine disease

9.2.5 Obstetrical Outcome

After conservative management and follow-up of 13 patients over a period of 30 years, as of the time of Gotlieb's report, 3 patients delivered 9 healthy babies, 2 more patients were pregnant, and 1 had a first-trimester abortion [Gotlieb et al. 2003].

Analyzing the group of 81 patients conservatively treated for endometrial cancer, Ramirez found out that 20 patients (24%) conceived at least once. However, it is not known how many patients actually attempted to become pregnant. Sixteen patients had 31 live births [Ramirez et al. 2004].

As the number of young women diagnosed with endometrial cancer is increasing, it is very likely that hormonal treatment will be a more accepted fertility-sparing approach in the future. The potential of both fatal and nonfatal recurrences, however, should not be underestimated.

In patients conservatively treated for early endometrial cancer, pregnancy should be achieved as soon as possible. Because of the high incidence of recurrent disease, it is reasonable to recommend hysterectomy once childbearing has been completed.

9.3 Ovarian Cancer

Up to 90% of ovarian tumors originate from epithelium, and about 10% are germ cell (OGCT) and sex cord stromal tumors (OSCST). The classification of ovarian epithelial tumors differentiates them into benign, borderline (BOT) and malignant tumors and according to whether adenomatous or fibrous elements are dominant. Approximately 10% of all epithelial ovarian tumors are malignant. Germinal cell tumors are more frequent among young women and adolescents. OGCT account for 20–25% of ovarian tumors, and only 3% of those are malignant.

9.3.1 Epithelial Ovarian Cancer

9.3.1.1 Epidemiology

More women die from ovarian cancer than from carcinoma of the cervix and endometrium combined. It is the second most common gynecologic cancer accounting for 26% of tumors but 52% of the total mortality. Although the incidence of epithelial ovarian cancer increases with age and is most common in women aged 55–59 years, it does occur in women of childbearing age as well. Several reports have estimated that 3%–17% of all epithelial ovarian cancer occurs in women younger than 40 years of age [Schilder et al. 2002]. According to the 25th FIGO Annual Report, 14.4% of epithelial ovarian cancer patients were younger than 40 [Pecorelli et al. 2003]. Borderline and early-stage invasive disease seem to be more frequent in women of childbearing age.

9.3.1.2 Risk Factors

A number of epidemiological risk factors are associated with ovarian cancer. Early menarche and late menopause increase the risk of ovarian cancer. Ovarian cancer has been associated with low parity and infertility. Oral contraceptive use, pregnancy, and lactation are associated with a reduced risk. All these factors, taken together, have led to the hypothesis that „incessant“ ovulation (through repeated stimulation of the epithelium of the ovarian surface) may be an important factor in pathogenesis of ovarian cancer, predisposing the epithelium to malignant transformation [Fathalla 1971]. Other factors such as talc use, galactose consumption, smoking, or childhood viruses have not been strongly correlated with epithelial ovarian cancer.

There is a family history in between 5% and 10% of women with epithelial ovarian cancers. These women have a higher risk of ovarian cancer than the general population. A woman with two first-degree relatives with breast or ovarian cancer has a lifetime risk of 30%–40%.

A strong family history of breast cancer, ovarian cancer, or both—sometimes occurring at an early age and in the same woman—may be related to the presence of an inherited mutation in one of two genes, known as *BRCA1* and *BRCA2.* A second familial disorder that carries with it an increased risk of ovarian cancer is referred to as Lynch syndrome II. Lynch syndrome II is caused by inherited germ line mutations in DNA mismatch repair genes, such as *MSH 2* (*mutS* homolog 2) or *MLH1* (*mutL* homolog 1) [Chung and Rustgi 2003]. Affected families have a predominance of hereditary nonpolyposis colon cancer, often on the right side of the colon and sometimes in association with other cancers, such as those of the endometrium, ovaries, or genitourinary tract. Hereditary ovarian cancers generally occur in women about 10 years younger than nonhereditary tumors [King et al. 2003]

9.3.1.3 Staging and Treatment

Many young women with an early-stage ovarian cancer wish to maintain reproductive capability. Fertility-sparing surgery is possible in borderline and early ovarian cancer, providing adequate staging has been accomplished.

Clinical staging is an important prognostic factor for ovarian cancer. It is based on findings at clinical examination and surgical exploration [Heinz et al. 2001]. Without careful and thorough surgical exploration, occult metastasis may be missed. Subclinical metastases are present in 5%–20% of suspected ovarian cancer, and if not detected by adequate staging, recurrence can be expected in up to 31% of patients [Young et al. 1986; DiSaia and Creasman 2002]. Recurrence rate for optimally staged patients is three times lower.

Surgical staging should include the following:

- Vertical incision is required for an adequate exploration of the upper abdomen.
- Any free fluid should be sent for cytologic evaluation.
- If no free fluid is present, peritoneal washings should be performed.
- Exploration of all peritoneal surfaces including the diaphragm, bowel serosa, and pouch of Douglas.

- Total abdominal hysterectomy and bilateral salpingo-oophorectomy or unilateral oophorectomy with biopsy of contralateral ovary.
- Biopsy of any suspicious areas or adhesions. If these is no macroscopic evidence of the disease, random peritoneal biopsies should be performed.
- Infracolic omentectomy.
- Adequate sampling of pelvic and para-aortic lymph nodes.

A truly localized disease is curable by surgery. The optimal surgical procedure for all epithelial ovarian carcinomas is total abdominal hysterectomy with bilateral salpingo-oophorectomy (adnexectomy) and surgical staging.

In the younger patient, when fertility is desired unilateral salpingo-oophorectomy with wedge biopsy of the other ovary, omentectomy, and ipsilateral lymph node sampling may be an appropriate solution, if the tumor is localized with favorable low-risk pathology.

9.3.2 Low-Malignant-Potential Ovarian Tumors

Low-malignant-potential (LMP) ovarian tumors (synonyms: atypically proliferating tumors, borderline ovarian tumors) constitute about 10%–15% of epithelial ovarian tumors. They are defined as those tumors that lack stromal invasion and are characterized by a less aggressive behavior than invasive epithelial tumors. Five-year survival exceeds 90.4% compared with invasive epithelial ovarian cancer (all stages), which accounts 46.4% [Pecorelli et al. 2003].

LMP tumors have been traditionally treated by hysterectomy with bilateral adnexectomy.

These tumors occur predominantly in premenopausal women, tend to remain confined to the ovary, and are associated with a very good prognosis. Patients with LMP tumors are usually 10–15 years younger than those with invasive ovarian cancer. LMP ovarian tumors are often diagnosed incidentally after ovarian cystectomies or unilateral oophorectomies in young women. The less aggressive nature of LMP tumors and their good prognosis have allowed fertility-sparing surgery for these young patients.

9.3.2.1 Oncological Outcome

One of the largest reported series of patients with LMP tumors treated conservatively was published in 2001 by Morice and colleagues [Morice et al. 2001]. Of 174 patients with LMP tumors treated at the Institute Gustave Roussy during the period of 32 years, radical treatment was performed in 125 patients (72%), while 49 patients (28%) underwent conservative treatment. The mean duration of follow-up was 109 ± 70 months (range 24–300 months). Five patients tretaed conservatively and eight treated with radical treatment were lost to follow-up. Nine of 44 patients (20.5%) who had conservative surgery and 6 of 105 patients (5.7%) who had radical surgery experienced tumor recurrence. No patients treated conservatively had recurrence in the form of invasive ovarian cancer. In all cases recurrences were diagnosed during routine follow-up and treated surgically. All these patients were alive and free of disease at the time of report.

Other reports have also shown that recurrence of LMP tumors is more frequent after conservative surgery (19%) compared to definitive surgery (5%) [Zanetta et al. 2001]. Recurrence rate reported in the literature after cystectomy was 12%–37.5% (up to 58%) and 0%–23% after unilateral oophorectomy [Morice et al. 2001]. However, overall survival is not significantly altered [Morris et al. 2000]). More recent data confirm that salpingo-oophorectomy and ovarian cystectomy are the procedures of choice, with recurrence rates of 2%–3% and up to 20% if a simple cystectomy is performed. Preservation of the contralateral ovary increases the risk of recurrence, but surgical resection is usually curative. Cystectomy should be reserved for patients with bilateral LMP tumors or for a recurrent LMP tumor in patients who have a history of adnexectomy and wish to preserve their fertility [Dexeus et al. 2006]. Type of surgical approach, laparoscopic versus laparotomic, does not seem to influence the outcome [Romagnolo et al. 2006].

One of the most recent studies conducted by Rao and co-workers confirmed that fertility-sparing surgery is an option for patients with LMP tumors. In that study 38 of 249 women (15%) with LMP tumors underwent fertility-sparing surgery. Thirty-three of these women (87%) had salpingo-oophorectomy and five patients (13%) had cystectomy. Six patients (16%) recurred after median follow-up of 26 months, and these patients were surgically retreated. No patient died from recurrent tumor [Rao et al. 2005]. Thus, even if conservative surgery increases the risk of recurrence of LMP tumors, recurrent disease is amenable to surgical treatment and patient survival is not affected by this conservative approach. Conservative surgery should therefore be considered safe only for treatment of young patients with LMP tumors who will comply with routine follow-up.

A much lower recurrence rate was reported in Boran's study of 142 patients surgically managed for LMP tumors. Sixty-two patients were treated by fertility-sparing procedures. The observed recurrence rates after radical and fertility-sparing surgery were 0.0% and 6.5%, respectively. Four patients from the conservative surgery group developed recurrence, in contrast to none of the patients from the nonconservative surgery group. No disease-related deaths occurred in any group. The mean duration of follow-up for the conservative surgery group was 44.3 months (range 3–128 months) Although much lower than in many other studies, the recurrence detected in this study was significantly higher after conservative surgical treatment compared to radical surgical approach, and thus close follow-up is recommended to detect recurrent disease [Boran et al. 2005].

9.3.2.2 Obstetrical Outcome

The first two studies evaluating obstetrical outcome of patients with LMP tumors treated with fertility-sparing surgery were published by Gotlieb and colleagues and Morice and colleagues [Gotlieb et al. 2003; Morice et al. 2001]. Gotlieb reported on 22 pregnancies in 15 patients treated conservatively, and Morice described 17 pregnancies occurring in 14 patients (11 pregnancies occurred in patients with stage Ia and 4 pregnancies in stage III disease). A few years later, in the conservatively managed group of 62 patients with LMP, Boran reported 10 women who had successful pregnancies, with a total of 10 live births and 3 abortions [Boran et al. 2005].

A French multicentric study included group of 360 women diagnosed with LMP tumors. One hundred and sixty patients from this group were conservatively treated. Out of all women wishing to conceive after the treatment, 32.3% became pregnant. Thirty conceptions resulted in 5 miscarriages, 8 elective terminations, 17 term deliveries, and 18 live births [Fauvet et al. 2005].

In an Italian multicentric study, 53 patients were conservatively treated for early ovarian cancer. Eight pregnancies obtained from this group of patients resulted in 7 healthy newborns [Romagnolo et al. 2006].

Eighteen patients (10%) in Morice's study were infertile before treatment and 4 patients had infertility after treatment. The question arises of how to treat infertility after conservative surgery, particularly by induction of ovulation. Induction of ovulation was attempted in a few patients with a history of LMP tumors, even stage III, and no recurrent disease was reported [Mantzavinos et al. 1992; Nijman et al. 1992; Chan et al. 2003]. Although there is a concern that high estrogen levels induced by superovulation might have a negative impact on oncological outcome, the experience of 16 patients who had undergone infertility procedures shows that ovulation induction is possible after conservative treatment of LMP tumors. In this group of patients, five pregnancies were achieved and no recurrence was detected [Madelenat et al. 1999]. Induction of ovulation can be discussed in patients with history of LMP, but only in patients with stage I disease and using a limited number of cycles. In patients with a history of adnexectomy for LMP tumors, cryopreservation of part of the ovary could be discussed if the disease recurs [Lobo 2005].

9.3.3 Early Epithelial Ovarian Cancer

Average survival time for epithelial ovarian cancer is 1.4 years, and overall total 5-year survival is 35%–40%. More than two-thirds of patients present with advanced disease, and in these stages 5-year survival is even lower (less than 30%) [Pecorelli et al. 2003]. Early ovarian cancer signifies localized disease and is equivalent to FIGO stage I, sometimes also including stage IIa disease. After a comprehensive laparotomy, only 10%–15% of all patients with epithelial ovarian cancer are diagnosed with an early-stage disease. The survival in an early-stage ovarian cancer reaches 90%, highlighting the importance of early diagnosis and adequate management of the disease (FIGO). Twenty percent of all malignant stage I epithelial tumors of the ovary occur in women under 40 years of age (FIGO). Many young women with early-stage ovarian cancer wish to maintain reproductive capability.

Standard treatment for ovarian cancer is bilateral salpingo-oophorectomy with hysterectomy and omentectomy. During the last decades, because of the improvement in molecular pathology, surgery, and randomized chemotherapy trials, low risk groups of patients were identified among those with gynecologic cancers. Low-risk patients have an excellent prognosis, can be primarily treated by surgery, and do not need any kind of postoperative chemo- or radiotherapy. This is the group of patients who could benefit from conservative surgery when family planning has not yet been completed [Makar and Trope 2001].

Conservative (fertility sparing) surgery is defined as the preservation of ovarian tissue in one or both adnexa and/or the uterus. The goal of conservative surgery in early ovarian malignant disease is preservation of reproductive and endocrine function with the cure of the disease. No definitive data exist to support traditional surgery over conservative surgery in young women with early epithelial ovarian cancers. Several studies have suggested that fertility-sparing surgery may be a viable option for selected patients of childbearing age with stage I ovarian carcinoma, after comprehensive surgical staging [Schilder et al. 2002; Gonzales-Lira et al. 1997; Monk and DiSaia 2005].

The fact that 15% with apparent stage I at the time of surgery have occult lymph node metastases warrants the complete surgical staging [Cass et al. 2001]. Also, coexisting endometrioid cancer of the endometrium was shown to be present in 14% of patients with endometrioid ovarian carcinoma. In patients with early endometrioid cell-type ovarian cancer wishing to retain their fertility, uterine curettage is recommended as a part of staging.

Multiple risk factors have been evaluated as to prognosis, and multivariate analyses have shown that only grade of differentiation, presence of ascites, and ovarian surface tumor were significant for relapse, but did not have an impact on survival. Therefore, the treatment approach is based on the presence of prognostic criteria (Table 9.2).

In the younger patient, when fertility is desired unilateral salpingo-oophorectomy with wedge biopsy of the other ovary, omentectomy, and ipsilateral lymph node sampling may be the appropriate solution, if the tumor is localized with favorable low-risk pathology.

Indications for adjuvant chemotherapy in patients with epithelial ovarian cancer treated with unilateral salpingo-oophorectomy should be based on these risk factors. A number of studies have concluded that the use of adjuvant chemotherapy offers no survival advantage to patients with well-differentiated stage Ia epithelial ovarian cancer.

Table 9.2 Early ovarian cancer risk groups

Low risk	High risk
Stage Ia or Ib	All stage Ic G 3
Grade 1 or grade 2	Grade 3
Non-clear cell histologic type	Clear cell histologic type
Intact capsule	Tumor growth through capsule
No tumor on external surface	Tumor on external surface
No ascites	Ascites
Negative washings	Positive washings
Unruptured capsule	Ruptured capsule
No dense adherence	Dense adherence
Diploid tumor	Aneuploid tumor

All incompletely staged patients with apparent early ovarian cancer should be considered high-risk patients. Patients with incompletely staged early ovarian cancer could be either surgically restaged or treated by adjuvant chemotherapy. The conclusion from ACTION/ICON1 studies was that in optimally staged patients adjuvant chemotherapy did not improve relapse-free or overall survival. In suboptimally staged patients adjuvant chemotherapy significantly improves both recurrence-free survival by 11% and overall survival by 7% at 5 years [ICON 1 and EORTC-ACTION Collaborators 2001].

Diagnosis of ovarian cancer in young women is often accidental at the time of laparotomy for an adnexal mass preoperatively misdiagnosed as endometriosis or benign tumor. Sometimes an acute abdomen due to torsion of pelvic mass requires immediate surgery. Unfortunately, it is not always a surgeon experienced in oncology who performs the initial operation. Therefore, it is important to stress that in all cases with suspicious findings, a two-step procedure is preferable: The first step should be cytologic washing with extirpation of ovarian tumor in toto, and if the definitive histopathology confirms the presence of malignancy a second surgery can be performed to obtain optimal staging before conservative treatment is allowed.

When evaluating a patient for fertility-sparing surgery, several requirements should be considered. The criteria for an ideal candidate include FIGO stage Ia disease, a patient of young age with low parity, an encapsulated tumor with no adhesions, and the ability for close follow-up. Such patients need no further therapy after surgery and comprehensive staging. In addition, a similar approach may be acceptable for women with stage Ia, grade 2 cancers, but experience in this area is limited. Finally, women with stage Ic disease, grade 3 tumors, or clear cell histology may still be candidates for conservative surgery, but adjuvant chemotherapy is generally recommended [Monk and DiSaia 2005].

9.3.3.1 Oncological Outcome

One of the most important conclusions of studies investigating fertility-sparing surgery in early ovarian cancer is that the patients with stage I ovarian cancer have excellent prognosis. The estimated survival was 98% at 5 years and 93% at 10 years [Schilder et al. 2002]. These rates compare favorably to the reported survival of patients with stage I ovarian cancer treated with more radical surgery [Pecorelli et al. 2003].

In one of the first studies of conservative surgical treatment in early invasive ovarian cancer, published in 1997, Colombo and her colleagues reported the results of conservative surgery in 56 of 99 patients with stage I ovarian cancer. In all these patients, careful staging was performed preoperatively. After a median follow-up of 75 months, no difference was observed between the patients treated conservatively and the group who underwent ablative surgery. The recurrence rate was similar: 3 of 56 in the conservative surgery group and 5 of 43 in the patients treated with ablative surgery [Colombo et al. 1997].

One of the largest studies evaluating the conservative approach was a multi-institutional retrospective investigation undertaken in the US to identify patients with stage Ia and Ic epithelial ovarian cancer who were treated with fertility-sparing surgery [Schilder et al. 2002]. Recurrence rate, survival, and reproductive outcome were evaluated. Fifty-two patients, at a mean age of 26 years (range 11–40 years) with stage I epithelial ovarian cancer, were treated by unilateral oophorectomy. Nineteen patients received adjuvant chemotherapy: 11 patients with stage Ia and 8 patients with stage Ic disease. The most common chemotherapy regimens were either cisplatin/taxol or carboplatin and oral melphalan. Duration of follow-up ranged from 6 to 426 months (median 68 months) Five patients developed tumor recurrence 8–78 months after initial surgery. Four of these patients had stage Ia and one had stage Ic disease.

It should be noted that two of the three patients who developed pelvic recurrence did so within 1 year of treatment and both had masses in the contralateral ovary detected on ultrasound. Therefore, all patients treated with conservative surgery for stage I ovarian cancer should be followed every 3 months with serum Ca 125 determinations and transvaginal sonography for a minimum of 2 years.

9.3.3.2 Obstetrical Outcome

Colombo's study was one of the first reported series of conservatively treated patients with early ovarian cancer. All patients who postoperatively received platinum-based chemotherapy maintained their menstrual function during treatment. All patients wishing to conceive succeeded without problems, and 25 conceptions yielded 4 miscarriages, 4 elective terminations, 2 ectopic pregnancies, and 15 term deliveries [Colombo et al. 1997].

After treatment 24 patients (22 stage Ia and 2 Stage Ic) from Schilder's study attempted pregnancy and 17 (71%) conceived. Six of these 17 patients had prior chemotherapy. These pregnancies resulted in 26 term deliveries and 5 spontaneous abortions. No congenital anomalies were noted in these or in the other term pregnancies reported in the literature. The findings of this investigation indicate that selected patients with completely staged stage I epithelial ovarian cancer who desire childbearing can be treated safely with unilateral salpingo-oophorectomy [Schilder et al. 2002].

In conclusion, the findings of the studies investigating the outcome of reproductive age women with stage I epithelial ovarian cancer who desire childbearing indicate that these patients can be treated safely with conservative surgery (unilateral adnexectomy). It is important to emphasize that complete surgical staging should be accomplished before fertility-sparing surgery is performed.

9.3.4 Malignant Nonepithelial Ovarian Tumors

Malignant ovarian germ cell tumors (OGCT) and sex cord stromal tumors (OSCST) are much less common than epithelial ovarian cancer. They account for less than 5% of all ovarian malignancies. OGCT and OSCST are:

- More frequent among young women
- Frequently limited to the ovary
- Extremely sensitive to chemotherapy

Today, the availability of effective chemotherapeutic agents has changed the option of traditional radical surgery to conservative surgery in the management of germ cell tumors. Such conservative surgery in early stages of the disease has been reported to result in 5-year survival of 90% or more [Gerhenson 1993].

One of the first reports of menstrual function and reproductive function after treatment with combination chemotherapy for malignant OGCR was Gershenson's study, which showed that 11 of 15 patients attempting pregnancy achieved pregnancy after combination VAC chemotherapy and delivered 22 healthy children [Gershenson 1988].

Several studies reported that conservative surgical approach in management of OGCT is equally effective when compared with more radical surgery. Tangir and colleagues published results of 122-month (24–384 months) follow-up of 86 patients with OGCT. All but five patients received chemotherapy postoperatively. Fertility-sparing surgery was performed in 64 patients. Thirty-eight of these patients have attempted conception and 29 (76%) of them, stages I–III, have achieved at least one pregnancy. Among the patients who conceived 20 patients were FIGO stage I, 1 was stage II, and 8 were stage III. A total of 38 children were born to these women. So, conservative surgery followed by chemotherapy became a standard care for early stages and selected advanced malignant OGCT [Tangir et al. 2003].

Zanetta and colleagues reported the largest series of young women with malignant germ cell tumors treated by conservative surgery [Zanetta et al. 2001]. Exploring the survival and reproductive function after treatment of 169 patients with malignant germ cell tumors, 138 (81%) of whom had conservative surgery, the survival rate of patients treated conservatively was exceeding 90%–100%, which did not differ from the survival rate of the entire group (89%–100%)

Thirty-two conservatively treated patients attempted to become pregnant, and 28 (88%) of them became pregnant. The total number of conceptions was 55, and in 38 (69%) of those full-term normal infants were born.

For all OGCT patients, except those with well-documented stage Ia pure dysgerminoma, postoperative chemotherapy is recommended.

Preservation of ovarian function, reproductive ability, and emotional attitudes in patients with malignant ovarian tumors were studied by Zanagnolo et al. [Zanagnolo et al. 2005]. The study included 75 women conservatively treated for stage I epithelial, BOT, OGCT, OSCST. Thirty patients from this group received adjuvant chemotherapy. Four patients (5.2%) had recurrence (35 months). Twenty patients attempted pregnancy, and 15 (75%) of them conceived. Twenty-three pregnancies resulted in 19 healthy newborns.

In conclusion, the results from several studies confirm that fertility-saving surgery is a safe approach in management of:

- Stage I (grade 1 and 2) epithelial ovarian cancer
- Any stage LMP tumor
- Malignant germ cell ovarian tumors
- Stage I sex cord stromal tumor

9.4 Summary

In a young woman with gynecologic cancer, preservation of fertility is possible. Fertility-sparing surgery may be safe in early ovarian cancer of certain histological subtypes such as ovarian tumors of low malignant potential, malignant ovarian germ cell tumors, and ovarian sex cord stromal tumors. For women with invasive epithelial ovarian cancer who have early-stage disease, fertility-sparing surgery may be an option. In some cases, fertility-sparing surgery may be followed by postoperative chemotherapy. The concept of fertility-preserving surgery in early cervical cancer has been adopted by several leading centers worldwide as an option for stage Ia and small Ib disease without the presence of lymphovascular involvement. Nonsurgical options such as hormonal therapy may be considered for women with early-stage, low-grade endometrial cancer.

Improvements in cancer cure rates and the development of conservative treatments mean that many young women with early gynecologic cancer can hope to start a new pregnancy after the treatment. Patients are generally advised to wait 2 years after treatment for any malignancy before attempting pregnancy, but the optimal interval between cure and conception must be carefully determined by a multidisciplinary team including oncologist and obstetrician. Gynecologic surgery and hemotherapy can have an impact not only on fertility, but also on the course of a next pregnancy (increased risk of miscarriage and premature delivery, etc.) These risks must be taken into account by the obstetrician.

Management of young women diagnosed with gynecologic cancer should be individualized, with the risk of conservative therapy balanced against the disadvantages of more radical treatment. The patient and the family should be extensively counseled. The alternatives to the traditional and standard radical procedures should be discussed, and the limitation of data regarding many conservative treatment options should be explained. The patients should be aware that by accepting fertility-sparing treatment they are assuming a small but undefined risk for recurrence of the disease. They need to know that these conservative therapeutic approaches are yet not considered "standard."

Furthermore, patients need to be assessed for the realistic probabilities of achieving conception on the basis on their age, history, and infertility evaluation. Some of them will require assisted reproduction technology (ARTS) to help achieve a pregnancy, especially in vitro fertilization (IVF). They may also consider ovarian tissue, oocyte, or embryo cryopreservation before definitive cancer therapies. And, finally, patients also need to understand the risk of premature delivery and the consequences of prematurity.

The care of the young patient with gynecologic malignancy is extremely complex and challenging. It necessarily requires a multidisciplinary approach with the close collaboration of gynecologist-oncologist, reproductive endocrinologist, and perinatologist.

References

Aburel E (1981) Colpohisterectomia largita subfundica. In: Sirbu P, editor. Chirurgica gynecologica. Bucharest, Romania: Editura Medicala Pub, p. 714–721

Amant F, Leunen K, Neven P, Berteloot P, Vergote I (2006) Endometrial cancer: predictors of response and preferred endocrine therapy . Int J Gynecol Cancer 16: 527

Benedet JL and Anderson GH (1996) Stage IA carcinoma of the cervix revisited. Obstet Gynecol 87: 1052–1059

Benedetti -Panici P, Greggi S, Colombo A, et al.(2002) Neoadjuvant chemotherapy and radical surgery versus exclusive surgery in locally advanced squamous cell cervical cancer: results from the Italian multicenter randomized study. J Clin Oncol 20: 179–188

Benshushan A (2004) Endometrial adenocarcinoma in young patients: evaluation and fertility-preserving treatment. Eur J Obset Gynaecol Reprod Biol 117: 132–137

Bokhman JV, Chepick OF, Volkova AT, Vishinevsky AS (1985) Can primary endometrial carcinoma stage I be cured without surgery and radiation therapy? Gynecol Oncol 20: 139–255

Boran N, Cil AP, Tulunay G, Ozturkolu E, Koc S, Bulbul D, Kose MF (2005) Fertility and recurrence results of conservative surgery for borderline ovarian tumors. Gynecol Oncol 97: 845–851

Bosch FX, Lorincz A, Munoz N, Meijer CJ, Shah KV (2002) The causal relation between human papillomavirus and cervical cancer. J Clin Pathol 55: 244–265

Boss EA, Van Gold RJT, Beerendonk CCM, Massuger LFAG (2005) Pregnancy after radical trachelectomy: a real option? Gynecol Oncol 99(3 Suppl 1): S152–S156

Chan JK, Lin YF, Loizzi V, Ghobriel M, DiSaia PJ, Berman ML (2003) Borderline Ovarian Tumors in Reproductive-Age Women. Fertility-Sparing Surgery and Outcome. J Reprod Med 48: 756–760

Carter J, Rowland K, Chi D, Brown C, Abu-Rustum N, Castiel M, Barakat R (2005) Gynecologic cancer treatment and the impact of cancer-related infertility. Gynecol Oncol 97: 90–95

Cass I, Li AJ, Runowicz CD, Fields AL, Goldberg GL, Leuchter RS, Lagasse LD, Kartan BY (2001) Patterns of lymph node metastases in clinically unilateral stage I invasive epithelial ovarian carcinomas. Gynecol Oncol 80: 56–61

Chung DC, Rustgi AK (2003) The hereditary nonpolyposis colorectal cancer syndrome: genetics and clinical implications. Ann Intern Med 138: 560–570

Colombo N, Chiari S, Maggioni A, Bonazzi H (1997) Controversal issues in the management of early epithelial Ovarian cancer: conservative surgery and role of adjuvant chemotherapy. Gynecol Oncol 55: 47–52

Creasman WT, Zaino RJ, Major FJ, et al.(1998) Early invasive carcinoma of the cervix (3 to 5 mm invasion): risk factors and prognosis. A Gynecologic Oncology Group study. Am J Obstet Gynecol 178 (1 Pt 1): 62–65

Dargent D, Brun JL, Roy M, Remy I (1994) Pregnancies following radical trachelectomy for invasive cervical cancer. Gynecol Oncol 52: 105 (abst.)

Dexeus S, Labastida R, Dexeus D (2005) Conservative management of epithelial ovarian cancer. Eur J Gynaecol Oncol 26: 473–478

Di Saia PJ, Creasman WT (2002) Epithelial ovarian cancer. In: Clinical Gynecologic Oncology, 6th ed. Mosby, p 289–350

Farhi DC, Nosanchuk J, Silberberg SG (1986) Endometrial adenocarcinoma in women under 25 years of age. Obstet Gynecol 68: 741–745

Fathalla MF (1971) Incessant ovulation—A factor in ovarian neoplasia? Lancet 2:163

Fauvet R, Poncelet C, et al. (2005) Fertility after conservative treatment of borderline ovarian tumors: a French multicenter study. Fertil Steril 83: 284–290

Ferlay J, Bray F, Pisani P, Parkin DM (2004). GLOBOCAN 2002: Cancer incidence, mortality and prevalence worldwide. IARC Cancer Base No. 5, version 2.0. Lyon: IARC Press, October 2004

Gerhenson DM (1988) Menstrual and reproductive function after treatment with combination chemotherapy for malignant ovarian germ cell tumors. J Clin Oncol 5: 270–275

Gerhenson DM (1993) Update on management malignant ovarian germ cell tumor. Cancer 71: 1581–1588

Gonzales-Lira G, Escudero-Le Los Rios, Salazar-Martinez E, et al. (1997) Conservative surgery for ovarian cancer and effect on fertility. Int J Gynaecol Obstet 56: 155–162

Gotlieb WH, Beiner ME, Shalmon B, Korach Y, Segal Y, et al. (2003) Outcome of fertility-sparing treatment with progestins in young patients with endometrial cancer. Obstet Gynecol 102: 718–725

Heinz AP, Odicino F, Maisonneuve P, et al. (2001) Carcinoma of the ovary. J Epidem Biostat 6: 107–138

ICON 1 and EORTC-ACTION Collaborators (2003) International Collaborative Ovarian Neoplasm trial 1 and Adjuvant Chemotherapy in Ovarian Neoplasm: two parallel randomized phase III trials of adjuvant chemotherapy in patients with early-stage ovarian carcinoma. J Natl Cancer Inst 95: 105–112

King MC, Marks JH, Mandell JB for the New York Breast Study Group (2003) Breast and ovarian cancer risk due to inherited mutations in BRCA 1 and BRCA 2. Science 302: 643–646

Kinkel K, Kaji Y, Yu KK, et al. (1999) Radiologic staging in patients with endometrial cancer: a meta-analysis. Radiology 212: 711–718

Lai CH, Huang HJ (2006) The role of hormones for the treatment of endometrial Hyperplasia and endometrial cancer. Curr Opin Obstet Gynecol 18: 29–34

Leitao MM Jr, Chi DS (2005) Fertility-sparing options for patients with gynecologic malignancies. Oncologist 10: 613–622

Lobo RA (2005) Potential options for preservation of fertility in women. N Engl J Med 353: 64–73

Lu KH, Burke TW (2000) Early cervical cancer. Curr Treat Options Oncol 1: 147–155

Madelenat P, Meneux E, Fernandez H, Uzan S, Antoine LM (1999) Place de l'ssistance à la procreation après taitment conservateur d'une tumour ovarienne : enquête multicentrique francaise. 10. Congrès de la Société Francaise d'Oncologie Gynécologique. Poitiers, France, Nov 5–6, 1999

Makar A, Trope C (2001) Fertility preservation in gynecologic cancer. Acta Obstet Gynecol Scand 80: 794–802

Mathews TJ, Hamilton BE (2002) Mean age of mother, 1970–2000. Natl Vital Stat Rep 51: 1–13

Monk BJ, DiSaia PJ (2005) What is the role of conservative primary surgical management of epithelial ovarian cancer: the United States experience and debate. Int J Gynecol Cancer 15, Suppl 3: 199–205

Morice P, Camatte S, El-Hassan J, Pautier P, Duvillard P, Castagne D (2001) Clinical outcomes and fertility after conservative treatment of ovarian borderline tumors. Fertil Steril 75: 92–96

Morris RT, Gershenson DM, Silva EG, et al. (2000) Outcome and reproductive function after conservative surgery for borderline ovarian tumors. Obstet Gynecol 95: 541–547

Munstedt K, Grant P, Woenckhaus J, Roth G, Tinneberg H-R (2004) Cancer of the endometrium: current aspects of diagnostics and treatment. Review. World J Surg Oncol 2:24 doi:10.1186/1477-7819-2-24 (http://www.wjso.com/content/2/1/24)

Nam J-H, Kim S-H, Kim J-H, Kim Y-T, Mok J-E (2002) Nonradical treatment is as effective as radical surgery in the management of cervical cancer stage Ia1. Int J Gynecol Cancer 12: 480–484

Palfalvi L, Ungar L, Boyle DC, Del Priore G, Smith JR (2003) Announcement of healthy baby boy born following abdominal radical trachelectomy. Int J Gynecol Cancer 13:250

Pecorelli S, Beller U, Heintz PA, Benedet LJ, Creasman WT, Peterson F (2003) The 25th FIGO Annual Report on the Results of Treatment in Gynecologic Cancer. Int J Gynaecol Obstet 83 (Suppl 1): 1–229

Plante M, Renaud MC, Harel F, Roy M (2004) Vaginal radical treachelectomy: an oncologically safe fertility-preserving surgery. An updated series of 72 cases and review of literature. Gynecol Oncol 94: 614–623

Plante M, Renaud MC, Hoskins IA, et al. (2005) Vaginal radical trachelectomy: a valuable fertility preserving option in the management of early-stage cervical cancer. A series of 50 pregnancies and review of the literature. Gynecol Oncol 98: 3–10

Plante M, Roy M (2006) Fertility-preserving options for cervical cancer. Oncology (Williston Park) 20: 479–88; discussion 491–493. Review

Ramirez PT, Frumovitz M, Bodurka DC, Sunn CC, Levenback C (2004) Hormonal therapy for the management of grade 1 endometrial carcinoma: a literature review. Gynecol Oncol 95 (1): 133–138

Rao GG, Skinner EN, Gehrig PA, Duska LR, Miller DS, Schorge JO (2005) Fertility-sparing surgery for ovarian low malignant potential tumors. Gynecol Oncol 98: 263–266

Ries LAG, Eisner MP, Kosay CL et al., eds (2004) SEER Cancer Statistics Review, 1975–2001. Bethesda, MD: National Cancer Institute. (http://seer.cancer.gov/csr/1975_2001)

Rodriguez M, Guimares O, Rose PG (2001) Radical abdominal trachelectomy and pelvic lymphadenectomy with uterine conservation and subsequent pregnancy in the treatment of early invasive cervical cancer. Am J Obstet Gynecol 185: 370–374

Romagnolo C, Gadducci A, Sartori E, Zola P, Maggino T (2006) Management of borderline ovarian tumors: results of an Italian multicentric study. Gynecol Oncol 101: 255–260

Schiffman MH, Brinton LA (1995) The epidemiology of cervical carcinogenesis. Cancer 76: 1888–1901

Schilder JM, Thompson AM, DePriest PD, Ueland FR, Cibull ML, et al. (2002) Outcome of reproductive age women with stage Ia or Ic invasive epithelial ovarian cancer treated with fertility-sparing therapy. Gynecol Oncol 87: 1-7

Seli E, Tangir J (2005) Fertility preservation options for female patients with malignancies. Curr Opin Obstet Gynecol 17(3): 299–308

Sivanesaratnam V (2001) Fertility and gynaecological malignancies. J Clin Gynaecol Res 27: 1-15

Smith JR, Boyle DC, Corless DJ, Ungar L, Lawson AD, et al. (1997) Abdominal radical trachelectomy: a new surgical technique for the conservative management of cervical carcinoma Br J Obstet Gynaecol 104: 1196–1200

Sonoda Y, Abu-Rustum NR, Gemignani ML, Chi DS, Brown CL, et al. (2004) A fertility-sparing alternative to radical hysterectomy: how many patients may be eligible? Gynecol Oncol 95: 534–538

Tangir J, Zelterman D, Ma W, Schwartz PE (2003) Reproductive function after conservative surgery and chemotherapy for malignant germ cell tumors of the ovary. Obstet Gynecol 101: 251–257

Ungar L, Smith JR, Palfalvi L, Del Priore G (2006) Abdominal radical trachelectomy during pregnancy to preserve pregnancy and fertility. Obstet Gynecol 108(3 Pt 2): 811–814

Whitney CW, Brunetto VL, Zaino RJ, et al. (2004) Phase II study of medroxyprogesterone acetate plus tamoxifen in advanced endometrial carcinoma: a Gynecologic Oncology Group study. Gynecol Oncol 92: 4–9

Young RC, Decker DG, Wharton JT, et al. (1986) Staging laparotomy in early epithelial ovarian cancer. Am J Obstet Gynecol 154: 282–286

Zanagnolo V, Saratori E, Trussardi E, Pasinetti B, Maggino T (2005) Preservation of ovarian function, reproductive ability and emotional attitudes in patients with malignant ovarian tumors. Eur J Obst Gynaecol Repr Biol 123: 235–243

Zanetta G, Bonazzi C, Cantu M, et al. (2001) Survival and reproductive function after treatment of malignant germ cell ovarian tumors. J Clin Oncol 19: 1015–1020

10 Leukaemia and Pregnancy

M. F. Fey, D. Surbek

Recent Results in Cancer Research, Vol. 178

10.1 Strategy of Literature Research

A PubMed search was undertaken using the grouped key words "leukaemia; pregnancy": 3,067 references were found, with the earliest (a case report in a Dutch journal) published in 1949 [1]. Only papers with clinical data were considered for this review, with the selection arbitrarily focussing on more recent papers; the majority of these were single case reports. Special consideration was given to case series (all of them retrospective in design). For obvious reasons, in this particular field no prospective series or randomised trials are reported in the literature. More recent literature was deliberately given preference over articles published before the 1980s, since some of the major advances in diagnosis and therapy of leukaemia were achieved as of the early 1990s.

10.2 Epidemiology and Biology of Human Leukaemia

Leukaemias are cancers of the haematopoietic system, derived from transformed haematopoietic stem cells within the bone marrow. They may occur within any age group, hence also in younger women of child-bearing age. In the general population, chronic lymphocytic B-cell leukaemia (CLL) is by far the most frequent type, with an incidence of about 15–20 cases/100,000 per year. Next in line are the myelodysplastic syndromes (MDS), which are characterised by profound disturbances of haematopoietic maturation often affecting many lineages. Acute myeloblastic leukaemia (AML) occurs at an incidence of 2–4 cases/100,000/year, followed down the line by chronic myelogenous leukaemia (CML), acute lymphoblastic leukaemia (ALL), which is much rarer in adults than in children, and a few other types of either myeloid or lymphoid neoplasms (Table 10.1).

In pregnancy, leukaemia occurs very rarely, at about a rate of 1 case in 75,000 pregnancies [2–7]. The frequency of the different types of leukaemias in pregnancy differs much from the distribution in the general population, but it corresponds to the age-specific incidence of the various types of leukaemia. AML and ALL are the most frequent types of haematological cancers diagnosed in younger adults aged between 20 and 40 years of age. Accordingly, the most frequent types of leukaemia found in pregnant women are acute leukaemias (two thirds of them AML), followed by CML, and CLL is very rare.

The aetiology of leukaemia in many cases remains unclear, but some AML may be linked to previous exposure to toxic substances, or ionising radiation. Patients cured for tumours who received alkylating agents and radiotherapy (for example, survivors of Hodgkin disease) are at increased risk of developing secondary AML.

Although rare families with hereditary predisposition to leukaemia (for example, CLL or AML) have been described [8, 9], the vast majority of cases are sporadic.

The molecular pathology of leukaemia follows a few basic rules:

a Acquired chromosomal abnormalities occur in haematopoietic stem cells that are pluripotent or committed to a particular lineage (myeloid or lymphoid);

b Chromosomal alterations in leukaemic cells are mostly reciprocal translocations in which genes residing on different chromosomes

Table 10.1 The salient features of most frequent types of human leukaemias

Diagnosis	Incidence (×/100,000/year) Median age at presentation (years)	Classification morphology, karyotype and molecular features	Clinical features	Typical treatment	Prognosis	Comments
Acute myeloid leukaemia (AML)	2–4 60 years	Heterogeneous WHO classification incorporating virtually all modern diagnostic techniques – AML with recurrent chromosomal alterations t[8;21], inv[16], t[15;17] see below – AML with multilineage dysplasia – AML with MDS – 50% AML with normal karyotype Most frequent molecular features (apart from fusion genes/chromosomal translocations) are FLT3 gene tandem duplications, or mutations in the nucleophosmin gene or in the C/EBPα gene	Chance finding or non-specific complaints such as fatigue, pallor, fever, bleeding or, rarely, organ infiltration (chloroma)	Induction therapy with anthracyclines and cytarabine (APL, see below); Followed by postremission therapy (generally postponed in pregnancy until after delivery) – Intensive consolidation chemotherapy – High-dose chemotherapy and autologous stem cell transplantation – Allogeneic stem cell transplantation with HLA-identical donor (preferably family, if not unrelated) Palliative treatment in patients unfit for intensive chemotherapy	5-year overall survival – 70%–80% in good-risk AML – 40%–50% in intermediate-risk AML – 0%–10% in poor risk and in patients under palliative treatment – 50% in patients undergoing allogeneic stem cell transplantation	Most frequent type of leukaemia in pregnancy

Table 10.1 *(continued)* The salient features of most frequent types of human leukaemias

Diagnosis	Incidence (×/100,000/year) Median age at presentation (years)	Classification morphology, karyotype and molecular features	Clinical features	Typical treatment	Prognosis	Comments
Acute promyelocytic leukaemia (APL)	0.2–0.5 30–40 years	Blasts exhibiting morphology of promyelocytes with heavy granules and Auer rods t[15;17]	As in AML, with a propensity to bleeding (coagulopathy) Mostly pancytopenic at presentation	Intensive chemotherapy as in other types of AML + all-trans retinoic acid (ATRA; differentiating agent)	5-year survival 75%	One of the more frequent leukaemias in pregnant women. Rapidly progressive and fatal if untreated, mostly due to coagulopathy and bleeding
Myelodysplastic syndromes (MDS) MDS include refractory anaemias and cytopenias, with or without excess of blasts, as well as chronic myelo-monocytic leukaemia	4–12 Mostly elderly patients (70 years)	Stem cell disorders with multilineage involvement WHO classification describes various categories of MDS with a wide range of prognostic implications Often presenting with refractory anaemia, eventually pancytopenia, may progress to AML Mostly chromosomal deletions, e.g. 5q- or 7- Complex karyotype aberrations signal adverse prognosis	Insidious onset of clinical symptoms often very gradual, in parallel to slow progression of marrow failure	Mostly managed with supportive care (transfusions, treatment of infections); intensive chemotherapy and allogeneic stem cell transplantation for younger age group only Some newer agents such as decitabine under clinical investigation	No curative treatment except for allogeneic stem cell transplantation. Median survival highly variable, ranging from many years in patients with refractory anaemia to a few months only in patients progressing to AML About 40%–50% of selected younger patients may enjoy long-term survival after allogeneic stem cell transplantation	Transition into frank AML

Table 10.1 *(continued)* The salient features of most frequent types of human leukaemias

Diagnosis	Incidence (×/100,000/year) Median age at presentation (years)	Classification morphology, karyotype and molecular features	Clinical features	Typical treatment	Prognosis	Comments
Chronic myelogenous leukaemia (CML)	1 55–65 years	t[9;22] = Philadelphia chromosome Massive leukocytosis including mature neutrophils and other types of blood cells Initially chronic phase, morphologically with maintained maturation, Progression to accelerated and then blast phase (resembling AML or ALL) after several to many years	Insidious onset Splenomegaly. Initially often few symptoms. General symptoms such as weakness, fever etc particularly in later phases	Imatinib mesylate (small molecule inhibiting the ABL kinase in the BCR-ABL fusion protein) Allogeneic stem cell transplantation in selected younger patients	Survival under imatinib mesylate approaching 85%–95% at 5 years	Molecular model disorder

Table 10.1 *(continued)* The salient features of most frequent types of human leukaemias

Diagnosis	Incidence (×/100,000/year) Median age at presentation (years)	Classification morphology, karyotype and molecular features	Clinical features	Typical treatment	Prognosis	Comments
Acute adult lymphoblastic leukaemia (ALL)	1.5 50 years in adults (4 > 5 years in children)	Mostly B-cell neoplasms, subdivided by immunophenotype, and molecular genetics CALLA+ ALL (CD10+) Progenitor B- ALL (CD10–) Phi+ ALL most frequent subtype in adults	Symptoms as in AML. Lymphadenopathy, spleno- and hepatomegaly more common than in AML	Induction based on cyclophosphamide, daunorubicin, vincristine and notably prednisone as well as L-asparaginase; less intensive than in AML Later therapy phases include early intensification chemotherapy, late intensification and finally maintenance (out-patient) chemotherapy In contrast to AML, ALL treatment programmes often last up to 2 years. CNS prophylaxis is required (in contrast to AML) Phi+ALL also receive imatinib mesylate Allogeneic stem cell transplantation is established in 1st remission in patients <60 years	Survival at 5 years – T-cell ALL 60% – Precursor B-cell ALL 30% – Phi+ ALL 0–10% – Elderly 10%	Prognosis in adults much worse than in childhood About 80% of children may expect cure

Table 10.1 *(continued)* The salient features of most frequent types of human leukaemias

Diagnosis	Incidence (×/100,000/year) Median age at presentation (years)	Classification morphology, karyotype and molecular features	Clinical features	Typical treatment	Prognosis	Comments
Chronic lymphocytic B-cell leukaemia (B-CLL)	12–15 70 years	Heterogeneous at molecular and clinical level Mostly chromosomal deletions, some undetectable in the karyotype	Often chance finding upon examination of peripheral blood smears. Splenomegaly and lymphadenopathy. Clinical outcome highly variable	Early stage CLL requires no treatment (often for many years) until progression Late stage CLL treated with various chemotherapy regimes, and/or antibodies (rituximab targeting the CD20 antigen, and alemtuzumab targeting CD52) Treatment palliative except perhaps for selected younger patients undergoing allogeneic stem cell transplantation	Highly variable with median survival between a few years and decades	Major efforts undertaken by cooperative groups to define risk-adapted treatment strategies
Hairy cell leukaemia (HCL)	0.1–0.2 Peak in 6th to 7th decade; mostly elderly males	Severe pancytopenia, typically with marked monocytopenia. Typical morphology of lymphoid cells with filamentous cytoplasmic projections, staining + for tartrate-resistant acid phosphatase B-cells expressing CD19 and CD20, as well as the monocytic antigen CD 11c	Often insidious. Splenomegaly	Current standard treatment consists of purine analogues (often no more than a single cycle); formerly interferon Indolent, with about 10% of patients never requiring therapy	Responses durable even after a single course of therapy in the great majority of patients, with median survival of many years	

or parts thereof are fused to form abnormal chromosomes, and in turn fusion genes, which are not present in any normal cells. CLL is an exception in that it harbours mostly chromosomal deletions rather than translocations;

c Additional gene mutations may comprise gene point mutations or gene deletions at the submicroscopical level that are not detected through cytogenetics;

d Genes involved in typical chromosomal alterations and genes otherwise mutated in leukaemia are often involved in molecular pathways which govern cell cycle control, apoptosis programmes (programmed cell death) and particularly cellular differentiation;

e These cytogenetic or molecular alterations in transformed leukaemic stem cells provide the molecular spark initiating, and the molecular drive maintaining, their clonal expansion.

Having acquired such chromosomal and molecular alterations, transformed haematopoietic stem cells show altered programmes of cellular proliferation, or differentiation, or both. As a rule of thumb, cellular differentiation is maintained in chronic leukaemias. For example, CML is characterised by massive expansion over time of the progeny of a transformed pluripotent haematopoietic progenitor cell, which has acquired a characteristic chromosomal aberration, the Philadelphia chromosome (i.e. the translocation t[9, 22]). Acute leukaemias are chiefly characterised by a block in either myeloid (AML) or lymphoid differentiation (ALL) which occurs at early stages of normal cellular maturation.

Given its systemic nature, not only does leukaemia involve the bone marrow (where it originates), but in most cases, leukaemic cells are spilled all over the body. One would therefore assume that, in contrast to solid tumours, there would be a particularly high risk of placental and hence fetal involvement if maternal leukaemia is present. Very few cases have been published in which the baby was found to harbour leukaemic cells in its organs or blood, or where leukaemic cells were detected in the placenta [10]. Thus, the placenta seems to be offering very efficient protection from spill-over of leukaemic cells into the fetus [11, 12], which is surprising, because bidirectional transplacental traffic of white blood cells has meanwhile been recognised to occur in most normal pregnancies [13]. Vertical transmission of maternal AML to the baby was demonstrated in a single case of acute monocytic leukaemia [14], where the boy was diagnosed with acute monocytic leukaemia at the age of 20 months. Interestingly, his leukaemic cells showed a female karyotype and their HLA type was consistent with that of the mother. HLA homozygosity of the mother might have played a role in inducing immunologic tolerance to maternal leukaemic cells present in the baby's system. No other such cases have been reported in the literature collected for the present article. However, most reports on leukaemia in pregnancy do not give any information on this particular issue.

10.3 Presentation and Diagnosis

Clinically the onset of leukaemia is often insidious. It may be a chance finding on a blood film requested for another reason, or patients may report non-specific complaints such as fatigue, pallor or dyspnoea and exhibit reduced performance status. Frequent presenting symptoms may be infections or bleeding. Occasionally, leukaemia is diagnosed as a chance finding on clinical examination when a large spleen or liver or enlarged lymph nodes are found and further investigated. The symptoms of leukaemia therefore often mimick frequent complaints in pregnancy, and thus the diagnosis of leukaemia is not suspected right away.

Table 10.1 provides a summary of the salient features of human acute and chronic leukaemias.

10.4 Treatment

Patients with leukaemia may be promised reasonable chances of cure, or at least worthwhile palliation with possible prolongation of survival over years rather than months only. The hallmarks of treatment are intensive chemotherapy programmes in acute leukaemias, targeted therapy in CML, and a variety of chemotherapies as well as antibody options for patients with CLL. In pregnancy-associated leukaemia, the same therapy principles apply as in non-pregnant patients [2–7].

10.5 Myeloid Neoplasms

10.5.1 Acute Myeloid Leukaemia

If left untreated, AML leads to death within a few months of the diagnosis. In pregnant women, it is therefore often not possible to postpone treatment until after delivery, except if the diagnosis is made very late in pregnancy, close to term. Even then, patients often present with profound cytopenia, and therefore the risk of caesarean section in a pregnant woman with the full haematological picture of AML must be weighed against the risks of treatment with the fetus still in utero.

Patients with newly diagnosed AML require intensive induction chemotherapy, usually combining anthracyclines and cytarabine given over several days [15]. In patients with excessive leukocytosis, particularly those with monocytic types of AML, leukapheresis may initially be necessary to prevent leukostasis. Chemotherapy leads to clearance of blasts from blood and bone marrow in the majority of cases, but also induces transient severe damage to the residual normal haematopoiesis. As a result patients suffer from treatment-induced severe pancytopoenia typically lasting for about 2–3 weeks. During this period they require supportive care. Neutropenia entails a considerable risk of infection, both bacterial and fungal, and hence intravenous broad-spectrum antibiotics are required in virtually all patients. Patients not responding to antibiotics may require antifungal treatment. In AML, granulocyte-colony stimulating factor is not routinely given during chemotherapy-induced bone marrow aplasia, since clinical trials have failed to demonstrate its unequivocal advantage over antibiotic treatment alone. Anaemia requires transfusions, as does thrombocytopenia to prevent or treat bleeding. Conditions such as neutropenic enterocolitis may call for parenteral intravenous nutrition. Once blast clearance has been achieved in a first induction cycle, subsequent treatment can be postponed for a week or two to allow for haematological recovery.

In case series where AML was diagnosed in the first trimester, many pregnancies were deliberately terminated or resulted in spontaneous abortion [5, 16]. In practice, chemotherapy during pregnancy is an option restricted to the second and third trimesters [5, 16, 17]. In a French series of cases, none of the babies exposed chemotherapy in utero during the second and third trimesters showed any malformations [16]. One case was reported in which the baby showed short digits and limbs as well as macrognathia, allegedly related to its exposure to chemotherapy in utero in the second trimester. Since every pregnancy carries a certain risk of the fetus suffering from developmental problems, notably malformations, it is difficult to establish firm links between exposure to potentially harmful substances and disturbed development in individual cases. Therefore, AML chemotherapy can and often must be initiated during the second or third trimester of pregnancy.

Depending on the stage of pregnancy, and the recovery of bone marrow function after initial treatment, caesarean section may be performed once the mother has obtained haematological remission, and her treatment can subsequently be resumed after her postoperative recovery. It is prudent to avoid periods of chemotherapy-induced cytopenias and infection during delivery [5].

In patients not responding to the initial induction, treatment must be continued with the fetus still in utero, since blast clearance is a prerequisite for normal bone marrow reconstitution. In such women, outcome is worse and delivery often must be postponed until remission is obtained. Ten to fifteen percent of all patients with AML are completely treatment-refractory, with a dismal outcome.

Patients achieving remission need consolidation treatment, which (depending on the AML risk profile) may consist of allogeneic stem cell transplantation with an HLA-identical donor, or high-dose chemotherapy with reinfusion of autologous stem cells harvested at the time of recovery from induction therapy, or intensive chemotherapy. Consolidation treatment can and should be postponed until after delivery.

The outcome and prognosis of AML much depends on patient age. The younger age groups enjoy a better prognosis, and pregnant women obviously belong to this subgroup of AML patients. Forty to fifty percent of patients under 40 years of age may enjoy long-term leukaemia-free survival, and such data have indeed been published for pregnant women with AML [16].

10.5.2 Acute Promyelocytic Leukaemia

Acute promyelocytic leukaemia (APL) is a special subtype of AML with specific clinical and haematological features, and special options for therapy (Table 10.1). Malignant blasts in APL are arrested at the promyelocyte stage of maturation. The molecular hallmark is the translocation t[15;17] (with a few rare variants described in the literature). Its fusion protein includes a part of the retinoic receptor α protein, partly responsible for the myeloid differentiation block. This block can be overcome by pharmacological doses of all-*trans* retinoic acid (ATRA), which has become essential in APL treatment. Induction with ATRA also greatly alleviates the risk of bleeding due to the typical coagulopathy often seen in this leukaemia, which can be rapidly progressive, and hence life-threatening. Retinoids are reportedly teratogenic, and therefore ATRA may not be considered safe in the first trimester (retinoid embryopathy) [19]. However, ATRA has been used in pregnancy as of the third week of gestation, with no malformation or any other teratogenic effects reported. In other cases, however, side effects ranged from fetal cardiac arrhythmias to premature induction of labour]19]. Thus, ATRA can safely be given as of the second trimester of pregnancy, but probably not before. In a single case in which ATRA levels were monitored in umbilical and neonatal serum, no serum levels were detectable [20]. Unfortunately, early hopes that ATRA in APL would obviate the need for intensive chemotherapy have been shattered, and current regimes foresee a combination of ATRA and chemotherapy based on anthracyclines as well as cytarabine which lead to transient, albeit severe, bone marrow damage. The prognosis of APL is on the whole good, with chances of leukaemia-free survival at 5 years in the range of 75% or higher. These treatment principles also apply to pregnant women with this particular leukaemia [21–24]. In pregnancy ATRA-chemo combination therapy can be administered as of the second trimester. If APL is diagnosed late in pregnancy and caesarean section is considered prior to starting anti-leukaemic treatment, haemostasis should be investigated very carefully. It may not be safe to undertake such surgical interventions in untreated maternal APL, since APL-triggered coagulopathy with severe bleeding may start very suddenly. In rare cases the diagnosis of maternal APL became apparent at the time of spontaneous full-term delivery, when the mother developed severe postpartum haemorrhage due to APL-related coagulopathy [25].

10.5.3 Chronic Myelogenous Leukaemia

CML often does not evolve very rapidly at the clinical and haematological levels. In historic series the median survival of patients with untreated CML was in the range of 30 months. Therefore, in pregnant women, careful monitoring of the clinical course may be an option, until a stage of pregnancy is reached at which delivery of the baby is feasible without too much risk for mother and child. In patients presenting with excessive leukocytosis and clinical signs of leukostasis, leukapheresis may be performed [26, 27], followed by systemic treatment. CML has become a paradigm for the success of targeted therapy in oncology. Since the fusion protein generated by the BCR-ABL fusion gene (an oncogenic tyrosine kinase) is the key molecular driving force behind the development and maintenance of the leukaemic clone, its specific blockade by a small molecule, the tyrosine kinase inhibitor imatinib mesylate (Gleevec), has turned out to be very effective. Imatinib mesylate is given orally, with few side effects, and virtually no suppression of normal haematopoiesis (unlike chemotherapy in the acute leukaemias). Imatinib mesylate is therefore the current treatment of choice in patients with CML, including pregnant women [28–33]. Whilst it is considered safe as of the second trimester, its risks in early pregnancy are uncertain. Interestingly, a cohort of women with CML have been reported who were taking imatinib mesylate when they conceived a child [29, 32–34]. In all of these cases exposure to imatinib mesylate had taken place during and after conception for a period of 4–9 weeks, until pregnancy was diagnosed. Imatinib mesylate was stopped in virtually all these pregnancies, and treatment was withheld until later in pregnancy, unless the women opted for therapeutic abortion. About two-thirds of these pregnancies were terminated early, but one-third were allowed to come to term. All but one of the babies born were healthy. One showed malformations (hypospadia). Although these cases might suggest that imatinib mesylate treatment during early pregnancy carries little risk of fetal damage, a decision to continue a pregnancy should be carefully discussed with the woman, since no firm guarantee for the safety of this drug during the first trimester can be given [29]. As the success of modern cancer treatments increases, and since newer targeted anti-cancer treatments (antibodies or small molecules such as imatinib mesylate) may be given over prolonged periods of time, pregnancies under such treatments may increasingly become an issue in young cancer patients.

Over time CML cells may become resistant to imatinib mesylate, but it is unlikely that this problem would occur during the relatively short time of pregnancy. More intensive treatment options such as allogeneic stem cell transplantation are not an issue during pregnancy.

10.5.4 Myelodysplastic Syndromes

Myelodysplastic syndromes (MDS) typically occur in elderly patients and are therefore very rare in pregnant women [35]. The diagnosis should be made by experienced haematologists, since it is not always easy to differentiate patients with refractory anaemia (one possible type of MDS according to the current WHO classification) from those with other types of anaemia or bone marrow dysfunction. The detection of clonal karyotype abnormalities may help greatly; MDS patients show typical chromosomal alterations such as the 5q- syndrome, loss of chromosome 7, or complex abnormalities. It has been suggested that MDS in pregnancy is more likely to evolve into frank AML [36], but the number of cases reported in the literature is too small to draw such conclusions.

Treatment of MDS is somewhat frustrating as there are no drugs which would easily induce a return to normal polyclonal haematopoiesis. Intensive chemotherapy is sometimes an option in younger patients, and its problems are much the same as in AML (see above), whilst the clinical efficacy is unfortunately less. In pregnancy, supportive care with transfusions and therapy of neutropenic infections is a firm recommendation, entailing little risk for the fetus and often allowing obstetricians to await a point in time at which the baby can be delivered by caesarean section [37].

10.6 Lymphoid Neoplasms

10.6.1 Acute Adult Lymphoblastic Leukaemia

Treatment protocols in adult ALL are typically risk-adapted, since ALL are a heterogeneous group of lymphoid leukaemias. In general their prognosis in adults is much less favourable than in children (where the majority of cases can nowadays be cured), and this holds true for pregnant women with these disorders. Philadelphia-positive ALL carries a particularly gloomy prognosis. It is not appropriate to describe the many complicated treatment protocols published for ALL subtypes here, but for pregnant women with ALL, a few rules can be outlined [7, 16]. Classical induction in ALL can be managed by relatively simple combinations of drugs, for example, combining vinca alkaloids and corticosteroids, topped up with anthracyclines [38]. These combinations may therefore be suitable to induce improvement of bone marrow function without too many side effects, and with relatively mild transient myelosuppression, and permit the pregnancy to reach a point at which delivery (mostly via caesarean section) can be envisaged. The more intensive consolidation and maintenance therapies in ALL can in most cases be postponed until after the baby is born. As in all types of oncological therapies, chemotherapy can be given relatively safely as of the second trimester, but not before. In patients with Philadelphia-positive ALL, imatinib mesylate is added to chemotherapy, although its ideal timing is currently unknown.

10.6.2 Hairy Cell Leukaemia

A few cases of hairy cell leukaemia (HCL) diagnosed in pregnancy have been reported [39–41].

HCL is an indolent B-cell neoplasm characterised by pancytopenia (notably monocytopenia) and splenomegaly, and a chronic course. Depending on the severity of pancytopenia, therapy may often be postponed. The standard treatment nowadays consists of purine analogues, for example cladribine, where a single cycle often suffices to induce remission. Safety is a concern in the first trimester, but the few case reports published suggest that in later pregnancy this type of treatment carries an acceptable risk.

10.6.3 Chronic Lymphocytic B-Cell Leukaemia

B-cell CLL is extremely rare in pregnancy. A handful of cases have been described [42–46], and in none of these was any cytostatic treatment necessary until delivery. Patients may need transfusions if anaemic. Autoimmune cytopenias (autoimmune haemolytic anaemia, or immune thrombocytopenia), which are more often seen in CLL than in other types of leukaemia, can be managed with corticosteroids. Although CLL is often marked by excessive leukocytosis, leukapheresis is rarely necessary, since the clinical features of hyperleukocytosis are often absent. Likewise, involvement of placenta or cord blood has not been found despite marked lymphocytosis in the maternal peripheral blood [44].

10.7 Outcome of Children Born to Mothers with Leukaemia Treated During Pregnancy

Leukaemia therapy during pregnancy implies a number of specific risks. Leukaemia as such may imply adverse pregnancy outcome including miscarriage, intrauterine growth retardation, prematurity and fetal death. Treatment of leukaemia imposes additional risks [2, 7]. Therapy in early pregnancy (whether given inadvertently or deliberately) carries a risk of fetal damage, including spontaneous abortion, intrauterine death and malformations [4]. Treatment during the second and third trimesters puts the fetus at risk of early premature birth, intrauterine death and disturbances of intrauterine growth and development. However, an outcome analysis of exposure to anthracyclines in utero indicated that during this period of pregnancy, the risk of fetal death, spontaneous abortion, or prematurity is consistently less than 10% [47]. Exposure to anthracyclines in utero may in rare instances lead to transient fetal heart toxicity, which shortly after birth may present as right ventricular failure, if the transition from fetal to postpartum circulation has not been completed [48, 49]. For these reasons, close monitoring of fetal growth and cardiac function by ultrasound including Doppler studies of fetal haemodynamics and fetal echocardiography is mandatory during chemotherapy [50]. In pregnancy there may be a risk for chemotherapy-induced bone marrow failure of the fetus. However, case reports in which umbilical cord blood samples were monitored during pregnancy failed to demonstrate any significant chemotherapy-induced fetal cytopenias [51, 52]. Nevertheless, if chemotherapy is administered near delivery, the newborn might be neutropenic or thrombocytopenic [16]. If premature delivery is planned by caesarean section, it may be necessary to promote fetal lung maturation with glucocorticoids. In women between 24 and 34 gestational weeks, betamethasone is advisable to induce fetal pulmonary maturation prior to leukemia treatment. If in such cases emergency delivery becomes necessary, for example, because of placental bleeding or infection, severe respiratory distress and intraventricular haemorrhage in the newborn would be prevented. Although women with leukaemia are at increased risk of infection, bolus injections of betamethasone do not unduly exaggerate this risk, and the advantages to the fetus largely overrule any small increase in the risk of maternal infection. After 34 gestational weeks, delivery of the baby might be indicated before starting leukaemia treatment, or after a first treatment course at the point of haematological recovery, because severe complications in the newborn are rare at this gestational age. After birth, breastfeeding should be avoided, if chemotherapy is to be initiated or continued, as significant haematological changes in breastfed newborns from women receiving chemotherapy have been reported.

In later childhood and in adolescence, offspring born to mothers who had received leukaemia treatment during pregnancy may perhaps develop late organ failure or secondary neoplasia

[53]. However, none of the children exposed to anthracyclines in utero were found to exhibit any signs of cardiac dysfunction on echocardiography performed at a median age of 17 years [54, 55]. Full-term children born to leukaemic mothers treated during pregnancy mostly show no long-term complications [5, 53]. However, these encouraging data do not account for the outcome of infants born prematurely or with a low birth weight, which may be much less favourable. Unfortunately, many of the case reports on leukaemia in pregnancy do not provide any such long-term data, and a valid systematic survey is not available in the literature [2].

10.8 Summary

In summary, the management of women diagnosed with leukaemia in pregnancy needs an interdisciplinary approach, including a careful oncological work-up as well as close monitoring of the pregnancy until delivery and beyond [56–58]. Patients with acute leukaemias normally must receive anti-leukaemic treatment at full dosage prior to delivery, except for selected women diagnosed very close to term. Treatment should be avoided in the first trimester. The prognosis of pregnant women with acute leukaemia corresponds to that of an age-matched and diagnosis-matched non-pregnant cohort of patients, provided appropriate treatment is given. If given as of the second trimester, the typical chemotherapy regimes used for acute leukaemias imply acceptable acute toxicities to the fetus, with a somewhat increased risk of premature birth or developmental retardation, but no clear evidence of late sequelae in children and adolescents who were exposed to cytostatic agents whilst in utero. In chronic leukaemias and MDS, treatment may often be delayed until after delivery. In CML targeted therapy with imatinib mesylate is safe as of the second trimester, and possibly even before. Obstetric care and monitoring of women with leukaemia are essential throughout the pregnancy to ensure the best possible outcome for mother and child.

Acknowledgements

Leukaemia research at our institution is supported by the Swiss National Foundation, the Swiss Cancer League (experimental), the Werner and Hedwig Berger-Janser Foundation for Cancer Research (experimental), as well as the Swiss Group for Clinical Cancer Research and the Dutch HOVON group (clinical).

References

1. Bult JA, Heinemann H (1949) [Title not available.] Ned Tijschr Geneeskd 93: 2976–2980
2. Cardonick E, Iacobucci A (2004) Use of chemotherapy during human pregnancy. Lancet Oncol 5: 283–291
3. Pentheroudakis G, Pavlidis N (2006) Cancer and pregnancy: poena magna, not anymore. Eur J Cancer 42: 126–140
4. Dilek I, Topcu N, Demir C et al. (2006) Hematological malignancy and pregnancy: a single-institution experience of 21 cases. Clin Lab Haem 28: 170–176
5. Greenlund L, Letendre L, Tefferi A (2001) Acute leukemia during pregnancy: a single institutional experience with 17 cases. Leuk Lymph 41: 571–577
6. Peleg D, Ben Ami M (1998) Lymphoma and leukaemia complicating pregnancy. Obstet Gynecol Clin North Am 25:365–383
7. Brell J, Kalaycio M (2000) Leukemia in pregnancy. Semin Oncol 27: 667–677
8. Segel GB, Lichtman MA (2004) Familial (inherited) leukemia, lymphoma, and myeloma: an overview. Blood Cells Mol Dis 32: 246–261
9. Song WJ et al. (1999) Haploinsufficiency of CBFA2 causes familial thrombocytopenia with propensity to develop acute myelogenous leukaemia. Nat Genet 23: 166–175
10. Sheikh SS, Mahmoud A, Khalifa et al. (1996) Acute monocytic leukemia (FAB M5) involving the placenta associated with delivery of a healthy infant: case report and discussion. Int J Gyn Pathol 15: 363–366
11. Potter JF, Schoenemann M (1970) Metastasis of maternal cancer to the placenta and fetus. Cancer 25: 380–388

12. Dildy GA, Moise KJ, Carpenter RJ et al. (1989) Maternal malignancy metastatic to the products of conception. A review. Obstet Gyn Surv 44: 535–540
13. Bianchi D, Romero R (2003) Biological implications of bi-directional feto-maternal cell traffic: a summary of a National Institute of Child Health and Human Development-sponsored conference. J Matern Fetal Neonatal Med 14: 123–129
14. Osada S, Horibe K, Oiwa K et al. (1990) A case of infantile acute monocytic leukemia caused by vertical transmission of the mother's leukemic cells. Cancer 65: 1146–1149.
15. Fey MF, Greil R, Jost LM (2005) ESMO Minimum Clinical Recommendations for the diagnosis, treatment and follow-up of acute myeloblastic leukemia (AML) in adult patients. Ann Oncol 16 (Suppl 1): i48–i49
16. Chelghoum Y, Vey N, Raffoux E et al. (2005) Acute leukaemia during pregnancy. Cancer 104: 110–117
17. Niedermeier DM, Frei-Lahr DA, Hall PD (2005) Treatment of acute myeloid leukemia during the second and third trimesters of pregnancy. Pharmacotherapy 25: 1134–1140
18. Ali R, Özkalemkas F, Özçelik T et al. (2003) Maternal and fetal outcomes in pregnancy complicated with acute leukemia: a single institutional experience with 10 pregnancies at 16 years. Leukemia Res 27: 381–385
19. Giagounidis AAN, Beckmann MW, Giagounidis AS et al. (2000) Acute promyelocytic leukemia and pregnancy. Eur J Haematol 64: 267–271
20. Terada Y, Scindo T, Endoh A et al. (1991) Fetal arrhythmia during treatment of pregnancy-associated acute promyelocytic leukemia with all-trans retinoic acid and favorable outcome. J Cell Biochem 46: 302–311
21. Consoli U, Figuera A, Milone G et al. (2004) Acute promyelocytic leukemia during pregnancy: report of 3 cases. Int J Hematol 79: 31–36
22. Lee DD, Park TS, Lee DS et al. (2005) Acute promyelocytic leukemia in late pregnancy with unusual secondary chromosomal change and its prognostic importance. Cancer Gen Cytogen 157: 92–93
23. Fadilah S.A.W, Hatta A.Z., Keng C.S et al. (2001) Successful treatment of acute promyelocytic leukemia in pregnancy with all-trans retinoic acid. Leukemia 15: 1665–1666
24. Carradice D, Austin N, Bayston K et al. (2002) Successful treatment of acute promyelocytic leukaemia during pregnancy. Clin Lab Haem 24: 307–311
25. Murrin RJA, Adjetey V, Harrison P et al. (2004) Acute promyelocytic leukaemia presenting as postpartum haemorrhage. Clin Lab Haem 26: 233–237
26. Bazarbashi MS, Smith MR, Karanes CH et al. (1991) Successful management of Ph chromosome + chronic myelogenous leukemia with leukapheresis during pregnancy. Am J Hematol 38: 235–237
27. Strobl FJ, Voelkerding KV, Smith EP (1999) Management of chronic myeloid leukemia during pregnancy with leukapheresis. J Clin Apheresis 14: 42–44
28. Hensley ML, Ford JM (2003) Imatinib treatment: specific issues related to safety, fertility, and pregnancy. Semin Hematol 40: 21–25
29. Prabhash K, Sastry PSRK, Biswas G et al. (2005) Pregnancy outcome of two patients treated with imatinib. Ann Oncol 16: 1983–1984
30. Ali R, Özkalemkas F, Özçelik T et al. (2005) Pregnancy under treatment of imatinib and successful labor in a patient with chronic myelogenous leukemia (CML) Outcome of discontinuation of imatinib therapy after achieving a molecular remission. Leukemia Res 29: 971–973
31. Heartin E, Walkinshaw S, Clark RE (2004) Successful outcome of pregnancy in chronic myeloid leukaemia treated with imatinib. Leuk Lymphoma 45: 1307–1308
32. Ault P, Kantarjian H, O'Brien S et al. (2006) Pregnancy among patients with chronic myeloid leukemia treated with Imatinib. J Clin Oncol 24: 1204–1208
33. AlKindi S, Dennison D, Pathare A (2005) Imatinib in pregnancy. Eur J Haematol 74: 535–537
34. Reichel RR, Linkesch W, Schetitska D (1992) Therapy with recombinant interferon alpha-2c during unexpected pregnancy in a patient with chronic myeloid leukaemia. Br J Haematol 82: 472–478
35. Steensma DP, Tefferi A (2001) MDS and pregnancy—the Mayo Clinic experience. Leuk Lymph 42: 1229–1234
36. Siddiqui T, Elfenbein GJ, Noyes WD et al. (1990) Myelodysplastic syndromes presenting in pregnancy. A report of five cases and the clinical outcome. Cancer 66: 377–381

37. Ikeda Y, Masuzaki H, Nakayama D et al. (2002) Successful management and perinatal outcome of pregnancy complicated with myelodysplastic syndrome. Leukemia Res 26: 255–260
38. Molkenboer JF, Vos AH, Schouten HC et al. (2005) Acute lymphoblastic leukaemia in pregnancy. Neth J Med 63: 361–363
39. Williams JK (1987) Hairy cell leukemia in pregnancy: a case report. Am J Obstet Gynecol 156: 210–211
40. Baer MR, Ozer H, Foon KA (1992) Interferon-alpha therapy during pregnancy in chronic myelogenous leukaemia and hairy cell leukaemia. Br J Haematol 81: 167–169
41. Alothman A, Sparling T (1994) Managing hairy cell leukaemia in pregnancy. Ann Int Med 120: 1048–1049
42. Ali R, Özkalemkas F, Özkocaman V et al. (2004) Successful labor in the course of chronic lymphocytic leukemia (CLL) and management of CLL during pregnancy with leukapheresis. Ann Hematol 83: 61–63
43. Christomalis L, Baxi LV, Heller D (1996) Chronic lymphocytic leukemia in pregnancy. Am J Obstet Gynecol 175: 1381–1382
44. Gürman G (2002) Pregnancy and successful labor in the course of chronic lymphocytic leukemia. Am J Hematol 71: 208–210
45. Kuroiwa M, Gondo H, Ashida K et al. (1998) Prolymphocytic transformation in chronic lymphocytic leukemia presenting a bilateral periorbital swelling. Am J Hematol 58: 98–102
46. Welsh TM, Thompson J, Lim S (2000) Chronic lymphocytic leukemia in pregnancy. Leukemia 14: 1155
47. Germann N, Goffinet F, Goldwasser F (2004) Anthracyclines during pregnancy: embryo-fetal outcome in 160 patients. Ann Oncol 15: 146–150
48. Achtari C, Hohlfeld P (2000) Cardiotoxic transplacental effect of idarubicin administered during the second trimester of pregnancy. Am J Obstet Gynecol 183: 511–512
49. Siu BL, Alonzo MR, Vargo TA et al. (2002) Transient dilated cardiomyopathy in a newborn exposed to idarubicin and all-*trans*-retinoic acid (ATRA) early in the second trimester of pregnancy. Int J Gynecol Cancer 12: 399–402
50. Meyer-Wittkopf M, Barth H, Emons G, Schmidt S (2001) Fetal cardiac effects of doxorubicin therapy for carcinoma of the breast during pregnancy: case report and review of the literature. Ultrasound Obstet Gynecol 18: 62–66
51. Morishita S, Imai A, Kawabata I et al. (1994) Acute myelogenous leukemia in pregnancy: fetal blood sampling and early effects of chemotherapy. Int J Gynecol Obstet 44: 273–277
52. Murray NA, Acolet D, Deane M et al. (1994) Fetal marrow suppression after maternal chemotherapy for leukaemia. Arch Dis Child 71: F209–F210
53. Reynoso EE, Shepherd FA, Messner HA et al. (1987) Acute leukemia during pregnancy: the Toronto leukemia study group experience with long-term follow-up of children exposed in utero to chemotherapeutic agents. J Clin Oncol 5: 1098–1106
54. Avilés A, Neri N, Nambo MJ (2006) Long-term evaluation of cardiac function in children who received anthracyclines during pregnancy. Ann Oncol 17: 286–288
55. Avilés A, Niz J (1988) Long-term follow-up of children born to mothers with acute leukemia during pregnancy. Med Ped Oncol 16: 3-6
56. Caligiuri MA, Mayer RJ (1989) Pregnancy and leukemia. Semin Oncol 16: 388–396
57. Su WL, Liu JY, Kao WY (2003) Management of pregnancy-associated acute leukemia. Eur J Gyn Oncol 24: 251–254
58. Zuazu J, Julia A, Sierra J et al. (1991) Pregnancy outcome in hematologic malignancies. Cancer 67: 703–709

11 Hodgkin and Non-Hodgkin Lymphomas During Pregnancy

P. Froesch, V. Belisario-Filho, E. Zucca

Recent Results in Cancer Research, Vol. 178

11.1 Epidemiology

Malignant lymphomas are classified into Hodgkin (HL) and non-Hodgkin lymphoma (NHL), which comprise 15%–30% and 70%–85% of all lymphomas, respectively.

HL accounts for less than 1% of all cancers. It is a disease of young adults, with a median age at diagnosis around 20–25 years, but in some countries another peak in the age-specific incidence of HL is described in older adults over 60 years. Although HL represents around 0.5% of all cancers, it is the second most commonly diagnosed cancer in people aged 15–29 years and the seventh most commonly diagnosed cancer in children under 15. The incidence has remained unchanged over the last 20 years, at about 3 per 100,000 males and 2 per 100,000 females [1]. The annually estimated incidence in the United States (US) is around 7,350–7,800 new patients (men and women) [2]. The disease is clinically characterised by painless, enlarged lymph nodes mainly in cervical areas, being detected as early stage in about 60% of cases, according to the modified Ann Arbor classification [3], and it does not seem to be affected by pregnancy, as we discuss below. Systemic symptoms (fever, weight loss, night sweats) can be described in one-third of patients at time of diagnosis. Because of improvements in therapy over the last 30 years, HL is today a highly treatable disease, with long-term survival rates above 80%–90%, especially in younger people [4].

NHLs account for 4%–5% of all cancers in western countries and represent the sixth most frequent tumour in men (after prostate, lung, colon and rectum, bladder and melanoma) and the fifth in women (after breast, lung, colon and rectum and uterine corpus) [5]. In western countries the incidence increased in the last 20 years of the previous century, only partly because of association with HIV infection. The frequency of NHL increases with age and around two-thirds of cases are diagnosed in people over 60 years [6]. However, from the mid-1990s the incidence of NHL in western countries appears somehow stabilised and no longer increasing. According to the American Cancer Society, since 1991 the increase in the incidence of NHL has only been in women, but this is more clearly evident in women older than 50 [7, 8]. Overall, in the US an estimated 71,380 new cases of lymphoma will occur in 2007, including 8,190 cases of HL and 63,190 cases of NHL, with an estimated 19,730 deaths (HL 1070 and NHL 18660 deaths) [9].

In contrast to HL, there is a high variability of clinical presentation and prognosis in patients with NHL; however, only a very few histological subtypes are commonly described in the lymphoma cases arising during pregnancy.

The coexistence of HL or NHL and pregnancy is a rare event, although lymphomas represent the fourth most frequent cancer diagnosis among pregnant women, behind cancers of the breast, cervix and ovary [10]. Taking into account data from the US Census Bureau and the age-adjusted lymphoma incidence statistics from the American Cancer Society, Pohlman et al. estimated that pregnancy-associated lymphoma incidence ranges from 1:1,000 to 1:3,000 deliveries for HL and up to 1:5,000 deliveries for NHL [11]. Despite the rarity of lymphoma in pregnancy, its management is a challenge for physicians. The harmful effects of lymphoma diagnostic and treatment procedures on foetal development and on pregnancy outcome should be taken into account, as well as the fact that lymphomas are most often curable diseases, although they can be rapidly fatal if not properly treated. Hence, best management needs a multidisciplinary approach which is ideally aimed to optimise the mother's chances of cure and yet allow deliver of a healthy child.

11.2 Impact of Pregnancy on HL

For a long time it was believed that HL was exacerbated by pregnancy and that HL itself can adversely affect the course of gestation and delivery. Since 1960, it has become clear that this is not the case; the actual prognosis of HL in pregnant women is similar to that of nonpregnant patients of childbearing age [12]. For instance, some reports found no difference in survival among women who had therapeutic abortion in comparison to those who did not [13–15], and only in a few studies was a higher incidence of advanced cases during pregnancy found [16–18]. In 1984, Gobbi et al. confirmed that survival of 21 pregnant women was comparable to that of 155 non-pregnant patients with HL despite a slightly higher incidence of advanced stage in pregnant patients [16]. The authors speculated that diagnosis may be delayed during pregnancy probably because early signs of HL may mimic pregnancy discomfort (fatigue, vomiting, loss of weight, abdominal pain). Interestingly, Lambe and Ekbom reported in 1995 a greater than expected HL incidence in the 6 months postpartum in a large population-based study from Sweden [18], most likely because the disease is sometimes first diagnosed after delivery.

11.3 Impact of HL on Pregnancy and Foetal Outcome

Maternal cells can reach the foetus; however, vertical transmission of HL from the mother to the product of conception is exceedingly uncommon. Foetal and placental involvement by HL are very rare, and only one case of placenta involvement with delivery of a normal foetus and another case of probable transmission from the mother to the foetus have been reported [13].

There are many studies about maternal and foetal outcome following HL in pregnancy, but there is no consensus on the impact of the disease on gestation course, incidence of spontaneous abortion, prematurity and foetal outcome.

11.3.1 Maternal Effects

Lishner et al. studied the effects of HL on the course and survival of 48 women who had HL and who were pregnant and compared their outcome with non-pregnant matched controls of similar disease stage and age at diagnosis and treatment in the same epoch [19]. Twenty-year survival of pregnant women with HL was not different from that of their matched controls [19].

11.3.2 Foetal Effects

Ebert et al. [20] identified 24 cases in the literature between 1983 and 1995 of women who received chemotherapy during pregnancy. Two women had spontaneous abortions after chemotherapy (MOPP, vinblastine and procarbazine) beginning in the first trimester; one foetus had multiple anomalies. Three women had therapeutic abortions; all received chemotherapy in the first trimester (MOPP, MOP, ABVD or cyclophosphamide plus radiotherapy in 1), and all three foetuses had multiple anomalies. One woman received MOPP during the first trimester, and the child was born with hydrocephalus and died 4 hours after birth. Another mother received single-agent cyclophosphamide beginning in the first trimester, and the infant was born with multiple anomalies, like the child of another woman who received vinblastine, vincristine and procarbazine beginning in gestational week 25 and died 2 days after delivery with atrial septum defect.

In contrast, 15 infants of mothers receiving chemotherapy (7 ABVD, 4 MOPP, 1 COPP, 3 MOPP/ABVD), 5 in the first trimester, were normal and remained healthy for a median of 9 (range 0–17) years after delivery [20].

In the retrospective study (median follow-up 18 years) of Aviles and Neri all 84 children who received chemotherapy in utero because of haematological malignancy of the mothers (including 26 women with HD treated with ABVD, ABD, EBVD or MOPP, 10 of them during first trimester) were born healthy and had normal growth without haematological, cardiac, renal, hepatic, neurological or psychological abnormalities [21].

Recently, Cardonick and Iacobucci wrote a review on the safety and efficacy of chemotherapeutic regimens in pregnancy by disease and trimester of exposure [22]. The ABVD regimen used for the 18 cases of HD was reported to be safe. Dacarbazine is the drug in the ABVD regimen with the least investigated safety profile in pregnancy, and some authors suggest omitting it because of the scarcity of studies [23]. However, the only patient in the series of Cardonick and Iacobucci with advanced-stage Hodgkin disease who was treated with ABVD without dacarbazine had recurrent disease within 1 year of delivery [22].

11.4 Impact of Pregnancy on NHL

Most women with non-Hodgkin Lymphoma (NHL) in association with pregnancy have an aggressive histological subtype and a disseminated disease, often with extra-nodal involvement at diagnosis; approximately two-thirds of cases present with stage IV disease [24, 25]. This may reflect the biology of lymphoma in young women of childbearing age, or may it be due to a delay in diagnosis and /or fear of radiological investigation during pregnancy.

The impact of pregnancy on lymphoma growth is unclear. During pregnancy the hormonal and increased blood flow changes may contribute to disseminate highly aggressive diseases (e.g. Burkitt lymphomas), with high incidence of breast, uterine and ovarian involvement. On the other hand, hormonal and immunologic changes occurring during pregnancy could stabilise the lymphoma's proliferation until delivery.

Years ago, a poor outcome was common because patients were not treated properly. For instance, in 1989 Ward and Weiss reported a series of 42 patients with only 13 survivors, but only 6 received multi-agent chemotherapy, 14 received a single agent and 22 received no treatment [26]. In another retrospective review of 96 patients, 47 died at a median of 6 months post-delivery [11]. In addition, as reported by Moore and Taslimi in 1992, delayed diagnosis in pregnant patients is frequent: From the 37 patients considered, 40% were diagnosed with more than 3 weeks' and 20% with even more than 3 months' delay [25].

In fact, if modern treatments were applied early in the course of the disease, responses and progression rates would be quite similar to those of non-pregnant women [23].

Although exceedingly rare, the haematogenous dissemination of leukemias and lymphomas to the placenta and foetus has been described as the second most common type of neoplasm involving the products of conception (placenta and foetus), with 11 documented cases among the 58 reported from 1866 to 1999 [10]. It is difficult to understand how the allogeneic foetus thrives and does not promote an immune rejection. One possibility is that the mother is homozygous for one of the foetus's HLA haplotypes (and in this situation the foetus would not recognise as foreign the major histocompatibility complex antigens on the mother's lymphoma cells). Another explanation is that maternal lymphoma cells might pass to the foetus early in gestation, when the foetus is immunologically immature. A third possibility is the presence of a congenital immunodeficiency [27]. The five cases with placental involvement by NHL published in the 1990s had very aggressive histological subtypes, and three of them were of T/NK cell origin. Only in one case (NK cell lymphoma) the maternal NHL dissemination involved the foetus [27].

11.5 Impact of NHL on Pregnancy and Foetal Outcome

In the study of Aviles and Neri all 29 mothers with diagnosis of NHL during pregnancy between 1970 and 1995 who received CHOP or a CHOP-like regimen (17 during first trimester) delivered babies without congenital malformations [21]. The birth weight, learning and educational performance were normal, and no congenital, neurological or psychological abnormalities were observed [21]. Similarly, Cardonick and Iacobucci reviewed 35 patients with non-Hodgkin lymphoma who were treated during pregnancy with multiple regimens, most of which included doxorubicin, cyclophosphamide and vincristine, and no malformations occurred, even with first-trimester treatment in 11 cases [22].

11.6 Management of Lymphoma in Pregnancy: General Considerations

The most common histologic subtypes during pregnancy are HL and aggressive NHL (diffuse large B cell and Burkitt). In women of childbearing age these conditions are most often curable. The management and the treatment must be individualised, and a multidisciplinary approach is needed. Whenever possible, treatment should be delayed until the end of the first trimester. A multi-disciplinary approach is mandatory and should involve a haemato-oncologist, a radiation oncologist, an obstetrician, a neonatologist, a paediatrician and a mental health professional. Treatment may be delayed in women with an indolent NHL until after delivery. Early delivery, when feasible, may minimise or avoid exposure to chemotherapy or radiation therapy.

Most common histological NHL subtypes during pregnancy are aggressive, and the delay of therapy until delivery appears to result in poor outcomes [26, 28, 29]. Consequently, many investigators favour immediate therapy despite pregnancy [30], but pregnancy termination in the first trimester might be an option to allow proper therapy for women with aggressive NHL [31, 25, 32].

11.7 Staging of Lymphoma During Pregnancy

Lymphoma staging in pregnancy must always include a history, a physical examination with routine blood tests, bone marrow biopsy and/or lumbar puncture.

The effects of ionising radiation on the embryo or foetus depend on the radiation dose and the gestational age at the time of exposure. Effects of ionising radiation on the embryo or foetus include miscarriage, foetal growth restriction, congenital malformation, mental retardation and increased cancer risk. This should be taken into account when planning the staging procedures in a pregnant woman with lymphoma. In general, radiation-induced health effects are not detectable for foetal doses below 50 mGy (= 5 rad). The estimated foetal doses during some common diagnostic imaging studies are reported in Table 11.1 [33, 34]. For non-ionising imaging modalities, there are at present no confirmed biologic effects associated with diagnostic ultrasound at standard power levels and there are no known risks to the foetus from an MR examination. In conclusion, chest X-ray (with adequate abdominal shielding) may be used. Abdominal ultrasound may identify gross disease in the abdomen or pelvis. Magnetic resonance imaging (without gadolinium) is the preferred tool for staging evaluation to avoid exposure to ionising radiation [35]. Tomographic and isotope scans (gallium scanning, PET scan, bone scan) are usually contraindicated. Echocardiography may be used to assess left ventricular function.

Table 11.1 Imaging procedures and associated average uterine/foetal doses

Procedure	Uterine/foetal dose (mGy)
Chest X-ray	0.0007–0.005
Pelvic-lumbar spine X-ray	0.45–3.6
Mammogram	0.2–4
Chest CT scan*	<1
Abdominal-pelvic CT scan*	18–26
Intravenous urography	14–45
Barium enema	36–40
99mTc-MDP bone scan	1.8–5

*10 slices with slice thickness = 10mm. Derived from Toppenberg et al. 1999 [33] and Pentheroudakis and Pavlidis 2006 [34]

11.8 Outline of Lymphoma Treatment Effects on Pregnancy

Standard treatments for HL and NHL comprise radiotherapy and chemotherapy (together with anti CD-20 monoclonal antibodies for B cell neoplasms). Recent reviews have addressed in detail the problems posed by radiotherapy and chemotherapy during pregnancy [22, 36]; here we just summarise the main issues related to lymphoma therapy.

11.8.1 Radiotherapy

The adverse effects of radiotherapy during pregnancy are well described, mainly in the critical phase of organogenesis. High incidence of developmental malformations and increased risk of lethality or intrauterine growth restriction are seen even with low doses of radiotherapy during these phases [37, 38]. However, with careful planning and supplemental shielding, radiotherapy can be a treatment option for specific tumours during pregnancy, with minimum risks to the foetus [36]. In pregnancy most cancers that are remote from the pelvis can be safely treated with radiotherapy. The effectiveness of radiotherapy during pregnancy in the treatment of supradiaphragmatic lymphoma lesions has been reported by many investigators [39]. Hodgkin disease most commonly presents as supradiaphragmatic lymphadenopathy. Patients with HL stage I and II are treated mainly with polychemotherapy followed by radiotherapy given only to the originally involved sites (involved-field radiotherapy). Termination of pregnancy is the individual's decision, and for foetal doses of less than 200 mGy in clinical practice there is no medical justification for termination (increased risk for foetal malformations begins at 100–150 mGy and is very high at 2,500 mGy) [10]. Foetal doses in excess of 200 mGy are rare for cancers which are remote from the pelvis and for which proper shielding has been applied.

11.8.2 Chemotherapy

Data regarding long-term effects on children in uterus exposed to most chemotherapeutic agents are incomplete. The toxic effects of chemotherapy depend on the timing of exposure, the dose and the characteristics of the drug to cross the placental barrier and affect the foetus. Generally, chemotherapy during the first 2 weeks after conception causes spontaneous abortion; from the 2nd to the 8th week of gestation (organogenesis) there is a high probability of congenital malformations and after the 3rd month an increased risk of growth retardation and low birth weight.

Bleomycin, doxorubicin, daunorubicin, vinblastine and vincristine have not been reported to cause adverse foetal outcome, whereas antimetabolites (methotrexate) and alkylating agents (cyclophosphamide), an integral part of regimens for treatment of NHL, should be avoided during the first trimester because of their properties of rapidly crossing the placenta and then carrying a high risk of malformations (absent toes, eye abnormalities, low-set ears, cleft palate).

During the second and third trimesters safe use of alkylating agents has been reported, with the exception of dacarbazine, which was not sufficiently investigated [22].

11.9 Treatment of HL in Pregnancy

HL has become one of the most curable human cancers, and overall about 80% of patients experience long-term disease-free survival. Therefore, current treatment strategies aim at further improving treatment outcome, while trying to minimise therapy-induced complications, such as infertility, cardiopulmonary toxicity and secondary malignancies. ABVD [doxorubicin (Adriamycin), bleomycin, vinblastine, and dacarbazine] [40] remains in most countries the standard therapy for patients with advanced HL, with eight cycles being the standard in Europe. Standard- or increased-dose BEACOPP (the latter known as BEACOPP-escalated, containing bleomycin, etoposide, doxorubicin, cyclophosphamide, vincristine, procarbazine, prednisone) [41] and Stanford V [42] are other commonly used treatments. Increased-dose BEACOPP may be particularly useful in patients with high-risk disease. However, increased-dose BEACOPP treatment is associated with higher rates of toxicity, including infertility and a higher risk of MDS/AML when compared to ABVD, and it is not the best choice if the patient wants to safely conclude her pregnancy.

The management of HL during pregnancy has been based on reports sometimes controversial about successful use of a variety of different therapies (Table 11.2). Furthermore, several controversies, for example about therapeutic abortion and better treatment for subdiaphragmatic or clinically advanced disease, still remain.

11.9.1 HL treatment During First Trimester

Therapeutic abortion must usually be avoided and is not justified except in inadvertent foetal exposure to teratogenic chemotherapeutic agents or to >10 cGy RT during the first 10 weeks. In case of low-intermediate risk (stage I–IIB) it should be delayed until the end of the first trimester.

If this is not possible a watch-and-wait approach until the second trimester, because of progressive disease or high-risk patients (bulky disease, B symptoms, visceral involvement, subdiaphragmatic disease), of vinblastine alone or ABVD without dacarbazine may be used (mechlorethamine, vincristine, procarbazine, prednisone).

11.9.2 HL treatment During Second and Third Trimesters

In localised or stable disease, treatment must be delayed as long as possible. In advanced cases with bulky disease, B symptoms, visceral involvement and/or subdiaphragmatic disease and rapid disease progression, ABVD (without dacarbazine) is the standard regimen because it is less toxic for the foetus while still maintaining a very good efficacy compared to other regimens. On the other hand, RT must normally be postponed after delivery except for localised low-dose irradiation (20 Gy) with proper shielding in stage I non-bulky supradiaphragmatic disease.

Table 11.2 Treatment recommendation for Hodgkin lymphoma during pregnancy

	Jacobs, 1981 [13]	Ward, 1989 [26]	Sutcliffe, 1986 [43]	Dhedin, 1993 [24]	Pohlman, 2000 [44]	Pereg, 2007 [53]
First trimester	TAB	Watch and wait if SD	TAB or no treatment until 2nd trimester	If possible, watch and wait, TAB in case of symptomatic disease	Wait until 2nd trimester	RT with abdominal shelding for stage I supradiaphragmatic
	IFRT for stage IA non-bulky (neck or axilla)	TAB for symptomatic and bulky disease. CT if abortion refused or PD (vinblastine alone)		if CT: vinblastine alone	TAB for symptomatic PD if CT: vinblastine alone or ABV	TAB for high risk/ advanced stage Wait until 2nd trimester or treat with single-agent if low risk / early stage
Second and third trimesters	- Stages I and II, watch and wait until delivery	Watch and wait if SD	CT for all patients	Watch and wait for localised disease until delivery	If possible, wait for delivery without therapy	ABVD
	- Stages III and IV, symptomatic, vinblastine alone, or, MOPP	Therapy for PD (vinblastine alone or combination CT)		ABV or CHOP-like for progressive disease	ABVD	Delay delivery to non-cytopenic period

TAB, therapeutic abortion; *IFRT*, involved field radiotherapy; *SD*, stable disease; *PD*, progressive disease; *CT*, chemotherapy; RT, radiotherapy

11.10 Treatment of NHL in Pregnancy

Many considerations presented above about HL obviously apply to the treatment of NHL in pregnant women.

11.10.1 Indolent NHL

Generally patients with indolent lymphoma can be just observed (wait and see) until after or at least until the end of first trimester, when appropriate treatment can be instituted.

11.10.2 Aggressive NHL

This group is represented by diffuse large B cell lymphomas (DLBCL), which comprise around 31% of all lymphomas, Burkitt and lymphoblastic lymphomas. Treatment should be based on the identified prognostic factors, according to the International Prognostic Index (IPI) [45]. Patients with early-stage disease (stage I or II non-bulky without adverse prognostic factors) have much better outcomes than those with advanced-stage disease. CHOP (cyclophosphamide, doxorubicin, vincristine, prednisone) has for long time been the standard treatment for NHL. Current standard practice is represented by a chemo-immunotherapy approach with CHOP in combination with the anti-CD20 monoclonal antibody, Rituximab (R-CHOP). This combination has been associated with higher response rates and prolonged overall survival for young and old patients [46, 47]. The therapy of early-stage disease usually consists of three cycles of R-CHOP followed by loco-regional RT. Alternatively, six to eight cycles of R-CHOP without RT may be an equally valid alternative [46].

For advanced-stage disease, although more complex regimens have been proposed, a significant treatment advantage over CHOP was not found. Increased dose CHOP-like regimens, shortening of the interval between courses to 2 weeks and combination with Rituximab have changed the modern therapeutic options. In general, the R-CHOP regimen given every 21 days is the current standard.

Most NHLs complicating pregnancy are aggressive and disseminated. Aggressive histology inevitably results in poor maternal outcome if proper treatment is not given as early as possible. Although prognosis had been reported to be poor, there is recent evidence to suggest that, when properly treated, pregnancy does not affect the course of lymphoma. The risk to the foetus can also be reduced by an appropriate therapeutic approach. A few recommendations are available [22, 24, 44], mostly derived from experiences of the pre-Rituximab era (Table 11.3).

Table 11.3 Treatment recommendation for aggressive non-Hodgkin' lymphoma during pregnancy

	Ward, 1989 [26]	Dhedin, 1998 [24]	Pohlman 2000 [44]	Pereg, 2007 [53]
First trimester	TAB during the first 8–12 weeks, followed by CT	TAB and systemic CT	TAB and systemic CT	TAB and standard CT
	IFRT for patients who refuse abortion	IFRT for selected cases stage IA	IFRT for selected cases stage IA	Short treatment delay for selected cases diagnosed near the end of first trimester
Second and third trimesters	Combination chemotherapy when early delivery is not possible	Full-dose chemotherapy	Full-dose chemotherapy (CHOP)	IFRT for selected cases stage IA
			High-dose CT for Burkitt' and lymphoblastic lymphoma	Full-dose standard chemotherapy

TAB, therapeutic abortion; *CT*, chemotherapy; *IFRT*, involved- field radiotherapy

11.10.3 NHL Treatment During First Trimester

During the first trimester the approach should be based on disease stage. In women with stage IA disease, an involved irradiation with proper shielding could be proposed, or a "watch and wait" attitude until the second trimester. In advanced-stage disease, therapeutic abortion must be discussed, to allow immediate initiation of a multidrug regimen. When therapeutic abortion is refused, a decision regarding treatment must be made which balances the prognosis of the mother and the hazard to the foetus.

11.10.4 NHL Treatment During Second and Third Trimesters

During the second and third trimesters the recommendations are to treat with full doses of the multidrug CHOP regimen. In the third trimester, if close to delivery, consider delivery before therapeutic intervention if foetal maturity has been established.

For localised disease Pohlman and Macklis [44] recommend three to eight cycles of CHOP, followed by involved-field radiotherapy (delayed until after delivery but no more than 9 weeks after the last cycle of chemotherapy). According to the GELA Group, radiotherapy is not indicated in the treatment [23].

CHOP is thought to be safe during the second and third trimesters of pregnancy. Data about R-CHOP are, however, quite scarce. Rituximab is a humanised IgG that passes the placental barrier and may interact with foetal B cells. Thus far, only a few case reports have been published on its use during pregnancy, all with short-term information regarding the clinical and immunological follow-up. In general, it seems that Rituximab can be safely given in pregnant women. Herold et al. [48] report a case of a 29-year-old pregnant woman with DLCL (CD20+), stage IIA bulky, treated with four R-CHOP cycles (full dose, without cyclophosphamide) in the second trimester. The patient achieved a very good partial remission and delivered a healthy girl. After delivery, two more cycles were given with complete remission. The child had a normal development, with a normal B cell population at 4 months.

Kimby et al. [49] report the case of a 37-year-old pregnant woman with relapsed indolent follicular NHL who was treated with Rituximab (unintentionally) during the first trimester. The treatment stabilised the disease. After an uncomplicated pregnancy, a healthy child was delivered and careful haematological and immunological monitoring revealed no adverse effects resulting from exposure to Rituximab. Friedrichs et al. [50] reported a case of a 35-year-old woman with Burkitt lymphoma who was treated with Rituximab and CHOP therapy early during pregnancy. Monitoring of Rituximab concentrations and B-cell counts in the child revealed a transient complete B-cell depletion associated with high Rituximab cord blood concentrations. B-cell recovery was fast, showing a regular immunophenotype without loss of CD20 antigen, no functional deficits and adequate vaccination IgG titer.

Decker et al. [51] reported a case of a 31-year-old woman who was diagnosed with a stage IIA diffuse large B-cell NHL (IPI low risk) at 15 weeks gestation. MRI showed an enlarged mediastinum and enlarged left supraclavicular nodes. The patient was given six cycles of R-CHOP-14. A complete response confirmed by MRI was achieved after the second cycle of treatment. In the 33rd week of pregnancy, the patient spontaneously delivered a healthy baby girl. The child's B cells were severely diminished (1% of normal) at birth but started to recover 6 weeks later, reaching the normal range after 12 weeks.

Very aggressive histological types (Burkitt lymphoma and lymphoblastic lymphoma) usually need a more aggressive therapeutic approach than R-CHOP and are best treated with high-intensity chemotherapy regimens including HD-MTX, which cannot be safely administered in pregnancy. The decision about treatment in these cases, especially if diagnosed during the first trimester, will necessarily involve a discussion of therapeutic abortion, and any treatment decision must be personalised, balancing the prognosis of the mother and the hazard to the foetus. No general guidelines can therefore be provided.

11.11 Conclusions

Although rare, HL and NHL during pregnancy require special consideration. It is a difficult situation in which the physicians need to provide the best approach to optimise the outcome for both mother and baby. Multidisciplinary care should always involve the mother, the foetus, and the family during the pregnancy, and long-term strict follow-up is advisable. In general, if possible, chemotherapy should be avoided during the first trimester, and whenever possible the pregnancy should be carried to term. Therapeutic abortion represents a complex issue with religious, ethical, psychological, social and cultural implications, which could not be addressed in this chapter. It does not appear to change the evolution of the disease and should be strictly reserved only for women who need urgent intervention. In fact, the published case reports with both maternal and foetal outcome support a pregnancy-conserving approach [52]. It is, however, likely that the use of therapeutic abortion is underreported. When treatment is necessary, mainly in the second and third trimesters, full doses of a properly chosen chemotherapy regimen can be administered, with curative intent. This rarely seems to carry consequences for the foetus. The same seems to be true for Rituximab with, however, still limited clinical experience. Radiotherapy should be delayed until delivery or, in selected cases, can be used with appropriate shielding to reduce the foetal exposure. Moreover, some authors suggest storing cord blood as a source of HLA-compatible stem cells that can be valuable for future therapy [52]. With the current management approach, most pregnant women with lymphoma can successfully carry the foetus to term and be successfully cured as well, often without fertility impairment.

References

1. UK Hodgkin's Lymphoma incidence statistics. Retrieved 13 Mar.2007, from http://info.cancerresearchuk.org/cancerstats/types/hodgkinslymphoma/incidence/
2. Jemal A, Murray T, Ward E, et al. (2005) CA Cancer J Clin 55(1): 10–30
3. Lister TA, Crowther D, Sutcliffe SB, Glatstein E, Canellos GP, Young RC, Rosenberg SA, Coltman CA, Tubiana M (1989) Report of a committee convened to discuss the evaluation and staging of patients with Hodgkin's disease: Cotswolds meeting. J Clin Oncol 7(11): 1630–1636
4. Draube A, Behringer K, Diehl V (2006) German Hodgkin's Lymphoma Study Group Trials: Lessons from the Past and Current Strategies. Clin Lymphoma Myeloma 6: 458–468
5. Jemal A, Siegel R, Ward E, Murray T, Xu J, Thun MJ (2007) Cancer statistics, 2007. CA Cancer J Clin 57: 43–66
6. Jost LM, Kloke O, Stahel RA (2005) ESMO Minimum Clinical Recommendations for diagnosis, treatment and follow-up of newly diagnosed large cell non-Hodgkin's lymphoma. Ann Oncol 16 Suppl 1: i58–i59
7. American Cancer Society (2007) Detailed Guide: Lymphoma, Non-Hodgkin's type: What Are the Key Statistics About Non-Hodgkin Lymphoma? Retrieved 13 Mar.2007, from http://www.cancer.org/docroot/CRI/content/CRI
8. SEER Fast Stats Results (2006) Trends (APC) of SEER Incidence Rates by Sex For Non-Hodgkin Lymphoma, Ages 50+, All Races SEER 13 Registries for 1994–2003 and 1999–2003 Age-Adjusted to the 2000 US STD Population. Retrieved 13 Mar 2007, from http://canques.seer.cancer.gov/cgibin/
9. American Cancer Society (2007) Cancer Facts & Figures 2007. Atlanta, American Cancer Society. Retrieved 13 Mar 2007, from http://www.cancer.org (http://www.cancer.org/downloads/STT/CAFF2007PWSecured.pdf)
10. Pavlidis NA (2002) Coexistence of pregnancy and malignancy. Oncologist 7: 279–287
11. Pohlman B, Lyons JA, Macklis RM (1999) Lymphoma in pregnancy. In: Trimble EL, Trimble CL, eds. Cancer Obstetrics and Gynecology. Philadelphia: Lippincott Williams & Wilkins, pp. 202–238
12. Barry RM, Diamond HD, Craver LF (1962) Influence of pregnancy in the course of Hodgkin's disease. Am J Obstet Gynecol 84: 445–454
13. Jacobs C, Donaldson SS, Rosenberg SA, et al. (1981) Management of the pregnant patient with Hodgkin's disease. Ann Intern Med 95: 669–675
14. Tawil E, Mercier JP, Dandavino A (1985) Hodgkin's disease complicating pregnancy. J Can Assoc Radiol 46: 133–137

15. Nisce LZ, Tome MA, He S, et al. (1986) Management of coexisting Hodgkin's disease and pregnancy. Am J Clin Oncol 9: 146–151
16. Gobbi PG, Attardo-Parrinello A, Danesino M, et al. (1984) Hodgkin's disease and pregnancy. Haematologica 69: 336–341
17. Jouet JP, Buchet-Bouverne B, Fenaux P, et al. (1988) Influence de la grossess sur le développement de la maladie de Hodgkin. Presse Med 17: 423–427
18. Lambe M, Ekbom A (1995) Cancers coinciding with childbearing: delayed diagnosis during pregnancy? BMJ 311: 1607–1608
19. Lishner M, Zemlickis D, Sutcliffe SB, et al. (1994) Non-Hodgkin's lymphoma and pregnancy. Leuk Lymphoma 14: 411–413
20. Ebert U, Loffler H, Kirch W (1997) Cytotoxic therapy and pregnancy. Pharmacol Ther 74: 207
21. Aviles A, Neri N (2001) Hematological malignancies and pregnancy: a final report of 84 children who received chemotherapy in utero. Clinical Lymphoma 2: 173–177
22. Carbonick E, Iacobucci A (2004) Use of chemotherapy during human pregnancy. Lancet Oncol 5: 283–291
23. Traullé C, Coiffier B (2006) Lymphoma and pregnancy. In: Canellos GP, Lister TA, Young B, eds The Lymphomas, second edition. Philadelphia: Saunders Elsevier, pp. 536–541
24. Dhedin N, Coiffier B (1993) Lymphoma and pregnancy. In: Canellos GP, Lister TA, Young B, eds. The Lymphomas. New York: Elsevier, pp. 549–556
25. Moore DT, Talismi MM (1992) Non-Hodgkin's lymphoma in pregnancy: a diagnostic dilemma. Case report and review of the literature. J Tenn Med Assoc 85: 467–469
26. Ward FT, Weiss RB (1989) Lymphoma and pregnancy. Semin Oncol 16: 397
27. Catlin EA, Roberts JD, Erana R, et al. (1999) Transplacental transmission of natural-killer-cell lymphoma. N Engl J Med 341: 85–91
28. Steiner-Salz D, Yahalom J, Samuelov A, Polliack A (1985) Non-Hodgkin's lymphoma associated with pregnancy: a report of six cases, with a review of the literature. Cancer 56: 2087
29. Spitzer M, Citron M, Ilardi CF, Saxe B (1991) Non-Hodgkin's lymphoma during pregnancy. Gynecol Oncol 43: 309
30. Gelb AB, Vanderijn M, Warnke RA, et al. (1996) Pregnancy associated lymphomas. A clinicopathologic study. Cancer 78: 304–310
31. Aviles A, Diaz-Maqueo JC, Torras V, Garcia EL, Guzman R (1990) Non-Hodgkin's lymphomas and pregnancy: presentation of 16 cases. Gynecol Oncol 37: 335
32. Nantel S, Parbbosingh J, Poon MC (1990) Treatment of an aggressive non-Hodgkin's lymphoma during pregnancy with MACOP-B chemotherapy. Med Pediatr Oncol 18: 143
33. Toppenberg KS, Hill DA, Miller DP (1999) Safety of radiographic imaging during pregnancy. Am Fam Physician 59: 1813–1818
34. Pentheroudakis G, Pavlidis N (2006) Cancer and pregnancy: poena magna, not anymore. Eur J Cancer 42: 126–140
35. Nicklas AH, Baker ME (2000) Imaging strategies in the pregnant cancer patient. Semin Oncol 27: 623–632
36. Kal HB, Struikmans H (2005) Radiotherapy during pregnancy: fact and fiction. Lancet Oncol 6: 328–333
37. Hall EJ (1994) Radiobiology for the radiologist, 4th ed. Philadelphia: JB Lippincott
38. Rugh R (1962) Low levels of x-irradiation and the early mammalian embryo. Am J Roentgenol 87: 559
39. Portlock CS, Yaholomon J (1999) The management of Hodgkin's Disese during Pregnancy. In Mauch PM, Armitage JO, Diehl V, Hoppe RT, and Weiss LM, eds. Hodgkin's Disease. Lippincott Williams & Wilkins, Philadelphia, Chapter 38
40. Bonadonna G, Valagussa P, Santoro A (1986) Alternating non-cross-resistant combination chemotherapy or MOPP in stage IV Hodgkin's disease. Ann Intern Med 104: 739–746
41. Diehl V, Sieber M, Ruffer U, et al. (1997) BEACOPP: an intensified chemotherapy regimen in advanced Hodgkin's disease. Ann Oncol 8: 143–148
42. Bartlett NL, Rosenberg SA, Hoppe RT, et al. (1995) Brief chemotherapy, Stanford V, and adjuvant radiotherapy for bulky or advanced-stage Hodgkin's disease: a preliminary report. J Clin Oncol 13: 1080–1088
43. Sutcliffe SB, Chapman RM (1986) Lymphomas and leukemias, in Allen HH, Nisker JA (eds): Cancer in pregnancy. Mt. Kisco, NY, Futura, pp. 135–189
44. Pohlman B, Macklis RM (2000) Lymphoma and pregnancy. Semin Oncol 27: 657–666

45. The International Non-Hodgkin's Lymphoma Prognostic Factors Project (1993) A predictive model for aggressive non-Hodgkin's lymphoma. N Engl J Med 329: 987–994
46. Pfreundschuh M, Trumper L, Osterborg A, et al. (2006) CHOP-like chemotherapy plus rituximab versus CHOP-like chemotherapy alone in young patients with good-prognosis diffuse large-B-cell lymphoma: a randomised controlled trial by the MabThera International Trial (MInT) Group. Lancet Oncol 7: 379–391
47. Coiffier B, Lepage E, Briere J, et al. (2002) CHOP chemotherapy plus rituximab compared with CHOP alone in elderly patients with diffuse large-B-cell lymphoma. N Engl J Med 346: 235–242
48. Herold M, Schnohr S, Bittrich H (2001) Efficacy and safety of a combined rituximab chemotherapy during pregnancy. J Clin Oncol 19: 3439
49. Kimby E, Sverrisdottir A, Elinder G (2004) Safety of rituximab therapy during the first trimester of pregnancy: a case history. Eur J Haematol 72(4): 292–295
50. Friedrichs B, Tieman M, Salwender H, et al. (2006) The effects of rituximab treatment during pregnancy on a neonate. Haematologica 91(10): 1426–1427
51. Decker M, Rothermundt C, Hollander G, et al. (2006) Rituximab plus CHOP for treatment of diffuse large B-cell lymphoma during second trimester of pregnancy. Lancet Oncol 7(8): 693–694
52. Habermann TM, Witzig TE (2003) Management of lymphoma during pregnancy. In Mauch PM, Armitage JO, Coiffier B, Dalla Favera R, and Harris HL, eds. Non-Hodgkin's Lymphomas. Lippincott Williams & Wilkins, Philadelphia, Chapter 38
53. Pereg D, Koren G, Lishner M (2003) The treatment of Hodgkin's and non-Hodgkin's lymphoma in pregnancy. Haematologica 92 (8): 1230-1237

12 Pregnancy and Thyroid Cancer

B. Gibelli, P. Zamperini, N. Tradati

Recent Results in Cancer Research, Vol. 178

12.1 Introduction

Thyroid cancer is the most common endocrine malignancy. More frequently diagnosed in women, it is a disease often detected in young patients. Therefore, about 10% of thyroid cancers occurring during the reproductive years are diagnosed during pregnancy or in the early postpartum period.

Thyroid cancer during pregnancy causes considerable anxiety about the optimal timing of recommended treatments and about both maternal and neonatal morbidity. However, thyroid cancer in young people generally has an excellent prognosis, and survival among women with thyroid cancer diagnosed during pregnancy may not differ from that in age-matched non-pregnant women with similar cancer.

Pregnancy faced after a carcinoma of the thyroid gland obviously needs both maternal and foetal controls. The main problems are: (1) to reach an adequate balance of maternal thyroid hormones which is absolutely required by the foetal central nervous system for a normal maturation, (2) to maintain the maternal levels of l-thyroxine in order to avoid possible recurrence or spread of the disease, and (3) to perform safe follow-up controls for the mother and plan further therapy when needed.

12.2 Maternal and Foetal Thyroid Physiology

The thyroid gland is the first endocrine gland to appear in embryonic development. At 10–12 weeks of embryo development, follicles containing colloid become visible, and the thyroid is able to incorporate iodine into thyroid hormones. The ultimobranchial body, arising from the inferior part of the fourth pharyngeal pouch, supplies follicular cells and C cells (parafollicular cells) to the lateral lobes of the thyroid, and the thyroglossal duct derives from the thyroid diverticulum. The post-embryonic persisting remnants of the ultimobranchial body and thyroid diverticulum, such as thyroglossal duct cysts and lingual thyroids, have for a long time been suspected to be rich in stem cells, contributing to both follicular cells and C cell tumours (Santisteban 2005).

Thyroid hormones are major factors for the normal development of the foetal brain, and until the end of the first trimester, when the hypothalamic-pituitary-thyroid axis becomes functional, the foetal brain is strictly dependent on local deiodination of maternal thyroxine (Pop et al. 2003; Morreale de Escobar et al. 2000; Glinoer et al. 2003; Shah et al. 2003; Alexander et al. 2004). Thyroid hormone deficiency may cause severe neurologic disorders, resulting from defects in neuronal cell differentiation and migration, axonal and dendritic outgrowth, myelin formation and synaptogenesis. The offspring of women with serum free thyroxine (fT4) concentration in the lowest decile of the reference range at 12 weeks of gestation may have significant delays in neurodevelopment. The mother is the sole source of the foetal supply of thyroid hormones from conception to approximately 13 weeks of gestation, when foetal thyroid function has developed. (Lazarus 2005; Lao 2005; Obregon et al. 1998).

Hypothyroidism must be absolutely avoided in every pregnant woman, especially in thyroid cancer patients; therefore, correct supplementation of thyroxine is of extreme importance.

During pregnancy the woman's thyroid physiology undergoes many well-defined changes, leading to an increase in the thyroid volume which is often associated with higher urinary iodine excretion. Also, such changes are related to the formation of new thyroid nodules with the histological features of nodular hyperplasia, and to an approximate doubling in thyroxine-binding globulin (TBG) concentrations due to an increase in oestrogen levels. The increased concentration of TBG as well as the increased capability to bind thyroxine (T4) can lead to augmented total T4 concentrations and reduced free fraction (see Table 12.1; Figs. 12.1 and 12.2). In healthy women, these changes lead to an increased TSH production with consequent increased production of total thyroid hormones (Glinoer 2005; Burrow et al. 1994; Neale and Burrow 2004). The final effect consists of a significant increase in the total thyroxine pool, mainly in the first trimester. This increment may be brought about largely by thyroid stimulation induced by human chorionic gonadotropin (HCG), thanks to its structural affinity with thyrotropin (TSH). It can be observed that a slight increase in fT4 and a reduction in TSH occur between the 9th and 12th weeks of gestation (see Fig. 12.1); subsequently, HCG level decreases and TSH reaches normal non-pregnant levels. The TSH concentration generally lies within the normal range after the 16th to 18th weeks (Santisteban 2005; Burrow et al. 1994; Shah et al. 2003) (see Figs. 12.1 and 12.2). In hypothyroid or thyroidectomised pregnant women, these physiological assessments obviously cannot happen and l-T4 requirement increases very early during pregnancy, reaching a plateau after the 16th to 20th weeks of gestation, with a required l-T4 dosage approximately 30%–50% higher than that administered before pregnancy.

Besides the well-known association between gestational hypothyroidism and impaired intel-

Table 12.1 Physiological changes in thyroid function during pregnancy

↑ TBG	↑ Serum total T4 and T3
↑ HCG (TSH effect)	↑ T3 and T4 pool size
↑ III 5-deiodinase	↑ T3 and T4 degradation
↑ Thyroid volume	↑ HTG (thyroglobulin)
↑ Iodine clearance	TSH ↓

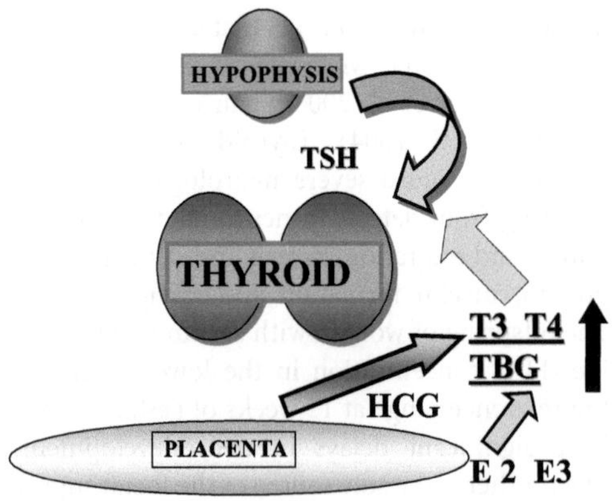

Fig. 12.1 Thyroid hormones in pregnancy: physiologic adaptation. (1) TBG (thyroid binding globulin) increases due to stimulation from placental E2 and E3 (oestradiol and oestriol) and to reduced hepatic clearance. (2) HCG (human chorionic gonadotrophin) has thyrotropin-like activity and stimulates total T4 secretion. (3) TSH may decrease between weeks 8 and 14 of gestation, inhibited by increased T4

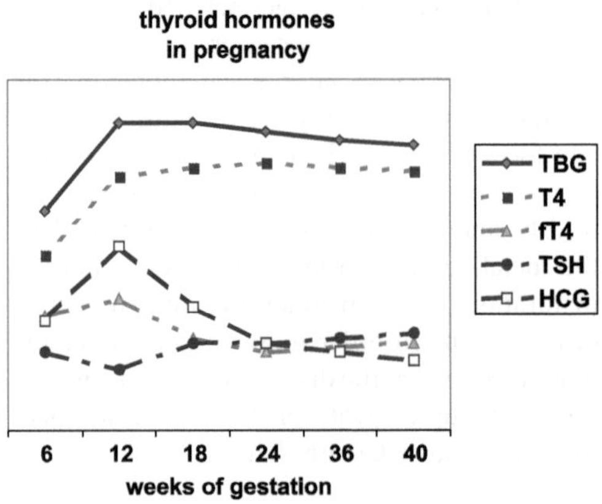

Fig. 12.2 Thyroid hormones in pregnancy: physiologic adaptation during gestational period

lectual and cognitive development in the offspring, untreated or inadequately treated and subclinical hypothyroidism is associated with foetal loss, anaemia, gestational hypertension and pre-eclampsia, abruptio placentae, increased risk of miscarriage, foetal growth retardation, perinatal mortality and neonatal morbidity (Blazer et al. 2003; Glinoer 2005; Haddow et al. 1999; Krassas 2000; Lao 2005; Morreale de Escobar et al. 2000; Obregon et al. 1998).

12.3 Thyroid Cancer

Thyroid cancer is the most common endocrine malignancy and is approximately 2.5 times more common in females than in males. Its incidence presents wide differences in various populations, ranging from 2 to 11 per 100.000 per year in developed countries. Those differences may be due to not only genetic but also environmental factors, mainly iodine deficiency. In the majority of autopsy studies no significant difference in the prevalence of occult microcarcinoma has been demonstrated between sexes, in contrast with clinically apparent papillary carcinoma, which is more common in women. These data could suggest the importance of growth factors (mainly TSH but also HCG) in growth, progression and spread of papillary tumours. In vitro oestrogens have been shown to down-regulate the NIS (sodium iodide symporter) gene and promote the production of HTG, increasing HTG gene expression via oestrogen receptors present in thyroid tissue, without stimulating rapid cell proliferation (Furlanetto et al. 1999; Bradley and Raghavan 2004; O'Connell and O'Doherty 2000). This could support the hypothesis that sex hormones and, therefore, menstrual and reproductive events may modify thyroid cancer risk in women (Truong et al. 2005), although these associations—which could indicate either a causal link or a surveillance bias—may reflect an aetiology shared by both the above-mentioned factors and thyroid cancer. This relation has not yet been confirmed.

The median age at diagnosis is low, below 40 years in most populations. For these reasons, differentiated thyroid cancer (DTC) is one of the most common cancers in women of reproductive age. Hence, thyroid cancer ranks among the most common cancers during pregnancy, with a prevalence of 3.6–14 per 100,000 live births, mirroring the population's incidence (Bradley and Raghavan 2004; Yasmeen et al. 2005; O'Connell and O'Doherty 2000; Hay 1999).

12.3.1 Differentiated Thyroid Cancer: Cancer Arising from Follicular Thyroid Cells

Mostly in young people, differentiated thyroid cancer (DTC) usually has a good prognosis, with an overall 90%–95% long-term disease-free survival for early-stage or low-risk tumours, representing the great majority of tumours diagnosed before 40–45 years of age. According to the current staging score (see Tables 12.2 and 12.3), DTCs of any dimension, even with nodal invasion, for patients below 45 years of age are classified as Stage I tumours, and pregnant patients are usually below 45 years of age.

Recent advances have improved our understanding of the pathogenesis of follicular-cell tumours as a classical model of multi-step carcinogenesis, in which cancer cells are produced from well-differentiated benign cells by transformation caused by accumulating damage to their genome. Some of these alterations have been clearly associated with radiation exposure.

Genetic alterations activating a common pathway of the RET-RAS-BRAF signalling cascade and other chromosomal rearrangements have been identified in most DTC (see Fig. 12.3), mainly in radioinduced tumours. The existence of common genomic changes between DTC and anaplastic carcinoma may provide convincing proof of the multi-step carcinogenesis hypothesis (see Fig. 12.3). Defects in transcriptional and post-transcriptional regulation of adhesion molecules and cell cycle control elements seem to affect tumour progression; thus mutations in the p53 gene do not seem necessarily responsible for the aggressive feature of anaplastic carcinoma (Kondo et al. 2006).

Although gene expression in thyroid cancer reveals highly consistent profiles, a second hypothesis has been proposed, which could possibly explain other "non-genetic non-RET" tumours: the hypothesis of foetal cell carcino-

Table 12.2 TNM classification (UICC, AJCC 2002)

T (primary tumour)	
Tx	Primary tumour cannot be assessed
T0	No evidence of primary tumour
T1	Tumour 2 cm or less in greatest dimension limited to the thyroid
T2	Tumour more than 2 cm but not more than 4 cm in greatest dimension limited to the thyroid
T3	Tumour more than 4 cm in greatest dimension limited to the thyroid or any tumour with minimal extra-thyroid extension (e.g. extension to sternothyroid muscle or perithyroid soft tissues)
T4a	Tumour of any size extending beyond the thyroid capsule to invade subcutaneous soft tissues, larynx, trachea, oesophagus or recurrent laryngeal nerve
T4b	Tumour invades prevertebral fascia or encases carotid artery or mediastinal vessels
All categories may be subdivided in solitary tumour and multifocal tumour (m) (the largest determines the classification)	
All anaplastic carcinomas are considered T4 tumours	
T4a	Intra-thyroid anaplastic carcinoma—surgically resectable
T4b	Extra-thyroidal anaplastic carcinoma—surgically unresectable
N (regional lymph nodes)	
Regional lymph nodes are the central compartment, lateral cervical and upper mediastinal lymph nodes	
Nx	Regional lymph nodes cannot be assessed.
N0	No regional lymph node metastasis
N1	Regional lymph node metastasis
	N1a metastasis to level VI (pretracheal, paratracheal and prelaryngeal/Delphian lymph nodes)
	N1b Metastasis to unilateral, bilateral or contra-lateral cervical or superior mediastinal lymph nodes
M (distant metastasis)	
Mx	Distant metastasis cannot be assessed
M0	No distant metastasis
M1	Distant metastasis

Table 12.3 Stage grouping for DTC

	≤45 years	>45 years		
	Papillary, follicular	Papillary, follicular, medullary		
Stage I	Any T, any N, M0	T1	N0	M0
Stage II	Any T, any N, M1	T2	N0	M0
Stage III	—	T1–T2	N1a	M0
		T3	N0-N1a	M0
Stage IVa	—	T1–T2–T3	N1b	M0
		T4a	N0–N1	M0
Stage IVb	—	T4b M0	any N	M0
Stage IVc	—	Any T	any N	M1

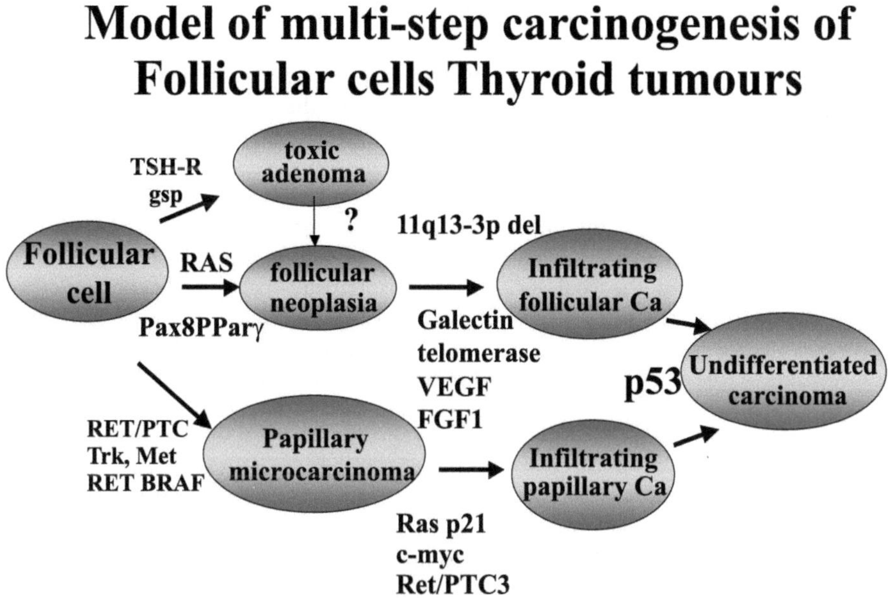

Fig. 12.3 Model of multi-step carcinogenesis of follicular cells thyroid tumours. TSH receptor gene: Activating mutations in part of the TSH-R gene have been demonstrated to result in increased amounts of cAMP stimulating proliferation and differentiation. Frequently found in hyperfunctioning adenomas, they are not found in thyroid cancers. RAS signalling pathway Point mutations in RAS activate the RAS molecule. Mutations in RAS have been shown in 50% of both benign and malignant thyroid tumours, indicating that RAS mutations are early events in thyroid tumourigenesis. Interaction between mutated RAS and other molecules such as IGF-I, PAX-8 and TTF1 have been postulated in differentiated thyroid cancers. TP53 gene: The p53 protein has a central role in cell cycle regulation. When genetic disruptions are recognised at the G/S checkpoint, p53 induces cell cycle arrest. The DNA repair systems are activated and, if repaired, the cell will proceed into the S phase and mitosis. However, if a cell is seriously damaged, p53 induces apoptosis. p53 mutations inhibit these protective mechanisms

genesis, according to which cancer cells are derived from the remnants of foetal thyroid cells rather than normal follicular cells (Takano and Amino 2005; Zhang et al. 2006; Thomas et al. 2006). Both hypotheses can be true and coexist; the second hypothesis (foetal cell carcinogenesis) could explain some cases of unusual rapidly growing DTC. Both hypotheses would suggest a higher thyroid neoplasm proliferation in stimulated thyroid tissue during pregnancy or adolescence, though even in growing tissues these cancers show a very good prognosis.

The best treatment for nearly all identified malignant thyroid neoplasm is surgery. Exceptions include some patients with anaplastic thyroid cancer or lymphoma. The aim of the primary treatment is an adequate excision of the primary tumour and any loco-regional extension. Considerable controversy exists as to the optimal extent of primary surgical resection. According to the extent of the disease, hemithyroidectomy or radical thyroidectomy is performed. As nodal spread is relatively common, initial surgical exploration should include careful examination of the central compartment nodes (paratracheal and tracheoesophageal) as well as dissection of clinically suspicious nodes for frozen section examination. Nodes in the jugular chains should also be carefully examined with ultrasound (US) before surgery and, when suspicious, fine-needle aspiration biopsy (FNAB) should be obtained. If nodal involvement is confirmed, total thyroidectomy and modified radical neck dissection are indicated. No convincing evidence justifies prophylactic multi-compartmental neck dissection in patients with PTC, especially in the absence of palpable metastatic lymphadenopathy.

12.3.1.1 Adjuvant Therapies

Thyroid Hormones

For endocrine therapy, post-operative oral administration of supraphysiologic oral doses of levothyroxine is used, assuming that the suppression of endogenous production of TSH deprives TSH-dependent DTC cells of an important growth-promoting influence and the goal for basal serum TSH should be in the 0.1–0.4 mIU/l range.

Radioactive Jodine

When radical thyroidectomy is performed, the second most frequently used post-operative adjuvant therapy for patients with DTC is *radioactive iodine* (RAI) therapy, with doses of I-131 administered in an attempt to destroy persistent neck disease or distant metastatic lesions. This adjunctive therapy is supposed to destroy occult microscopic carcinoma within the thyroid remnant by being actively trapped both by normal and pathological thyroid cells, and to facilitate follow-up because serum thyroglobulin (Tg) measurements are more reliable after the destruction of residual normal thyroid tissue.

External Irradiation

External irradiation is rarely used as adjunctive therapy in the initial management of patients with DTC, which is known to be poorly radiosensitive. It may be useful, however, in patients with poorly differentiated (higher histologic grade) tumours that do not concentrate RAI.

Chemotherapy

In patients with DTC, chemotherapy is restricted to those tumours that are surgically unresectable, are unresponsive to RAI and have been treated with external irradiation.

Unfortunately, no actual treatment protocol has yet resulted in constant tumour regression or stabilisation.

12.3.1.2 Follow-Up

Follow-up is planned according to the stage of the disease and the extent of the surgery performed.

Every patient undergoes neck ultrasound and serum assay for thyroglobulin, HTG antibodies, fT4 and TSH. For thyroidectomised high-risk patients, I-131 scan is also indicated, and serum HTG measurement—performed either with thyroxine therapy deprivation or under recombinant human TSH (rTSH) stimulation—has been proven to be a useful and reliable marker of disease progression or persistence.

In our own experience, the best follow-up method to detect loco-regional recurrences is, without doubt, neck sonography followed by a meticulous physical examination by experienced personnel and, if indicated, ultrasound-guided FNA to confirm clinical suspicion of neck recurrence.

12.3.2 Medullary Thyroid Cancer: Cancer Arising from Parafollicular Thyroid Cells

Medullary carcinoma of the thyroid (MTC) constitutes approximately 5%–10% of thyroid cancers, though there are no precise figures available for both incidence and survival rates because of the great geographic variations mainly due to its familial pattern. Although uncommon, MTC is interesting because of its biochemical and genetic features and clinical association, both in the autosomal-dominant inherited syndromes with incomplete penetrance (MEN IIA and IIB) and in the non-MEN forms.

Familial cases account for about 30% of MTCs (see Fig. 12.4). Sporadic or non-familial forms, which usually occur after the age of 40, are more malignant than follicular carcinoma. The occurrence of MTC in both sporadic and familial forms makes the clinical approach to this tumour different from that for other thyroid tumours. First, patients with MTC should always be suspected of carrying the genetic form of the disease. Secondly, the possible presence of associated conditions, such as pheochromocytoma, should be recognised before submitting patients to thyroidectomy. Finally, since MTC clinical behaviour is extremely variable, this type of tumour represents a true therapeutic challenge.

MTC arises from C cells secreting calcitonin, a 32-amino acid peptide. Calcitonin is the most clinically useful biochemical marker for these tumours, and C cell hyperplasia represents a pre-cancerous stage. These neuroendocrine cells are believed to be of neural crest origin, thus having a separate lineage from the endoderm-derived follicular thyroid cells. For this reason, in addition to calcitonin gene products, such as calcitonin CGRP (calcitonin-gene-related-peptide) and C-CAP (katacalcin), MTC cells express several other biochemical markers that reflect the APUD features of those cells present in the diffuse neuroendocrine system (see Table 12.4), implicated in the pathogenesis of the symptoms that may occur in patients with advanced disease. Such symptoms include flushing, diarrhoea, carcinoid syndrome or Cushing syndrome. These cells can also produce prostaglandins and other neuroendocrine markers such as chromogranin A, now used with calcitonin and CEA in MTC patient follow-up.

When dealing with MTC, we should always bear in mind that these patients may be the index case for one of the familial forms of the disease: Pre-symptomatic screening of relatives of MTC patients enables early diagnosis of this malignancy. Early diagnosis rather than more extensive surgery may improve survival and reduce recurrences, mostly in the MEN IIB form of MTC, which is highly aggressive. In MEN IIB carriers, routine thyroidectomy is justified in childhood, regardless of serum calcitonin level.

Table 12.4 Medullary thyroid cancer

Secretion products and tumour markers
Calcitonin
Katacalcin (= C-pro-calc) pro-calcitonin
CGRP (calcitonin-gene-related peptide)
CEA,
Chromogranin A, amyloid, melanin, NSE
Catecholamines, dopa-decarboxylase, histaminase, serotonin, prostaglandins, kallikreins, kinins
ACTH and CRF, MSH , nerve growth factor, somatostatin, β-endorphin, substance P, VIP, prolactin-releasing hormone, neurotensin, gastrin-release peptide

Biochemical screening of familial disease consists of serum calcitonin evaluation both in the basal state and after pentagastrin stimulation. After the identification of a mutation in the RET proto-oncogene, both in MEN IIA and B and in non-MEN forms, genetic screening of individuals with a RET mutation may be performed. Screening studies should begin shortly after birth in infants at risk for MEN IIB, and by 1 year of age in children at risk for MEN IIA.

In inherited forms, the initial germline mutation produces multiple foci of cells—the so-called C-cell hyperplasia—that are susceptible to tumour formation, and each MTC is the result of a second cell transformation in one of these susceptible clones (see Fig 12.4).

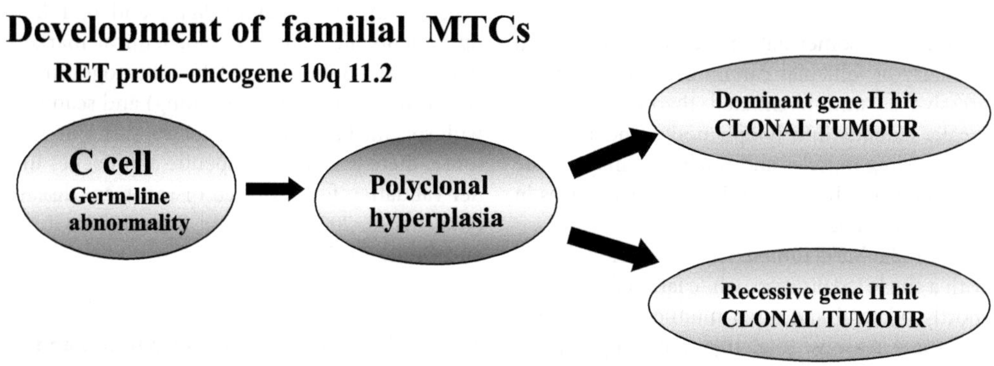

Fig. 12.4 Model of multi-step carcinogenesis of medullary thyroid cancer

Primary MTC lesions become visible at echography as solid masses; dense calcifications may appear on plain film radiography. Fine needle aspiration shows a mixture of round, polyhedral and spindle-shaped cells which may seem undifferentiated and look like a variable amount of extra-cellular amyloid.

The cells of C-cell hyperplasia are rich in mature neurosecretory granules containing calcitonin; the foetal marker CEA is expressed only at low levels. In microscopic MTC, however, CEA levels are increased and the pattern of staining for calcitonin is homogeneous. Very aggressive tumours stain for calcitonin less intensely, and with a heterogeneous pattern. Calcitonin immunostaining and circulating CEA levels are now used as prognostic factors. Somatostatin, secreted by thyroid C cells, seems to play an important role in the regulation of normal calcitonin secretion. MTCs, like other neuroendocrine tumours, usually express somatostatin receptors. Follow-up of MTC patients can therefore be performed by using the somatostatin analogue octreotide scintigraphy (octreoscan) also. Imaging of recurrent MTC with an octreotide scan should be employed to determine the presence of somatostatin receptors: The presence of these receptors provides the basis for treatment with long-acting analogues of somatostatin or with Y-octreotide (DOTATOC).

Another useful marker is chromogranin A, a glycoprotein present in a variety of polypeptide-secreting endocrine cells including cells from the adrenal medulla, parathyroids and thyroid C cells. Tumours staining for chromogranin A can be subsequently monitored with chromogranin assay.

MTC is somewhat more aggressive than papillary or follicular carcinoma, but not as aggressive as undifferentiated thyroid cancer. It locally extends into lymph nodes and into the surrounding muscles and trachea. It may invade lymphatic and blood vessels and metastasizes in lungs, bones and liver.

Sporadic MTC tumours are often monolateral with a single localisation, while familial forms are mostly bilateral and often multifocal or diffuse. For these reasons, total thyroidectomy appears to be the appropriate approach to MTC, even in paediatric and adolescent patients. Central neck and upper mediastinum clearance and, in addition, mono- or bilateral node dissection (depending on the extent of nodal involvement) would be also advisable. The most appropriate treatment for clinical N0 tumours is still a matter of debate, but most surgeons prefer performing prophylactic node dissection because MTC metastasizes in regional lymph nodes at a very early stage.

Surgery is the only treatment which is considered potentially curative for metastatic or recurrent medullary carcinoma. The role of radiotherapy is controversial, as MTC is generally thought not to be radio-sensitive, but only few studies have reported a favourable response with external radiotherapy in patients with inoperable or recurrent disease. Therapy with octreotide (a long-acting somatostatin analogue) has been tested in metastatic disease, without consistent effects in most patients, perhaps owing to the low density of somatostatin receptors in advanced disease. Radioactive iodine is ineffective because I-131 uptake by MTC cells is negligible. Radiometabolic therapy with Y-DOTATOC, radioactive yttrium linked to octreotide, has shown favourable effects in less than 20% of metastatic patients. No reliably effective chemotherapeutic regimen has yet been identified. Various agents have been tested, but none appears to be able to lead to long-lasting remission. The administration of dacarbazine plus 5-FU has been proposed: these drugs seem to have acceptable activity and are well-tolerated, though the natural history of MTC is so variable that these results should be considered provisional. Moreover, new drugs with anti-angiogenetic, anti-tyrosine kinase and anti-VEGF effects are currently under observation.

In conclusion, there are several new ways to expedite the diagnosis of MTC and to follow up patients after surgery: biochemical markers (CEA, calcitonin, katacalcin, cromogranin-A, etc. according to tumour staining) and scanning with specific ligands such as octreotide. Furthermore, there are new therapeutic approaches under validation for advanced or recurrent disease (Gagel et al. 2005; Raue and Raue 2005; Gimm and Dralle 2005).

12.3.3 Other Tumours in the Thyroid Gland

Less common histological types such as insular, poorly differentiated or undifferentiated thyroid cancers are extremely uncommon in young people. They are very aggressive, poor-prognosis tumours and deserve different treatment, from debulking to demolitive surgery according to stage, local spread and histology.

Lymphomas, sarcomas and angiosarcomas or metastasis from distant tumours are sometimes found in the thyroid gland, but prognosis and therapy are the same as for these tumours with different localisation.

12.4 Thyroid Cancer and Pregnancy

Pregnant women with malignant thyroid nodules are twice as likely to be asymptomatic as non-pregnant women, because of physiological thyroid increase during pregnancy. For this reason, thyroid cancers found in pregnant women are often larger than in non-pregnant patients. Clinical and ultrasound findings are often enough to suspect a malignancy. Skilled examiners and good-quality images with grey-scale and power Doppler US seem more reliable than any other technique in detecting and differentiating malignant and benign solid thyroid nodules, especially for small lesions. This is crucial if we have to give up other control methods such as I-131 scan or CT scan because of pregnancy. Even during pregnancy, US-guided FNAB is the investigation of choice, thanks to its reliability and safety.

Papillary thyroid cancer is the most common histological type detected in pregnant women, and in most series 90%–95% of thyroid carcinomas diagnosed are Stage I disease, most of them found in the first trimester of pregnancy at the first antenatal visit. The predominance of papillary cancer may be an important factor favouring localised disease, as these cancers metastasizes slowly and mostly in the lymphatic system, whereas less common follicular cancers tend to spread via angioinvasion with a higher frequency of distant metastasis. Although thyroid cancer during pregnancy may have a faster growth (Rosen et al. 1997; Kobayashi et al. 1994) since hormonal factors (mainly HCG) could accelerate tumour progression, the real impact of pregnancy seems to be minimal. As a matter of fact, the rates of recurrence or the disease-free period do not differ between pregnant and non-pregnant women affected by the same disease (Hod et al. 1989; Yasmeen et al. 2005; Chloe and McDougall 1994; Rosen et al. 1997; Mestman et al. 1995). Hod et al. did report one single case of accelerated tumour growth during pregnancy, but this would appear to be an exception rather than the rule (Hod et al. 1989).

In a large retrospective study on 595 pregnancy-associated thyroid cancers, Yasmeen et al. detected no difference in outcome, disease-free survival and morbidity when compared to age-matched non-pregnant women (Yasmeen et al. 2005). In contrast to what is observed in other pregnancy-associated cancers, no metastasis of DTC to placenta or foetus has yet been reported. An association between thyroid cancer and parity or full-term pregnancy has been investigated in many studies without significant or conclusive results (Truong et al. 2005).

In a large study conducted by Truong et al., a history of miscarriage was associated with a slightly increased risk of DTC (odds ratio 1.4) while voluntary abortion was associated with an odds ratio of 3.1. Voluntary abortion was more strongly associated with papillary microcarcinoma than with larger tumours. The mechanism linking miscarriage to thyroid cancer has not been explained yet, though, besides HCG stimulating effect, it is likely that miscarriage may be induced by thyroid disorders (mainly autoimmunity often associated with thyroid cancer) or hormonal dysfunction such as hypothyroidism. The study of Truong et al. demonstrated a stronger association between voluntary abortion and thyroid cancer. However, this may reflect a surveillance bias, since these women may also be more actively screened for thyroid disorders. This hypothesis is supported by the strong association with microcarcinomas and by the short time span between abortion and cancer diagnosis (Truong et al. 2005; Krassas 2000).

During pregnancy, cellular immunity changes, as reflected by a decrease in the T-cell number. Pregnancy-associated immune tolerance, designed for foetal survival, could enhance disease progression, though, according to bibliographic searches and our own experience, pregnancy after thyroid cancer has shown no significant effect on morbidity, disease-free period or survival time, and pregnant women with thyroid cancer had favourable outcomes regardless of the timing of diagnosis (Moosa and Mazzaferri 1997; Bradley and Raghavan 2004).

Guidelines for the evaluation and treatment of thyroid cancer must consider the gestational age but also the individual patient's wishes. Detection of a thyroid cancer during pregnancy should not be the reason for termination of pregnancy, and in the large majority of cases it does not require urgent surgery.

The problem of thyroid cancer and pregnancy can affect three groups of patients:

1. **Patients with no prior history of cancer** in whom a malignant thyroid nodule is suspected or diagnosed during pregnancy. For these patients, surgery could be safely performed during the middle trimester or delayed until delivery without worsening the prognosis (Chloe and McDougall 1994; Tan et al. 1996). Thyroidectomy during pregnancy has not been associated with adverse maternal or neonatal outcomes (Harmer and McCready 1996; Vini et al. 1999) There are no indications for termination of pregnancy (O'Connell and O'Doherty 2000). When surgery is planned during pregnancy, it is important to consider both gestational age and the type of general anaesthesia. Whenever possible, the operation should be performed during the second trimester or after delivery. During the first trimester, that is the organogenesis period, general anaesthetic agents may have some teratogenic potential or may rise the risk of miscarriage. In the third trimester, surgery may induce premature labour. Physiological changes of pregnancy, such as increased heart rate and blood volume, may complicate general anaesthesia, and hypotension caused by vena cava compression of the uterus during a prolonged supine position may cause foetal hypoperfusion (Bradley and Raghavan 2004). Postponing surgery to at least 6–7 months after diagnosis of DTC in the first trimester has not adversely affected prognosis; on the other hand, thyroidectomy can be safely performed in the second trimester of pregnancy or after delivery (Lao 2005). Thyroxine therapy should be started immediately after surgery because untreated hypothyroidism may expose the mother to a higher risk of disease recurrences as well as having an adverse effect on cognitive functions and on the regular growth of the offspring. Regular assessments of TSH and fT4 level every 6/8 weeks during pregnancy and breast-feeding are indicated to ensure an adequate dose of l-thyroxine. Follow-up may be carried out on a regular basis with ultrasound techniques and thyroglobulin assay, as in non-pregnant women. Radioiodine therapy, when needed, can be safely postponed until after breast-feeding.
2. **Pregnant patients with a history of previously treated** DTC with no evidence of recurrent or persistent disease by imaging and by thyroglobulin measurement *("cured" patients).* Whether women treated for thyroid cancer should become pregnant is a matter of concern, but current evidence suggests that DTC should not discourage intended pregnancy, with the usual recommendation to postpone it to at least 6 months after radioiodine therapy. Despite the theoretical proliferative stimulation caused by HCG and placental growth factors, published data show that there is no evidence that thyroid cancer can be influenced by pregnancy. Also, follow-up studies have shown no significant increase in risk. Usually, patients are recommended to postpone pregnancy to 6–12 months after radioiodine (I-131) treatment, to avoid a possible higher risk of miscarriage noted in the first few months after radioiodine therapy and to allow time enough to exclude residual disease requiring further treatment (Lazarus 2005; Schlumberger et al. 1996; O'Connell and O'Doherty 2000). The mutagenic effect of radiation and the theoretical possibility that it may affect germ cells, thereby causing genetic damage, congenital abnormalities and malignancy in the offspring, miscarriages or premature birth, have raised concerns about the use of radioactive iodine during childbearing age. Virtually any person treated with any dosage of I-131 is at potential risk, but current information based on experimental evidence in animals and follow-up studies on humans failed to reveal statistically significant effects of I-131 on chromosomal abnormalities, congenital malformation and childhood cancers. In a large retrospective study, Dottorini et al. evaluated fertility and long-term effects of

I-131 therapy in 815 women. Among children born from I-131-treated women, the authors found only one case of ventricular septal defect and patent ductus arteriosus (Bal et al. 2005; Dottorini et al. 1995; Krassas 2000). A possible increase in the rate of miscarriages has been reported to occur in the early period after therapy, but it remains uncertain whether abortion can be caused by I-131 per se or by the thyroid autoimmunity often associated with the disease, or by the hypothyroid-hyperprolactinemic status accompanying I-131 therapy. At present, a consensus has been reached on the fact that radioiodine treatment of DTC does not affect pregnancy outcome and does not appear to be associated with any genetic risk, with the usual recommendation to delay pregnancy for 6–12 months after radioiodine exposure, even if there is no evidence that pregnancy before this period could lead to a less favourable outcome (Krassas 2005).

3. **Pregnant patients with evidence of persistent disease despite therapy.** Management of these patients and providing evidence-based advice are obviously extremely difficult tasks. Patients with active DTC can be reassured that, as mentioned above, pregnancy itself does not appear to increase disease progression; therefore a gap in treatment during pregnancy is not contraindicated. When simple increase in serum HTG levels are observed, further therapy is not necessary. For patients with local recurrent disease, ultrasound examination by skilled hands is of utmost importance, both to help surgeons in selecting tissues to be removed and to perform local therapy, such as alcoholisation of small lesions. For patients with advanced disease, ultrasound control of tissue growth can help in therapeutic decisions such as timing of surgery. As mentioned above for the first diagnosis of thyroid cancer, whenever possible, surgery should be carried out during the second trimester or after delivery.

For any patient, both with first diagnosis or recurrent disease, post-operative therapy for DTC is based on the administration of supraphysiologic "suppressive" oral doses of l-thyroxine. This treatment has been widely used for more than 40 years, with the assumption that suppression of endogenous TSH deprives TSH-dependent DTC cells of the most important growth factor. Therefore, thyroxine therapy aims at suppressing pituitary secretion of TSH, as indicated by serum TSH levels below 0.05 mIU/l. In univariate analyses, thyroxine therapy apparently helps decrease cancer-related death rates among patients with PTC. Many series have reported reduced rates of tumour recurrence both in PTC and in FTC. Doses of l-thyroxine greater than 150/200 μg (at least 2 μg/kg/day) are usually needed to maintain the maternal serum free thyroxine concentration within the upper third of the reference range and to suppress TSH levels. Usually, the dosage needs to be increased as early as during the fifth week of gestation, and fT4 TSH control is recommended every 6 weeks for adequate adjustment of the dosage. After delivery, thyroxine dose can be gradually reduced to the pre-pregnancy level, while TSH concentration should be constantly monitored (Glinoer 2003; Lao 2005).

Patients with MTC, whose tumours deriving from C cells are not TSH-dependent, do not require suppressive therapy but only thyroxine replacement therapy after surgery, and the dosages are those used for hypothyroidism.

The pregnancy status requires much more accuracy in assessing l-thyroxine dosage to protect the foetus from maternal hypothyroidism because, as mentioned above, the mother is the sole source of thyroid hormones for the embryo in the first trimester of pregnancy. As regards pharmacokinetics, oral dosing produces therapeutic effects within 3–5 days. Approximately 40%–80% of oral doses is absorbed, with peak serum levels measured within 2–4 h, the half-life of an administered dose being approximately 1 week. The extent of absorption is increased in fasting status and decreased in inadequate intestinal absorptions, often caused by other drugs, such as ferrous sulphate. Therefore, during pregnancy, thyroxine and ferrous sulphate dosages should be spaced at least 4 hours apart. There is limited but still important placental transfer of maternal T4 to the foetus (Burrow et al. 1994), while placental type III deiodinase catalyses the conversion of T4 to the more active form reverse-T3, which crosses the placental barrier, and to less active

3,3'-diiodothyronine (T2). This represents a homeostatic mechanism for maintaining T3 production in the placenta when maternal serum T4 concentrations are modified (Burrow et al. 1994; Dussault et al. 1969; Fisher et al. 1964). Frequent monitoring and adjustment of l-T4 dosage are then important because of large fluctuation of T4 metabolism during pregnancy.

12.5 Concluding Remarks

When treating thyroid cancer in pregnancy, three factors should be considered:

1. **The effect of cancer on pregnancy:** → no metastasis to placenta or foetus; no IUGR. Pregnancy seems not to be compromised by thyroid cancer.
2. **The effect of pregnancy on cancer:** → in vitro accelerated cell growth; no effect seen in vivo Survival and disease-free interval seem identical in pregnant and non-pregnant women.
3. **The effects of management modalities on pregnancy outcome:** → no I-131 l-T4 requirement. Critical monthly adjustment of l-thyroxine therapy.

References

Alexander EK, Marqusee E, Lawrence J, Jarolim P, Fisher GA, Larsen PR (2004) Timing and magnitude of increases in levothyroxine requirements during pregnancy in women with hypothyroidism. N Engl J Med 351: 241–249

Bal C, Kumar A, Tripathi M, Chandrashekar N, Phom H, Murali NR, Chandra P, Pant GS (2005) High-dose radioiodine treatment for differentiated thyroid carcinoma is not associated with change in female fertility or any genetic risk to the offspring. Int J Radiat Oncol Biol Phys 63(2): 449–455

Blazer S, Moreh-Waterman Y, Miller-Lotan R, Tamir A, Hochberg Z (2003) Maternal hypothyroidism may affect fetal growth and neonatal thyroid function. Obstet Gynecol 102(2): 232–241

Bradley PJ, Raghavan U (2004) Cancers presenting in the head and neck during pregnancy. Curr Opin Otolaryngol Head Neck Surg 12(2): 76–81

Burrow GN, Fisher DA, Larsen PR (1994) Maternal and fetal thyroid function N Engl J Med 331(16): 1072–1078

Chloe W, McDougall IR (1994) Thyroid cancer in pregnant women: diagnostic and therapeutic management. Thyroid 4: 433–435

Dottorini ME, Lomuscio G, Mazzucchelli L. Vignati A. Colombo L (1995) Assessment of female fertility and carcinogenesis after I-131 therapy for differentiated thyroid cancer J Nucl Med 36(1):21–27

Dussault J, Row VV, Lickrish G (1969) Studies of serum triodothyronine concentration in maternal and cord blood: transfer of triiodothyronine across the human placenta. J Clin Endocrinol Metab 29: 595–606

Fisher DA, Lehman H, Lackey C (1964) Placental transport of thyroxine. J Clin Endocrinol Metab 24:939–940

Furlanetto TW, Nguyen LQ, Jameson JL (1999) Estradiol increases proliferation and down-regulates the sodium/iodide symporter gene in FRTL-5 cells. Endocrinology 140(12): 5705–5711

Gagel RF, Hoff AO, Cote GJ (2005) Medullary thyroid carcinoma. In: Werner & Ingbar's The Thyroid : A Fundamental And Clinical Text. Braveman, Utiger eds. 9th ed., pp. 967–989

Gimm O, Dralle H (2005) Therapy for medullary thyroid cancer. In: Thyroid Cancer. Biersack, Grunwald eds. Springer, Berlin, pp. 335–347

Glinoer D (2005) Thyroid disease during pregnancy. In: Werner & Ingbar's The Thyroid : A Fundamental and Clinical Text. Braveman, Utiger eds. 9th ed., pp. 1086–1108

Glinoer D (2003) Management of hypo- and hyperthyroidism during pregnancy. Growth Horm IGF Res 13 (suppl A): S45–S54

Haddow JE, Palomaki GE, Allan WC, Williams JR, Knight GJ, Gagnon J, O'Heir CE, Mitchell ML, Hermos RJ, Waisbren SE, Faix JD, Klein RZ (1999) Maternal thyroid deficiency during pregnancy and subsequent neuropsychological development of the child. N Engl J Med 341(8): 549–555

Harmer CL, McCready VR (1996) Thyroid cancer: differentiated carcinoma. Cancer Treat Rev 22: 161–177

Hay I (1999) Nodular thyroid disease diagnosed during pregnancy: how and when to treat. Thyroid 9: 667–670

Hod M, Sharony R, Friedman S, Ovadia J (1989) Pregnancy and thyroid carcinoma: a review of incidence, course and prognosis. Obstet Gynecol Surv 44: 774–779

Kobayashi K, Tanaka Y, Ishiguro S et al.(1994) Rapidly growing thyroid carcinoma during pregnancy. J Surg Oncol 66: 61–64

Kondo T, Ezzat S, Asa SL (2006) Pathogenic mechanism in thyroid follicular-cell neoplasia Nat Rev Cancer 6(4): 292–306

Krassas GE(2000) Thyroid disease and female reproduction. Fertil Steril 74 (6): 1063–1070

Lao TT (2005) Thyroid disorders in pregnancy. Curr Opin Obstet Gynecol 17: 123–127

Lazarus JH (2005) Thyroid disorders associated with pregnancy etiology, diagnosis and management. Treat Endocrinol 4: 31–41

Mestman JH, Goodwin M, Montoro MM (1995) Thyroid disorders of pregnancy. Endocrinol Metab Clin North Am 24: 41–71

Moosa M, Mazzaferri EL (1997) Outcome of differentiated thyroid cancer diagnosed in pregnant women. J Clin Endocrinol Metab 82: 2862–2866

Morreale de Escobar G, Obregon MJ, Escobar del Rey F (2000) Is neuropsychological development related to maternal hypothyroidism or to maternal hypothyroxinemia? J Clin Endocrinol Metab 85: 3975–3987

Nam KH, Yoon JH, Chang HS, Park CS (2005) Optimal timing of surgery in well-differentiated thyroid carcinoma detected during pregnancy. J Surg Oncol 91(3): 199–203

Neale D. Burrow G (2004) Thyroid disease in pregnancy. Obstet Gynecol Clin N Am 31: 893–905

Obregon MJ, Calvo RM, Escobar del Rey F, Morreale de Escobar G (1998) Thyroid hormones and fetal development. In: The thyroid and age. Pinchera A., Mann K. Hostalec U, eds. Schattauer Verlagsgesellschaft mbH Stuttgart, Germany, pp. 49–73

O'Connell TB, O'Doherty MJ (2000) Differentiated thyroid cancer and pregnancy. Nucl Med Commun 21: 127–128

Pop VJ, Brouwers EP, Vader HL et al. (2003) Maternal hypothyroxinaemia during early pregnancy and subsequent child development: a 3-year follow-up study. Clin Endocrinol (Oxf) 59: 282–288

Rago T, Vitti P, Chiovato L, Mazzeo S, De Liperi A, Miccoli P, Viacava P, Bogazzi F, Martino E, Pinchera A (1998) Role of conventional ultrasonography and color flow-Doppler sonography in predicting malignancy in 'cold' thyroid nodules. Eur J Endocrinol 138(1): 41–46

Raue F, Raue FK (2005) Diagnosis of medullary thyroid cancer. In: Thyroid Cancer. Biersack, Grunwald eds Springer, Berlin, pp. 297–310

Rosen IB, Korman M, Walfish PG (1997) Thyroid nodular disease in pregnancy: current diagnosis and treatment. Clin Obstet Gynecol 40: 81–89

Rossing MA, Voigt LF, Wicklund KG, Daling JR (2000) Reproductive factors and risk of papillary thyroid cancer in women. Am J Epidemiol 151(8): 765–772

Santisteban P(2005) Development and anatomy of the hypothalamic-pituitary-thyroid axis. In: Werner & Ingbar's The Thyroid: A Fundamental and Clinical Text. Braveman, Utiger, eds. 9th ed., pp. 8-26

Schlumberger M, De Vathaire F, Ceccarelli C, Delisle MJ, Francese C, Couette JE, Pinchera A. Parmentier C (1996) Exposure to radioactive iodine-131 scintigraphy or therapy does not preclude pregnancy in thyroid cancer patients. J Nucl Med 37: 612–615

Shah MS, Davies TF, Stagnaro Green A (2003) The thyroid during pregnancy: a physiological and pathological stress test. Minerva Endocrinologica 28: 233–245

Smith LH, Danielsen B, Allen ME, Cress R (2003). Cancer associated with obstetric delivery: results of linkage with the Californian cancer registry. Am J Obstet Gynecol 189: 1128–1135

Takano T, Amino N (2005) Fetal cell carcinogenesis: a new hypothesis for better understanding of thyroid carcinoma. Thyroid 15(5): 432–438

Tan GH, Gharib H, Goellner JR et al. (1996) Management of thyroid nodules in pregnancy. Arch Intern Med 156: 2317–2320

Thomas T, Nowka K, Lan L, Derwahl M (2006) Expression of endoderm stem cell markers: evidence for the presence of adult stem cells in human thyroid glands. Thyroid 16(6): 537–544

Truong T, Orsi L, Dubourdieu D, Rougier Y, Hemon D, Guenel P (2005) Role of goiter and of menstrual and reproductive factors in thyroid cancer: a population-based case-control study in New Caledonia (South Pacific), a very high incidence area. Am J Epidemiol 161(11): 1056–1065

Vini L, Hyer S, Pratt B, Harmer C (1999) Management of differentiated thyroid cancer diagnosed during pregnancy. Eur J Endocrinol 140: 404–406

Weisz B, Schiff E, Lishner M (2001) Cancer in pregnancy: maternal and fetal implications. Hum Reprod Update 7(4): 384–393

Yasmeen S, Cress R, Romano PS, Xing G, Berger-Chen S, Danielsen B, Smith LH (2005) Thyroid cancer in pregnancy. Int J Gynecol Obstet 91: 15–20

Zhang P, Zuo H, Ozaki T, Nakagomi N, Kakudo K (2006) Cancer stem cell hypothesis in thyroid cancer. Pathol Int 56 (9): 485–489

13 Gastrointestinal, Urologic and Lung Malignancies During Pregnancy

G. Pentheroudakis, N. Pavlidis

Recent Results in Cancer Research, Vol. 178

13.1 Introduction

As postponing childbearing to later reproductive ages constitutes a trend in developed societies and cancer incidence increases with age, the occurrence of malignancy during pregnancy is likely to become an increasingly common phenomenon [1]. Still, gastrointestinal (GI), renal and pulmonary malignancies usually affect patients of older age, making their association with pregnancy rare. The experience accumulated suffices for the formulation of clinical guidelines only in the case of colorectal cancer, while in the case of other GI, renal and pulmonary tumours one must resort to application of standard clinical practice adapted to the peculiarities of pregnancy. In any case, the clinical expertise of the multidisciplinary management team, the extent of disease and the prognosis, coupled to feedback from the patient and family, will define the therapeutic approach.

13.2 Gastrointestinal Cancer

13.2.1 Colorectal Cancer

13.2.1.1 Epidemiology

Colorectal cancer (CRC) is the third leading cause of cancer death in women, though it is uncommon in women aged less than 40 years. The cumulative risk of developing colorectal cancer in women before their forties is 1:2,000 [2]. The incidence of colorectal cancer during gestation appears to be 1 in 13,000 pregnancies, with a median patient age of 31. Up to the year 2003 three hundred cases of gestational colorectal cancer have been reported in the medical literature [3].

Colorectal cancer in young patients is occasionally associated with genetic syndromes or chronic inflammation. Familial adenomatous polyposis, Lynch syndromes, familial colorectal cancer syndrome and long-standing inflammatory disease of the bowel are present in young patients with CRC more often than in those older than 50 years. Still, in a series of 19 pregnant women with CRC, only 4 had recognisable genetic syndromes or inflammatory bowel disease [4]. It appears that existing data for geographic variation of CRC incidence in the general population are no different in pregnant women. A higher incidence is seen in industrialised societies of Western Europe and North America, while it is 15 times lower in Africa, South America and Asia [5].

An intriguing finding is the high incidence of rectal cancers in pregnant women. Only 20%–25% of large intestine tumours are located in the rectum in the general population, as opposed to 80% of tumours in 205 pregnant patients reported by Bernstein et al. [6]. This phenomenon may reflect a different biology of the malignancy or could simply be due to easier diagnosis of the occasional rectal tumours because of exacerbation of rectal symptoms from uterine pressure or frequent gynaecological examinations.

Adenocarcinoma is by far the most frequent histologic type of cancer of the colon and rectum. Several case reports and patient series provide hints for predominance of poorly differentiated mucinous tumours in pregnant women. However, other published reports lack such data and the relative proportion of high-grade adenocarcinomas during pregnancy cannot be safely estimated [7, 8]. Data on lymphatic/vascular invasion, perineural invasion, aneuploidy, microsatellite instability and thymidylate synthase levels are lacking as well.

13.2.1.2 Presentation

Symptoms and signs such as abdominal cramps, rectal bleeding, diarrhoea, constipation, weight loss, nausea-vomiting, abdominal mass and anaemia make up a clinical picture common to both the general population and pregnant CRC patients [9]. However, the co-existence of pregnancy may mask some of these or prompt the patient and physician to attribute them to gestation. Nausea is often misdiagnosed as a normal manifestation of pregnancy, though it should wane after the first trimester. Anaemia may be attributed to pregnancy-associated iron/folate deficiency and haemodilution, while weight loss and abdominal masses are masked by the foetus. Haemorrhoids, often present in pregnancy, are taken as the sole source of rectal bleeding and hormonal changes with pressure from the gravid uterus as the cause of altered bowel habits.

Laboratory investigations reveal microcytic anaemia, hypoalbuminaemia and deranged liver function tests in the presence of hepatic metastases. Ironically, the first two along with elevated serum alkaline phosphatase levels are seen in normal pregnancies, because of iron/folate deficiency, increase of plasma volume and enhanced placental synthesis of alkaline phosphatase. Overall, symptoms and signs commonly associated with pregnancy are unlikely to worry patient and physician enough to embark on a diagnostic work-up which is potentially hazardous for the embryo. Therefore, pregnant women are diagnosed with locally advanced or metastatic colorectal tumours more often than their non-pregnant counterparts [10]. Epidemiological and clinicopathological differences between colorectal tumours affecting pregnant and non-pregnant patients are shown in Table 13.1.

13.2.1.3 Diagnosis and Staging

Diagnosis and staging of a solid tumour require its imaging, histological documentation and study for invasion of surrounding tissues/organs and distant spread. Computerised tomography (CT) readily detects the latter two and has therefore become standard in the diagnostic approach of patients with colorectal cancer. However, plain abdominopelvic radiographs and CT are contraindicated in pregnant women because of the relative increase in the risk of abortion, growth defects and teratogenesis [11]. Ultrasound of the abdomen/pelvis is cheap and safe for the foetus and can detect hepatic metastases larger than 1 cm with 75% sensitivity. Transrectal ultrasound is also safe and more sensitive than physical examination for the study of intestinal wall infiltration and regional lymphadenopathy (sensitivity 75%–85%) [12]. In addition, transrectal ultrasound may identify those cases of bulky

Table 13.1 Epidemiological and clinicopathological differences between CRC of pregnant and non-pregnant women

Parameter	General population	Pregnancy
Age	>45	Usually <40
Incidence	Cumulative risk 1:17	1 in 13,000 gestations
Risk factors	Very rare association with genetic syndromes or known predisposing conditions	Occasional association with genetic syndromes and strong predisposing conditions
Symptom duration	Variable	Often prolonged because of late diagnosis
Primary site	Large intestine in >75% of cases	Rectum in 60%–80% of cases
Pathologic stage	Variable	Usually locally advanced or metastatic stage
Mucinous histology	Rare	More common
Ovarian metastases	Rare, 3%–8% of cases	More common, 25%–30% of cases

rectal tumours of the anterior wall which cause stenosis of the vaginal canal and will, therefore, be problematic for vaginal delivery.

Magnetic resonance imaging (MRI) of the abdomen seems to be safe, as foetal exposure to powerful electromagnetic fields has not been associated with abortion or congenital malformations. Still, many authors advocate against the use of paramagnetic enhancing agents during gestation and advise avoiding abdominopelvic MRI altogether during the first trimester of pregnancy, a period crucial for organogenesis [13]. Non-contrast-enhanced MRI is equally effective to CT in depicting pelvic and hepatic lesions, with a reported sensitivity of 80%.

Colonoscopy is probably the most definite diagnostic modality which provides tumour imaging as well as biopsy material in patients with CRC. It also picks up the 5% of patients who have a synchronous second tumour of the large intestine. In theory, colonoscopy in pregnant women carries the risks of uterine pressure and placental detachment, intestinal perforation and foetal injury from maternal hypotension/hypoxia or diazepam or midazolam administration. These risks are probably quite low: In 28 colonoscopies performed, Cappell et al. reported no adverse events for mother or foetus. Rectosigmoidoscopy or partial colonoscopy is even safer, as shown by a series of 59 cases [14]. Overall, only partial colonoscopy and rectosigmoidoscopy for left-sided tumours should be considered routine in pregnant women in view of the more abundant cumulative experience in the literature. When colonoscopy is necessary for the diagnosis/biopsy of right-sided tumours, avoidance of abdominal pressure, positioning in a left lateral decubitus position to avoid the supine hypotensive syndrome, gentleness of manipulations, suppression with meperidine instead of benzodiazepines, administration of nasal oxygen to the mother and vital sign monitoring by means of cardiac monitoring/oxymetry and sphygmomanometry are necessary to minimise associated risks.

Serum carcinoembryonic antigen (CEA) levels are not elevated by pregnancy; accordingly, CEA monitoring may be used after diagnosis of CRC for follow-up of pregnant women with resected early tumours as well as for evaluation of response to therapy of pregnant women with advanced disease [15]. Either the AJCC-TNM or the modified Astler-Coller Dukes staging classification may be used. In one of the larger reported series of 39 pregnant patients, none had Dukes A disease, 41% had malignant infiltration of the whole thickness of the bowel wall without nodal involvement (Dukes B disease), whereas 59% of patients had either locoregional nodal involvement or distant metastases [6]. As mentioned above, this advanced stage of CRC in pregnant women has been attributed to late diagnosis rather than aggressive biology. An intriguing clinical feature of pregnancy-associated CRC has been the relatively high frequency of ovarian deposits (25% of cases), in contrast to their rarity (3%–8%) in women older than 40 years [16]. Metastases to the placenta or embryo are exceedingly rare (one reported case only). Guidelines for the diagnosis, staging and non-surgical management of the pregnant woman with colorectal cancer are shown in Table 13.2.

Table 13.2 Guidelines for diagnosis, staging and non-surgical management of pregnant patients with colorectal cancer in comparison to general population

Diagnostic/ therapeutic modality	General population	Pregnancy
Serum CEA	Pre-surgical level evaluation for definition of prognosis and post-surgical monitoring for diagnosis of relapse	Similar use as CEA serum levels are not falsely elevated in gestation
CT of abdomen/pelvis	Indicated for imaging of extracolonic spread and intra-abdominal metastases	Contra-indicated because of increased risk for abortion, mutagenesis and teratogenesis
Abdominal ultrasound	Less sensitive than CT, with the exception of transrectal ultrasound	Sensitive for the imaging of hepatic metastases and lympadenopathy >1–2 cm

Table 13.2 *(continued)* Guidelines for diagnosis, staging and non-surgical management of pregnant patients with colorectal cancer in comparison to general population

Diagnostic/ therapeutic modality	General population	Pregnancy
MRT of abdomen/pelvis	As effective as CT, more expensive	May replace CT. Its use in the 1st trimester and gadolinium administration are relatively contra-indicated
Rectosigmoidoscopy	Total colonoscopy preferred	Safe during gestation
Colonoscopy	Routinely indicated for diagnosis of primary and synchronous cancers and biopsy	Probably quite safe, though experience is limited. Performed with special precautions for right-sided tumours
Adjuvant 5-FU-based chemotherapy	Routinely indicated for Dukes C and high-risk B2–B3 tumours	Contra-indicated during the 1st trimester, may be administered during the 2nd, 3rd trimesters or post-partum for Dukes C tumours
Adjuvant pelvic radiotherapy	Indicated for Dukes B2–B3, C rectal tumours either before or after surgery	Contra-indicated during pregnancy. May be administered for Dukes B2–B3, C rectal tumours either post-partum or after pregnancy termination. Causes permanent ovarian ablation

13.2.1.4 Surgical Management

Surgical resection of the intestinal tumour with adequate clear margins and locoregional lymphadenectomy is the mainstay of therapy for tumour control and provides significant prognostic information for the risk of malignant relapse. When distant metastases are present, a palliative by-pass operation for prevention or relief of obstruction/perforation is sometimes indicated. In pregnant women, the timing and type of surgery depend on the gestational stage, extent of disease, prognosis and wishes of the patient. Any surgical operation of a pregnant woman beyond the 20th week of gestation should take into consideration the "supine hypotensive" syndrome, caused by compression of the inferior vena cava by the enlarged uterus and resulting in reduction of cardiac preload, hypotension and sympathetic activation. A left lateral tilt position of the patient may be used to minimise this risk.

When CRC is diagnosed during the first 20 weeks of gestation, surgical resection is indicated so as to minimise the risk of locoregional tumour progression and metastases [17]. Older surgical series from the 1970s had reported an unacceptably high risk of foetal loss (as high as 23%), but advances in surgical techniques and supportive care resulted in superior outcomes in the 1990s: The rate of embryonal mortality has been reported as low as 3.8%, with the incidence of premature delivery and low birth weight remaining double that of the general population [18, 19]. Hysterectomy is required only for improved access to the rectum in difficult cases, upon uterine infiltration by tumour or when maternal life expectancy is shorter than the time needed for birth of a viable foetus [20].

When CRC is diagnosed during the second half of gestation (weeks 21–40), the operation is delayed until a viable foetus can be delivered. Ninety-five percent of embryos are viable by the 32nd–34th weeks; accordingly, induction of vaginal delivery is indicated at that time point [21]. After an intervening period of 1–2 weeks, necessary for the involution of the uterus and resolution of vascular congestion of pelvic structures, surgical resection of the intestinal tumour and lymph nodes takes place [3].

An emergency laparotomy may be necessary

upon occurrence of acute intestinal bleeding, perforation or obstruction for resection of tumour and management of the acute complication: This should take place immediately at any gestational stage. Visual inspection and biopsy of the ovaries has been advocated by some authors, in view of the high frequency of ovarian deposits. If the uterus is to be left in situ and the ovaries look normal, ovariectomy should not be performed [22]. The indications for delivery by means of caesarean section are identical to those of the general population, with two additional indications: the presence of a bulky rectal cancer which compromises the birth canal and the risk for extension of the perineotomy wound into a large anterior rectal carcinoma. When a caesarean section is planned, tumour resection may take place during the same operative procedure [22].

13.2.1.5 Chemotherapy and Radiotherapy

Metastatic colorectal cancer is an incurable disease, with a median survival of 14–20 months and a 5-year survival rate of 2%–5%. The pregnant woman with metastatic CRC should be informed of the perspectives for long-term disease control and the realistic aims of therapy, which are symptom control and modest survival prolongation. A primary decision which must be reached is whether continuation of pregnancy is feasible and/or desirable. Factors such as gestational stage, tumour burden and rate of disease progression as well as the patient's cultural, religious, ethical and personal beliefs will define the decision made. If the diagnosis is set during the 1st trimester and immediate institution of chemotherapy is warranted because of symptomatic, high-volume or rapidly progressing malignancy, pregnancy termination should be implemented. Foetal exposure to cytotoxic agents during the first trimester carries a high risk of malformations and abortion (15%–25%) [23]. If metastatic CRC is diagnosed during the 2nd trimester chemotherapy administration is relatively safe, as stillbirth or congenital defects are seldom seen (2%–3% of pregnancies). Premature delivery, growth retardation and low birth weight are seen in 15%–20% of such cases, though they are usually mild and reversible. A retrospective review of 355 pregnancies in 205 women concurrently receiving 5-fluorouracil (5-FU)-based chemotherapy reported delivery of healthy infants in all cases [24]. Advanced CRC diagnosed during the third trimester may be managed either with immediate chemotherapy or by withholding treatment until after the birth of a viable foetus (34th week of gestation). Chemotherapy should not be administered after the 35th week so as to avoid occurrence of spontaneous delivery when the mother is myelosuppressed [25].

Adjuvant 5-FU-based chemotherapy reduces the risk of locoregional or distant malignant relapse and improves survival of patients with resected Dukes C colorectal cancer (absolute survival benefit at 5 years of 10%–20%). Patients with resected high-risk Dukes B2 or B3 tumours (perforation, obstruction, T4 disease, grade 3, lymphatic/vascular invasion) probably derive a survival benefit, though a smaller one. Any cytotoxic agent should not be administered during the first trimester of pregnancy (period of organogenesis). After that period, the pregnant patient who had her Dukes C CRC resected during the first 20 weeks of gestation may be commenced on adjuvant 5-FU-based chemotherapy, provided she accepts a low risk of adverse effect to the foetus (probably lower than 5%–6%) [25]. Diagnosis of CRC during the latter 20 weeks of pregnancy is usually managed by follow-up, delivery in the 32nd–34th weeks and institution of adjuvant chemotherapy afterwards.

5-FU combined with calcium folinate (leucovorin) is the most widely prescribed chemotherapeutic regimen for the management of patients with advanced or early colorectal cancer. No mutagenic or teratogenic effects have been found in humans or animals for leucovorin; consequently, the 5-FU-leucovorin regimen is the safer choice when chemotherapy is administered to pregnant women within the first trimester [26]. Data on the effects and safety of DNA-topoisomerase I inhibitors (irinotecan), platinum analogues (oxaliplatin) and biological modifiers (bevacizumab, cetuximab) are either absent or scant. Their use is contraindicated during pregnancy.

Pelvic radiotherapy, before or after surgery,

reduces the risk of locoregional relapse of rectal tumours with extracolonic spread. Pregnant women with rectal cancer are deprived of this therapeutic modality as pelvic radiotherapy to a cumulative dose of 40–45 Gy will invariably lead to abortion, stillbirth, congenital malformations or severe growth retardation, depending on gestational stage. Any pregnant patient with localised rectal cancer requiring adjuvant radiotherapy to the pelvis should either discontinue pregnancy or defer radiotherapy until after delivery. Some surgical groups with high expertise in total mesorectal excision have reported locoregional relapse rates of 5% or less when the circumferential resection margins are clear, making radiotherapy unnecessary. In any case, pelvic radiotherapy administered either during or after delivery will cause permanent ovarian ablation and infertility, an effect quite devastating in young patients [27]. The pregnant patient with locally advanced, irresectable rectal cancer should terminate gestation in order to be managed immediately with induction pelvic radiotherapy with or without chemotherapy.

13.2.1.6 Prognosis

Retrospective data on the outcome of pregnant patients with colorectal cancer from the 1960s and 1970s created the impression that the carcinoma follows an aggressive course characterised by frequent relapse, early dissemination and fulminant progression. Several investigators have reported the presence of oestrogen and/or progesterone receptors in 5%–27% of colorectal tumours [28]. These hormones stimulated cellular proliferation in neoplastic cell cultures in vitro, an observation which created fears for accelerated cellular turnover in CRC of pregnant women under the influence of high serum oestrogen levels. More recent experimental data, however, with more sound methodological backgrounds reported a lack of oestrogen/progesterone receptors in colorectal cancer [29]. Oestrogens and progestogens do not seem to modify the risk of CRC development, as its incidence is not influenced by number of gestations or contraceptive use [30].

The initial conclusions from older series have been challenged by findings of more recent patient series. The most important prognostic factor which defines patient outcome seems to be the TNM tumour stage, in accordance with CRC in the general population. Other clinicopathologic factors that affect prognosis in both pregnant and non-pregnant women with CRC are presentation with obstruction or perforation, initial CEA serum levels, clear resection margins, histological grade and mucinous differentiation. Both young non-pregnant patients and pregnant women aged less than 40 share a modest to poor prognosis, a fact attributed to diagnostic delays leading to advanced cancer stage at presentation [31]. Several investigators have published relatively small patient series with 5-year survival rates around 40%. The common presence of ovarian metastases, the frequent mucinous histology associated with chemoresistance, the rapid cell turnover of the malignant clone due to gestational hormones and a fulminant biologic behaviour of the tumour, characteristic of young patients, have been proposed as alternative explanations for the adverse prognosis associated with pregnancy. Still, the 5-year survival of pregnant women with CRC is no different from that of general population patients with CRC of matched TNM or Dukes stage and number of involved lymph nodes (Table 13.3) [6, 31, 32]. Delayed diagnosis seems to be the most probable cause of pregnant patient presentation with advanced stage, high-volume CRC, while aggressive disease behaviour in young ages may be a minor contributor.

Table 13.3 Outcome of pregnancy-associated CRC by stage

Stage	5-year overall survival rate
Rectal cancer	
Dukes B	83%
Dukes C	27%
Dukes D	0%
Colon cancer	
Dukes B	75%
Dukes C	33%
Dukes D	0%
Number of patients	41

13.2.2 Other Gastrointestinal Tract Carcinomas

13.2.2.1 Gastric Cancer

Only 1% of gastric cancers are diagnosed in patients aged less than 30 years, and 3.5%–6.5% in those aged less than 40 years [33]. Based on the incidence of pregnancy in these age groups in Western societies, the expected annual incidence of gastric adenocarcinoma in pregnant women is nine new cases in the US and one to two in Germany, the UK, and France [34]. Despite these calculated figures, only 131 cases of gestational stomach cancer have been reported over the last 50 years.

Presenting symptoms consist of nausea, vomiting, anorexia, weight loss and epigastric pain, with common signs being chronic iron-deficiency anaemia, haematemesis and melena. Attribution of symptoms to the pregnancy or peptic ulcer disease is the rule, resulting in diagnostic delays. Commonly, the diagnosis of malignancy is made post-partum, when symptoms and signs persist. The median symptom duration has been found to exceed 6 months in pregnant patients, in comparison to less than 4 months in non-pregnant women with gastric cancer [35]. In two large reviews of reported cases, 65%–80% of gastric tumours had been diagnosed after the 30th gestational week. As a result, most patients are diagnosed with locally advanced or metastatic gastric cancer. Women with gastric tumours confined to the mucosa or submucosa made up only 3% of the Japanese review of 103 pregnant patients and 0% of the Western review of 31 pregnant patients. The rest of the patients harboured tumours infiltrating through the serosa (T3–4), involving locoregional lymph nodes (N1–3) or metastasising in distant sites (M1) in more than three-quarters of cases [36, 37].

In contrast to the general population, the majority (74%–95%) of gastric cancer cases associated with pregnancy are high-grade tumours, diffuse type according to the Lauren classification. Tumour growth follows a diffuse scirrhous pattern (Borrmann type III or IV). The histological features carry adverse prognostic information but characterise young, rather than pregnant, patients. Young women (<35–40 years of age) with gastric cancer develop ovarian, mesenteric-para-aortic nodal and peritoneal deposits in 20%–40% of cases, but rarely do so in the liver (<10% of cases, in contrast to 55% of gastric cancer cases diagnosed in patients older than 40). This metastatic behaviour has been reported as characteristic of diffuse-type gastric carcinomas [35, 38].

The reported survival of pregnant patients with adenocarcinoma of the stomach has been rather poor. Barely 30% of women survive longer than 6 months and 4% are alive 5 years after the diagnosis. In the Japanese review, a laparotomy was done in 77% of women and a potentially curative resection in 48%. The overall survival rates of operated women at 1, 3 and 4 years were 32%, 21% and 5%, while no woman with inoperable tumour survived longer than 6 months. In the much smaller Western review, laparotomy and gastrectomy were carried out in 93% and 60% of pregnant women, respectively. Overall survival rates at 1 and 3 years were 33% and 8%, respectively. The poor prognosis of pregnant gastric cancer patients is attributed to the diagnostic delay which results in disease presentation at advanced stages. An aggressive biologic behaviour of the tumour in younger patients cannot be ruled out, though no consensus exists regarding the latter in published retrospective series and case-control studies: Younger patients with gastric cancer have been reported to fare better than older patients in some series, while their outcome was similar to that of older patients in other series [33, 35, 38, 39].

Oestrogen and progesterone receptors have been found in 23% of gastric adenocarcinomas and in vitro experiments established the stimulatory effect of oestrogens/progestogens in neoplastic cell cultures and gastric tumour xenografts implanted in mice [37, 40]. As a consequence, the hypothesis of enhanced tumour cell proliferation in pregnant women due to the favourable hormonal milieu was put forward several decades ago. To test this hypothesis, Furukawa et al. analysed the clinical course of 20 young women with gastric cancer and a history of pregnancy during the previous 2 years in comparison to 44 young women diagnosed with the same tumour but without a history of gestation and 57 young male patients with gastric cancer [41]. Tumour stage was more advanced and survival was poorer in the group of patients with a history of pregnancy, a finding which was attributed to hormonal influences and immunosuppression. Those findings have not been confirmed by other investigators; in fact, several reported absence of hormonal receptors in 80%–90% of gastric tumours and identical clinical outcome of patients with and without a gestational history [37]. To conclude, only the delay of diagnosis and resulting presence of high-volume disease upon institution of therapy are convincingly responsible for the dismal prognosis of patients harbouring gastric cancer during pregnancy.

Early diagnosis of gastric cancer upon appearance of symptoms or signs is mandatory and the definite diagnostic modality is oesophagogastroscopy with biopsies. The safety of oesophagogastroscopy in pregnant women has been established by cumulative clinical experience. Cappell et al. conducted a large case-control study comparing 83 pregnant women undergoing upper GI endoscopy with matched pregnant (not undergoing the procedure) and non-pregnant (undergoing the same procedure) women as control subjects [42]. With appropriate monitoring of vital signs, avoidance of excessive doses of sedatives (meperidine and low or no midazolam doses safer) and expertise, the study reported no increase in adverse events in the pregnant patient group. Barium upper GI studies and CT of the abdomen are contraindicated because of the risks to the embryo. Unfortunately, the endoscopic study of the most common symptoms associated with gastric cancer would result in performance of 1,000,000 gastroscopies for the diagnosis of the nine malignant cases that occur annually in the United States [43]. The reason is the normal manifestation of these symptoms in 50%–70% of healthy pregnant women. Pregnancy-associated nausea and vomiting usually subside after the 12th to 16th gestational weeks; accordingly, its persistence during the second or third trimesters combined with other suspicious signs and symptoms should be investigated.

The management of the pregnant patient with gastric cancer is defined by the stage of malignancy, the stage of gestation and the patient's wishes. The general principle that the patient's life takes precedence over the embryo's life, when both cannot be preserved, should be discussed with the patient and family. Upon acute gastric bleeding, perforation or obstruction, surgical correction of the complication along with tumour resection according to oncologic principles should be carried out immediately, irrespective of the gestational stage. If the malignancy is diagnosed during the first 24 weeks of pregnancy, surgical resection of the tumour with parallel avoidance of disruption of the gravid uterus is advised. When diagnosis of malignancy occurs after the 24th week, the therapeutic choices are (a) observation until a viable foetus can be delivered (32nd–34th weeks) and then gastrectomy, (b) pregnancy termination and immediate gastrectomy and (c) attempt at gastectomy and continuation of pregnancy. The latter choice incurs risks for embryonal integrity and surgical as well as anesthesiological expertise are mandatory. When birth takes place via vaginal delivery or caesarean section, the surgical management of gastric cancer may take place immediately after birth or a few days later [36].

Adjuvant chemotherapy is of no clear survival benefit and should not be administered during pregnancy. Recent clinical trials demonstrated a statistically significant survival benefit with either three courses of pre-operative chemotherapy followed by surgery and three courses of post-operative chemotherapy or by post-operative administration of combined chemoradiotherapy. Of course, adjuvant post-operative chemoradiotherapy is only an option for pregnant women diagnosed with gastric cancer during the third trimester and can only be administered postpartum. Pre- and post-operative adjuvant chemotherapy can theoretically be given in pregnant patients after the first trimester, though the narrow risk-benefit ratio of such a therapy renders it unlikely to be implemented in clinical practice.

Metastatic gastric cancer is an incurable disease and chemotherapy only has a palliative intent. Its diagnosis during pregnancy should lead to pregnancy termination if it is estimated that the mother's life expectancy is shorter than the time required for foetal maturation and delivery. When birth of a viable infant is possible, the maternal prognosis and the prospects for therapeutic interventions of the metastatic malignancy should be discussed with the patient and her family. Only then should she be able to take some crucial decisions jointly with the family and treating physician regarding the fate of the pregnancy and the timing of initiation of chemotherapy. As discussed in earlier chapters, administration of the most active compounds (5-FU, cisplatin) is relatively safe for the mother and embryo (risk of congenital malformations less than 5%, growth retardation, low birth weight, premature delivery 15%–35%), provided it starts after the first trimester (organogenesis) [23].

When pregnancy is not terminated, the foetal prognosis is good. Of 134 pregnant patients with gastric cancer, 72% gave birth to healthy infants. When the diagnosis of cancer was established after the 30th week, viable foetuses were delivered in 88% of Japanese cases and 100% of Western cases [36, 37]. The baby is safe from malignant deposits, as only two cases of placental metastases and none of embryonal metastases have been reported in the literature to date [44]. Among curatively resected women, abstinence from further child-bearing for 3 years is advised, as more than 75% of malignant relapses occur during that time period.

13.2.2.2 Pancreatic Cancer

Adenocarcinoma of the pancreas usually affects elderly patients, while endocrine pancreatic neoplasms may affect younger patients. The vast majority of patients are older than 50 years and as a result its coexistence with pregnancy is very rare. To date, only seven cases of pancreatic adenocarcinoma and 19 of pancreatic insulinoma diagnosed antepartum have been published [45]. Tumour symptoms are often masked by pregnancy or falsely attributed to it (nausea, vomiting, weight loss, epigastric discomfort). Moreover, pancreatic cancer quite often has minimal symptoms and signs until late in its natural history. As a consequence, diagnosis of cancer at advanced stages was usually seen. Cancer of the pancreas has been linked to obstructive jaundice, pre-eclampsia, HELLP syndrome (haemolysis, elevated liver enzymes, low platelets) and intractable hypoglycaemia during the first trimester (insulinoma) in pregnant patients. Such a clinical picture or pregnancy-associated symptoms of excessive intensity should be investigated with a high degree of suspicion, especially in women older than 35 years. Of note, the patient age in the seven reported cases of gestational pancreatic cancer ranged from 37 to 45 years [6, 45, 46]. The biological behaviour of exocrine pancreatic cancer is similar to that affecting the general population, as Targarona et al. did not find expression of hormone receptors in a series of 15 biopsied pancreatic adenocarcinomas [47]. Moreover, large series evaluating the association of endocrine factors with pancreatic cancer mortality in 387,981 patients failed to find any, apart from a reduced relative risk of death (0.80) in women with five or more births [48].

The diagnostic approach consists of physical examination, full serum biochemistry, full blood counts, an ultrasound of the abdomen and a chest X-ray. Cytologic/biopsy diagnosis should be pursued by means of endoscopic retrograde cholangiopancreatography (ERCP), guided fine-needle aspiration or open biopsy. This is particularly important as space-occupying lesions of the pancreas may be benign cystadenomas, solid pseudopapillary tumours, lymphomas, neuroendocrine tumours or insulinomas, all of which are commoner than pancreatic adenocarcinoma in young pregnant women. In the case of diagnosis of malignancy, serum CEA and CA 19-9 levels may be used for follow-up and for monitoring response to therapy, as they are not influenced by pregnancy. On the contrary, serum alkaline phosphatase may normally increase two- to fourfold during gestation because of placental synthesis [15]. Instead of a CT, a non-enhanced MRI scan of the abdomen/pelvis may be used for tumour imaging and staging after the first trimester of pregnancy [13].

The management of the occasional pregnant woman with pancreatic cancer should be based on the same oncological principles which apply to the general population. In most cases, the malignancy is inoperable (80%–90% of the patient population) and the only realistic aim is symptom palliation. If the life expectancy of the affected patient is likely to be shorter than the time needed for delivery of a viable infant, pregnancy should be terminated. If the woman feels strongly in favour of pregnancy continuation, bile drainage for relief of obstructive jaundice and dietetic support should be implemented until delivery.

The few available data show that ERCP stenting or percutaneous transhepatic cholangiography and drainage are feasible and safe in pregnant women. The radiation dose to which mother and foetus are exposed during an ERCP procedure (contrast agent and serial X-rays) is 1–1.2 cGy, but increases sharply to 30–50 cGy when prolonged fluoroscopy is used. Although doses in excess of 100 cGy are needed to cause abortion, doses as low as 10–15 cGy in the first trimester may cause teratogenesis. Accordingly, bile stenting or drainage procedures under real-time fluoroscopic guidance are safe only during the second and third trimesters of pregnancy. During the first trimester, ultrasonic guidance and serial X-rays may be used instead. Alternatively, a palliative surgical procedure allows relief of obstructive jaundice and gastrointestinal obstruction and is safe for the embryo [49].

In the rare instances in which an operable pancreatic tumour is diagnosed during the first 24 weeks of gestation, a potentially curative surgical resection should be carried out. Accumulating experience with gastric and colorectal cancer cases shows that such an operation is compatible with continuation of pregnancy. Two case reports of successful outcome of distal pancreatectomy and of pancreaticoduodenectomy in pregnant women have been published [50, 51]. If pregnancy is more advanced, the choice of strategy must be individualised: Termination of pregnancy and surgery, attempt at surgical tumour resection with pregnancy continuation, observation until the 32nd–34th week for delivery and surgery post-partum are choices that carry risks and benefits. These need to be thoroughly discussed by the patient, family and managing team. The future mother should understand, though, that withholding surgical treatment until delivery of a viable foetus is not safe, as it may allow tumour progression and inability for subsequent surgical extirpation. On the other hand, she should also be aware of the low chances for long-term remission even in the face of a curative tumour resection. When pregnancy proceeds to delivery, the infant does not seem to be endangered by malignant deposits, as the experience with other, more common gestational tumours has shown. The first case of placental metastases from pancreatic cancer was reported as late as in 2006 [52].

In most cases, pancreatic cancer causes severe pain. The analgesic management of a pregnant patient is important for her quality of life, though difficult. Almost all medicinal agents should be avoided during the first trimester of pregnancy, a period crucial for organogenesis. When pregnancy is continued, paracetamol is safe during the second and third trimesters, though usually inadequate for pain control. Non-steroidal antiinflammatory agents and opioids, such as the safer agents pethidine and fentanyl, are relatively contraindicated during gestation as they have been linked to developmental disorders and embryonal respiratory depression [53]. Neurolytic blocks of the coeliac plexus and epidural analgesia are safer for the embryo and may diminish the patient's need for pain-killers, but experience is lacking. The need for aggressive analgesic management of the patient may well necessitate termination of pregnancy.

13.2.2.3 Hepatocellular Cancer

Hepatoma is seldom diagnosed in pregnant women. Up to 2005, 40 cases were published in the medical literature [54, 55]. This tumour more commonly affects men (male-to-female ratio 7:1 in Asia and 5:1 in Western countries) and ages older than 45 years, parameters that explain its rare association with pregnancy. In large patient series from Hong Kong and the United Kingdom, only 12%–17% of the patients were women and 2%–4% were of child-bearing age [56]. The most common risk factors incriminated for development of hepatocellular cancer are chronic viral hepatitis B or C: HCV infections make up 60%–70% of Western hepatoma cases, while HBV infection is widespread in Africa and Southeast Asia (60%–80% of cases of hepatoma). Alcoholic cirrhosis is responsible for 20% of hepatomas, while haemochromatosis, Wilson disease, primary biliary cirrhosis, autoimmune hepatitis, prolonged contraceptive use and chronic aflatoxin exposure make up the minority of remaining cases. It must be emphasised that women with hepatic cirrhosis due to chronic viral HBV or HCV infections or alcoholism usually have impaired fertility [57]. This epidemiological observation constitutes one additional reason for the rare coexistence of hepatoma with pregnancy. Other hepatic tumours that are occasionally diagnosed in pregnant women are hemangiomas, focal nodular hyperplasia, liver cell adenomas and an indolent variant of hepatoma, fibrolamellar carcinoma [58]. Imaging with ultrasound or MRI of the abdomen, serum AFP level determination and guided fine-needle aspiration biopsy of these lesions will establish the diagnosis, with the exception of hemangiomas, which should not be biopsied because of the risk of bleeding.

From a total of 40 reported hepatoma cases, more than half of the patients were of African or Far East descent. The median patient age at diagnosis was 31 years, 80% of patients had a history of two or more gestations while chronic hepatitis B or C was present in half of them. In 10% of women, a history of prolonged (more than 5 years) contraceptive use was present. Fatigue, ascites, nausea/vomiting, right upper quadrant dull pain and hypoglycaemia (probably via secretion of insulin-like growth factor) were the most common presenting symptoms. Occasionally, the tumour manifests itself as a medical emergency, when it causes intrahepatic or peritoneal bleeding or when it ruptures into the peritoneal cavity, or instead it may be an incidental finding during serum AFP level determination as part of routine screening for neural tube defects and Down syndrome. The diagnosis of hepatoma was established after the 20th gestational week in three-quarters of reported cases, in the vast majority of which the disease was either metastatic or locally advanced. The median tumour diameter exceeded 3 cm. Only four women had normal AFP levels, eight had serum AFP between 80 and 400 ng/ml while 26 had a serum AFP in excess of 400 ng/ml. In 40% of cases pregnancy was terminated either because of the poor maternal life expectancy or in order to allow immediate institution of hepatic resection, hepatic arterial chemoembolisation or palliative management. In 60% of cases a viable foetus was born, as the diagnosis had been set in advanced stages of pregnancy. In those cases, treatment was withheld for a few weeks until delivery; however, the patient's prognosis remained poor. Only four mothers were alive 6 months after diagnosis [59, 60].

A study of the epidemiological characteristics of the 40 reported cases leads to interesting insights into the disease and its natural course. The lag time from HBV/HCV infection until the development of hepatoma may be quite short in young pregnant women (5–15 years), in contrast to the prolonged time period (20–30 years) seen in the general population [57]. Young patients with HBV/HCV cirrhosis often have near-normal fertility, with infertility being restricted to those patients with long-standing, advanced cirrhosis. The prolonged use of contraceptives increases the risk of fibrolamellar carcinoma, a hepatocellular cancer with indolent behaviour and no association with chronic viral hepatitis [58, 61]. In five reported cases, earlier diagnosis and slow tumour progression allowed curative surgical resection resulting in superior prognosis for the patients.

The impact of the hormonal milieu in the pathogenesis and course of hepatoma has been debated for a long time. Mucci et al. conducted a case-control study of 50 hepatoma cases and 62 female controls and reported that women with hepatoma had a lower mean age at menarche and a higher mean age at menopause, with the risk of development of hepatocellular cancer increasing by 24% for each later year of menopause [62]. Other investigators calculated the relative risk for hepatoma as 3.5 in women with four or more previous pregnancies [63]. Oestrogen and progesterone receptors are commonly seen in hepatocellular carcinoma cells (20%–40%). Despite these hypothesis-generating data, the effect of pregnancy and its hormones in hepatoma is still not clear. Patient immunosuppression from placental steroids and cell cycle stimulation by high levels of gestational oestrogen/progesterones may contribute to rapid tumour growth [64, 65]. However, the delayed diagnosis due to the low-grade nature of symptoms and the masking of symptoms from pregnancy suffices in order to interpret the dismal prognosis of pregnant women with hepatoma. Moreover, a meta-analysis of 7 trials randomising 689 patients with unresectable hepatoma to best supportive care or treatment with tamoxifen failed to show any survival benefit for the anti-oestrogen [66].

A localised hepatocellular cancer diagnosed during the first half of pregnancy should be managed surgically (hepatic segmental resection) with a concurrent attempt at pregnancy continuation, provided surgical/anaesthesiological expertise and patient hepatic reserves are satisfactory. Quite often, though, these conditions are not met and pregnancy is terminated. Pregnancy termination is also advised when more radical treatment modalities are contemplated, such as liver resection and orthotopic liver transplantation. When hepatoma is diagnosed during the third trimester of pregnancy, the patient together with her physician may opt for withholding treatment until the 32nd–34th gestational weeks, when delivery of a viable foetus is feasible, provided her general condition, the hepatic reserves and the rate of progression of the tumour allow such a strategy [60, 67]. Locally advanced tumours may be palliated by locoregional nonsurgical therapies, such as percutaneous ethanol injection, radiofrequency ablation, chemoembolisation via the hepatic artery or systemic chemotherapy. The safety of these approaches for the foetus is not known. Consequently, when they have to be implemented before delivery, termination of pregnancy is advised. The time of institution of therapy, the options for terminating or continuing pregnancy and the life expectancy of a pregnant woman with unresectable liver cancer should be discussed with the patient and family so as to reach joint, informed decisions.

13.3 Urologic Malignancies

13.3.1 Renal Cancer

13.3.1.1 Epidemiology

The most common tumours affecting pregnant women are cancer of the cervix uteri, breast cancer, melanoma, lymphomas and leukaemias. Urologic cancer is extremely rare in gestation, despite the current tendency of women to bear children at more advanced ages. Renal cancer constitutes 3% of all malignancies seen in adults, with an annual incidence of 8.7:100,000 in the general population. A slight male predominance has been observed (male-to-female ratio 3:2) [68–70]. The environmental factor which increases the risk of renal cancer is smoking, while other factors such as chronic diuretic use, diet rich in animal fat, hypertension, diabetes and a female body mass index (BMI) higher than 35 in the age group 35–50 carry weak associations with development of renal carcinoma [71–73].

No clear picture on the association of renal cancer with female sex hormones has emerged to date from available epidemiological studies. The use of contraceptives or hormone replacement therapy does not seem to increase the risk of renal tumours. Women with delayed puberty and first pregnancy were reported to be at a lower risk of renal cancer, while another study found an inverse relationship between the number of pregnancies and this risk [73]. Still other investigators reported that the risk of renal cancer in women increases as the number of gestations increases [74]. Experimental animal models showed development of renal adenocarcinoma after ostrogen administration and tumour regression with progestogens or testosterone. Mundy et al. evaluated immunohistochemically the proliferation indexes Ki67 and PCNA, the apoptotic markers p53 and BCL2 and oestrogen/progesterone receptors in renal tumours and normal tissues of two pregnant patients with renal adenocarcinoma and five healthy pregnant women. No differential expression of PCNA, BCL2 or hormonal receptors was found between tumour and normal tissues, or between patients and healthy women. In normal tissues, increased expression of p53 was seen in the patient group, and of Ki67 in healthy women [75].

Older publications reported the incidence of gestation-associated urologic malignancies to be as high as 1 in 1,000 pregnancies, a figure which seems to be exaggerated and has not been confirmed [76]. Genetic factors, such as loss of genetic material in the 3p chromosome, carry an increased risk of tumorigenesis in the kidney. The tumour suppressor gene VHL in 3p25–26 is lost in the von Hippel–Lindau syndrome, resulting in overexpression of the vascular endothelial growth factor (VEGF) and dysregulation of the cell cycle. The net effect is the development of clear cell renal adenocarcinomas with abundant neovasculature [77–79]. The incidence of Von Hippel-Lindau syndrome in pregnant patients with renal cancer has not been studied, but a hypothesis has been postulated: Pregnancy is normally characterised by intense new tissue and vascular structure formation. This hormonal, cytokine and vascular milieu may contribute to the development and rapid growth of angiogenic tumours. Moreover, pregnancy incurs a natural "immunosuppressive" state, in order to protect the foetus from immune rejection by the maternal organism, an environment which could protect maternal tumours from immune surveillance. Still, this relative immune suppression is directed towards avoidance of rejection of the embryo only and pregnant women were shown to elicit normal immune responses against viral, bacterial and neoplastic antigens. The low number of cases of gestational urologic malignancies does not allow any safe conclusions to be drawn on the impact of pregnancy on the course of cancer.

13.3.1.2 Presentation

The first review of the literature on co-existence of renal neoplasms with gestation was reported in 1986 by Walker and Knight [80]. In total, 70 cases were reported, in 35 of whom a diagnosis of renal adenocarcinoma was established. In 16 patients an angiomyolipoma was found. Although these tumours are benign, their growth along with rich perfusion and increased intra abdominal pressure during pregnancy occasionally lead to rupture and massive bleeding. The histological diagnosis was nephroblastoma in five patients, adenoma in three, angiosarcoma in two and carcinoid tumour, fibroma, renal pelvis carcinoma, paraglomerular apparatus tumour and capsular osteoadenocarcinoma in one patient each. Four patients did not have a biopsy. An online search identified 69 cases of renal cancer in pregnant women from 1984 to 2004 (Table 13.4) [81–141]. Thirty-one pregnant women harboured renal adenocarcinomas, 27 angiomyolipomas, three nephroblastomas, three lymphomas and the rest oncocytomas, angiomas and paraglomerular apparatus tumours.

The classical triad of pain, haematuria and palpable mass was not present in any of the

Table 13.4 Primary renal neoplasms in pregnancy

Tumour type	1980–1986 [80]	1984–2004 [81–141]
Benign		
Angiomyolipoma	16	27
Adenoma	3	-
Paraglomerular apparatus tumour	1	1
Fibroma	1	2
Lymphoma	-	2
Oncocytoma	-	1
Angioma	-	1
Unbiopsied	4	-
Malignant		
Renal adenocarcinoma	35	31
Nephroblastoma	5	3
Angiosarcoma	2	-
Carcinoid	1	-
Capsular osteoadenocarcinoma	1	-
Renal pelvis carcinoma	1	-
Lymphoma	-	1

1984–2004 cases. In two patients, the diagnosis was incidental upon routine ultrasonographic follow-up of the embryonal formation. Flank/abdominal pain was the main symptom in half of the cases, while haematuria was present in 22%. Other symptoms and signs present in the clinical picture at diagnosis were anaemia, haemolysis, palpable abdominal mass, hypertension with proteinuria, recurrent urinary tract infections, suprapubic pain and dry cough in a patient with pulmonary metastases. In sharp contrast, the Walker review reported that a palpable mass was the presenting sign in 88% of cases with presence of haematuria in 47%. In a quarter of cases, the diagnosis of renal tumour was set after delivery. These differences between older and more recent patient series reflect the impact of high-precision modern imaging modalities (real-time ultrasound and magnetic resonance scans). Almost all cases in the 1984–2004 era were diagnosed by means of abdominal ultrasound. A supplemental MRI scan was done in 76% of cases. In 58% of cases the left kidney was affected by tumour, the diagnosis being established in the second and third trimesters in most cases.

13.3.1.3 Diagnosis and Staging

Older series suggested that the radiation exposure of the embryo should not exceed 5–10 cGy during the first trimester or 50–100 cGy during the second and third trimesters. However, the relationship between radiation exposure and risk of foetal mutagenesis/teratogenesis is not deterministic but statistic, meaning that no radiation dose carries a zero risk of foetal injury [142, 143]. Nowadays, a chest X-ray with appropriate abdominal lead shielding exposes the uterus/embryo to an extremely low dose of 0.0004 mGy and is considered safe. On the contrary, intravenous urography is not cost-effective, as the foetal radiation exposure is 10–45 mGy and small tumours may not be visualised, as they do not distort the pelvic/calyceal contour or draining structures [144].

Ultrasonography of the abdomen/pelvis is a routine staging procedure, frequently performed during pregnancy. It carries no risk for the foetus and has a sensitivity of 82% in the diagnosis of renal space-occupying lesions. Computerised tomography of abdomen/pelvis exposes the uterus to 18–25 mGy and should be avoided, unless a medical emergency warrants it (massive rupture and bleeding of renal tumours). MR imaging should be considered the radiologic procedure of choice when ultrasonography is not adequate for diagnosis or design of surgical approach. The method provides valuable information on tumour size, site, extension to adjacent tissues, cystic or solid appearance of tumours, lymph nodal status, vascular invasion and peritoneal/abdominal tumour spread. However, widespread use and repeated and prolonged scans should be avoided, as the absence of deleterious effects on the embryonal development cannot be firmly established. Several investigators recommend its avoidance during the period of organogenesis (1st trimester). Gadolinium, the paramagnetic contrast agent used, is taken up by the embryo, excreted via its urinary tract and swallowed with the amniotic fluid, and thus is absorbed again in the embryonal systemic circulation. In animal models, its administration in high doses caused embryonal defects and growth retardation. The drug is also secreted in maternal milk in low concentrations. Consequently, though gadolinium-enhanced MR scans provide valuable imaging details of tumour vasculature as well as of the urinary draining tract, its administration should be avoided either throughout pregnancy or at least during the first 24 weeks [145–147].

Urinary cytologic examination is advised, though its sensitivity is low and false-negative results are common. Cystoscopy and ultrasound-guided fine-needle aspiration biopsy of renal neoplasms are relatively safe and should be performed when indicated. Angiomyolipomas have a characteristic radiological appearance and may bleed when biopsied [76, 80].

13.3.1.4 Treatment and Prognosis

The proposed therapy of pregnant women with localised resectable renal carcinoma is radical nephrectomy. The decision on the timing of operation should be individualised according to the gestational period, the cancer stage and the patient's wishes. From a surgeon's and anaesthetist's point of view, pregnancy is not a contraindication for operation [148, 149]. Of course, the subtle adaptations of the cardiovascular, nervous, respiratory and metabolic systems of mother and embryo should be taken into consideration. Respiratory support and avoidance of hypotension/intravascular volume depletion are pivotal for preventing foetal hypoxia. The risks of suppression of the embryonal cardiovascular and nervous systems from excessive anaesthesia should be kept in mind. When the operative positioning of the mother is supine, especially in the second and third trimesters of pregnancy, the enlarged uterus may compress the aorta and inferior vena cava with adverse effects for the foetus and the mother; appropriate measures should be taken, such as adequate hydration and lateral positioning of the mother. The postoperative period may be complicated by premature uterine contractions when there is intense pain. Adequate analgesia is important and paracetamol, codeine with sparse administration of meperidine or fentanyl for severe pain is safe on a short-term basis. If the patient is diagnosed with localised non-bulky renal cancer after the 24th gestational week, follow-up until delivery of a viable foetus via caesarean section in the 32nd–34th weeks followed by radical nephrectomy either during the same operation or 2–3 weeks later is also an option which would minimise the risks of disturbing pregnancy at the cost of some delay in therapeutic intervention.

When the tumour is not resectable because of development of metastases, the mother's life expectancy and wishes should determine the proper course of action. Termination of pregnancy is advised, though some patients may feel strongly about having their child. Though not harmful to the foetus, hormonal therapy with progestogens has been abandoned as ineffective. Interferon therapy has been administered in pregnant women with hepatitis C, chronic myeloid leukaemia and hairy cell leukaemia without reported untoward effects for the embryo and seems to be safe for use during pregnancy [150, 151]. Interleukin-2 has been shown to cause placental detachment in pregnant rats and increased serum levels have been found in women with recurrent spontaneous abortions [152, 153]. As no experience of its safety exists in pregnant women, it should not be administered during gestation. Thalidomide is teratogenic and is absolutely contraindicated. There are no data whatsoever regarding the use of multi-targeted kinase inhibitors (sunitinib, sorafenib) in human pregnancy; accordingly they should not be administered. Radiotherapy cannot be administered during gestation; in addition, renal cancer is a radioresistant tumour. Palliative radiotherapy to bony metastatic deposits distant from the uterus (thoracic spine, skull, arms) may in theory be administered in pregnant patients in experienced centres with appropriate dosimetry and shielding, as successful outcomes have been reported by some centres treating pregnant women with lymphomas [154]. However, the lack of such expertise, the fear of litigation and the dismal maternal prognosis would in most instances necessitate termination of pregnancy.

In the cases reported from 1984 to 2004, the tumour was diagnosed at operable stages in the majority of women. In one case only, termination of pregnancy was chosen because of presence of pulmonary metastases. In one other case, an abortion occurred. After radical nephrectomy, at least 13 women continued their pregnancies and gave birth to healthy children via vaginal delivery. A caesarean section occurred in five patients, resulting in delivery of healthy infants. In two of those cases, caesarean section and radical nephrectomy were performed simultaneously while in another case nephrectomy was performed metachronously. One patient with locally advanced disease underwent tumour regional embolisation, while another had a partial nephrectomy, in both cases the pregnancy continuing normally. Overall, the accumulating evidence suggests that thanks to frequent ultrasonographic screening renal cancer is diagnosed without delay during pregnancy and radical nephrectomy is safely performed with good curative potential. Maternal and foetal prognosis is excellent, no different from that of non-pregnant patients with renal cancer. In fact, in a published series patients with renal cancer diagnosed during pregnancy had a better than expected survival [80].

13.3.2 Urothelial Cancer

13.3.2.1 Epidemiology

From 1966 to 2001, 24 cases of non-bilharzial bladder cancer were reported in the English medical literature and reviewed by Wax et al. [155]. Since 2001, seven more cases have been published [156–159]. Bladder cancer is the eighth most common cancer in women and most such tumours affect elderly patients in the sixth and seven decades. Urothelial tumours in women aged under 40 are typically low-grade superficial, non-invasive transitional cell tumours. One-third of these malignancies are associated with cigarette smoking, additional risk factors being frequent urinary tract infections, phenacetin use and exposure to naphthylamines, benzidine, nitrosamines, dyes, petroleum derivatives, aluminum. Squamous cell bladder cancer is related to urinary calculi, catheters and schistosomiasis. In pregnancy, the average age of affected patients was 30 years. Histological features of urologic gestational cancers are similar to those of tumours affecting the general population: 90% are transitional cell cancers, three-quarters of which represent papillary superficial disease, mostly grade 1–2 [155]. Squamous cancer is associated with schistosomiasis, while adenocarcinomas are rare (<1%). Transitional urothelial tumours affecting young patients should urge clinicians to study their family history and, in the presence of suspicion for a genetic background, to check the tumour for microsatellite instability (MSI). Presence of MSI would establish the diagnosis of hereditary non-polyposis colorectal cancer syndrome (HNPCC, Lynch syndrome). If this is the case, screening of the patient and family for MLH1, MSH2 and MSH6 mutations is mandatory [158].

13.3.2.2 Presentation, Diagnosis and Staging

The most common presenting complaint of pregnant and non-pregnant women is total gross painless haematuria and attention is needed so as not to confuse it with vaginal bleeding. If the source of bleeding is uncertain, a urine specimen obtained by catheterisation should be sent for analysis. Initial confusion of haematuria with obstetrical haemorrhage was reported in 7 of 24 pregnant women with bladder cancer. Irritative symptoms such as frequency, urgency and dysuria do not eliminate the possibility of malignancy. Urine cultures, microscopic analysis and cytology should supplement the diagnostic workup. Most pregnant patients with bladder cancer present in the second and third trimesters.

Imaging studies are helpful in detecting bladder tumours and nodal and distant metastases. Ultrasound is safe and visualises bladder filling defects larger than 2 cm, hydronephrosis/hydroureter, renal calculi, renal solid and cystic masses and hepatic deposits >1–2 cm. Despite the diagnostic difficulty created by the physiologic hydronephrosis of pregnancy, most recently reported bladder tumours in pregnancy were detected by ultrasound [155]. Intravenous urography is usually avoided during pregnancy because of the high ionising radiation doses delivered to the foetus. Cystoscopy is considered the most useful test, as it can be performed in the office with a flexible endoscope under local anaesthesia. In the pregnant cancer patients reported, the entire urethral/bladder mucosa was inspected without complications. When needed, cystoscopic biopsy or resection of tumour with underlying muscle is performed under regional or general anaesthesia [76]. A chest X-ray with abdominal lead shielding is safe and can show or rule out lung metastases>2 cm. Radioisotope bone scans and CT scans should be avoided during pregnancy. MRI avoids foetal X-ray exposure and is not contraindicated after the first trimester. MRI may be used for the detection of gross nodal metastases and local extension to muscle wall/perivesical fat or surrounding organs.

13.3.2.3 Management and Prognosis

Superficial tumours are resected cystoscopically with safety during pregnancy. Such an approach was implemented in 18 of 24 pregnant women with bladder cancer, with excellent tumour control [155]. Alternatively, such treatment of low-grade superficial tumours may be deferred until after delivery. The risk of non-invasive recurrence is related to the number and size of primary tumours, grade, lymphatic invasion and carcinoma in situ. However, follow-up approaches and adjuvant intravesical chemotherapy or immunotherapy may preoccupy the patient and her physician after delivery. Only one report described the use of adjuvant bacille Calmette-Guerin (BCG) immunotherapy during pregnancy (2nd trimester), without any problems encountered for the mother or foetus [159].

Radical cystectomy with pelvic lymph node dissection is the standard therapy for patients with muscle-invasive bladder cancer localised to the pelvis. In women, this procedure includes en bloc removal of the bladder, urethra, anterior vaginal wall, uterus, ovaries and pelvic peritoneum. Few such cases of invasive bladder cancer have been described in the literature [160, 161]. Some investigators suggest termination of pregnancy if invasive cancer is diagnosed during the first or early second trimester, followed by definitive treatment. If tumour is detected in the late second or third trimester, caesarean delivery at or beyond 32 weeks of gestation should be followed by radical cystectomy immediately. Hendry suggested early pregnancy termination and definitive therapy if the tumour was poorly differentiated and invaded the muscle wall [162]. Clearly, no consensus exists and few data are available to support any specific action plan. The managing team should individualise care for the patient, while respecting the woman's wishes with respect to the foetus. Adjuvant pelvic radiotherapy or systemic chemotherapy may improve locoregional tumour control and survival of patients with node-positive or perivesical fat-extending tumours, but in view of the toxicity and their marginal benefit, they should be administered post-partum.

Overall, the outcome of pregnant women with bladder cancer published in the literature does not seem to be worse than reported survival rates for non-pregnant patients with age- and stage-matched tumours. Accordingly, when diagnosis is set after the 24th gestational week, the urgency to definitively treat pregnant patients as soon as invasive bladder carcinoma is established is not supported by the available evidence.

13.4 Lung Cancer

13.4.1 Epidemiology

Lung cancer constitutes the first cause of cancer death in both sexes in developed societies [163]. The incidence of lung cancer increases with age and peaks in the sixth and seven decades of life. Only 1%–6% of patients are younger than 40 years, while 7%–12% are aged 40–50 [164–168]. The proportion of female lung cancer patients in the less than 40 age group is 24%–46%, clearly higher than the ratio of women in ages more than 40 years (12%–30%) [169–172]. The most common histologic type in younger ages in both sexes is adenocarcinoma, a type of tumour that is only weakly associated to smoking history [173, 174]. Studies in US colleges showed that smoking increased in frequency by 31% in females compared to a 23% increase seen in males over the last decade of the twentieth century [175]. This tendency, along with the delayed child-bearing in later reproductive ages, may lead to commoner diagnosis of lung cancer in pregnant women. Lung cancer ranked second in the causes of cancer death affecting women of reproductive age [176].

Smoking is the main risk factor incriminated for development of lung cancer. Tobacco smoke contains 500 volatile substances, such as aromatic hydrocarbons, aromatic amines, nitrosamines and more than 3,500 corpuscles. The risk of lung cancer increases with the tar content of the cigarette, the number of cigarettes consumed daily and the number of smoking years. Passive smoking also increases this risk (odds ratio 1.6) in a dose-dependent manner. Other risk factors with a weaker association are asbestos exposure, environmental pollution from SO_2, ozone, radon and wood or coal smoke.

The coexistence of lung cancer with pregnancy is exceedingly rare: only 25 cases have been described in the literature from 1953 until 2006 [177–201]. Affected women were aged 25 to 46 years (median 36 years). Only 56% of pregnant patients were smokers, a fact that emphasise the predominance of non smoking-related tumours in this patient group, as well as the importance of passive smoking. Non-small cell lung carcinomas (NSCLC) were diagnosed in 72% of patients, the rest harbouring small cell lung cancer (SCLC). The most common NSCLC histological types encountered were adenocarcinoma and large cell undifferentiated carcinoma. The median gestational age at diagnosis was 29 weeks (range 16–37 weeks).

13.4.2 Presentation

The clinical picture in pregnant women seem to be no different than those of the sex and age-matched patients of the general population. Signs and symptoms may be due to the primary tumour, locoregional extension, distant metastases and paraneoplastic syndromes.

Cough, haemoptysis, thoracic pain and dyspnoea are among the most common presenting symptoms related to the primary tumour. In occasional cases, the diagnosis is made by an incidental finding seen on a chest x-ray of an asymptomatic patient. Hoarseness of voice due to infiltration of the retrograde laryngeal nerve, dysphagia and superior vena cava syndrome due to esophageal and vena caval compression are seen, the latter mostly in small cell lung cancer. Horner`s syndrome is caused by involvement of the cervical sympathetic plexus by tumour. Pericardial and pleural effusion, infiltration of the upper ribs leading to pain (Pancoast`s syndrome) have been reported in pregnant patients as well. The presence of distant metastases may cause hepatic capsular pain, headaches, vomiting, seizures and bone pain. Paraneoplastic syndromes in the form of Cushing`s syndrome (ectopic ACTH production by tumour), hypercalcemia (secretion of PTHrP by squamous cell lung cancer), inappropriate antidiuretic hormone secretion (small cell lung cancer) and neurologic syndromes have not been described in pregnant women to date.

13.4.3 Diagnosis and Staging

The diagnosis/staging of lung cancer in a pregnant woman necessitates imaging of the tumour, definition of its locoregional and distant extent and biopsy. Physical examination, medical history and full serum biochemistry as well as blood counts are the sine qua non first steps. Serum alkaline phosphatase, LDH and beta-chorionic gonadotropin may be physiologically elevated by pregnancy, while anaemia and erythrocyte sedimentation rate (ESR) will be affected as well. A chest x-ray is associated with exceptionally low ionising radiation doses to the foetus and can be safely performed, whereas a CT of the chest should be avoided. Ultrasonography or MRI of the abdomen/pelvis will provide the necessary information regarding presence of distant deposits. Radioisotope bone scans should be avoided and work up of painful bony sites should be restricted to plain x-rays. Tissue diagnosis should be obtained by means of ultrasound-guided fine needle aspiration or bronchoscopy.

The current published knowledge about flexible bronchoscopy (FB) in pregnant patients is limited to a few case reports and one review article [202]. Maternal respiratory function adapts to gestation by an increased central respiratory drive, a decrease in functional residual capacity of the lungs, an increase of tidal volume, increased arterial oxygen levels and tissue oxygen consumption, increased airway mucosal oedema and limited diaphragmatic mobility. Available evidence shows that FB and endobronchial/transbronchial biopsy can safely be performed during pregnancy, provided certain conditions are met: It is always preferable to defer it until after delivery or after the 28th gestational week (when a viable foetus can be delivered if urgently required). When medically indicated, bronchoscopy should be performed by an experienced bronchoscopist with the patient in the left lateral decubitus or seated position. The patient`s medical history and physical condition should be assessed carefully. The procedure should be as brief as possible and done under maternal cardiac monitoring/oxymetry/sphygmomanometry in a well-equipped hospital with ready access to anesthesia, obstetric and neonatology services. Nasal oxygen should be given to keep maternal oxygen saturation at 97–100% levels. For conscious sedation, low doses of meperidine with or without midazolam is used judiciously, though benzodiazepine use is safer under foetal heart monitoring.

13.4.4 Management and Prognosis

Twenty-five cases of pregnancy-associated lung cancer have been published during the last 50 years [177–201]. Characteristics of these cases are shown in Table 13.5. All cases were diagnosed during the second and third trimesters, the median gestational week at diagnosis being 29 weeks. This fact probably allowed deferral of any antineoplastic therapy until after delivery of a viable foetus in the 32nd week and beyond, in those cases in which continuation of pregnancy was selected. In 21 of 25 cases, lung cancer was either locally advanced or metastatic at the time of diagnosis (stage IIIB/IV). Only two women received therapy during gestation, one radiotherapy and another cisplatin/vinorelbine chemotherapy after the 26th gestational week. No foetal toxicity was reported.

Fourteen women received therapy after delivery. Three underwent thoracotomy for surgical extirpation of malignancy; one of them also received adjuvant radiotherapy. Three patients were managed with definitive radiotherapy only, while one received concurrent chemoradiotherapy. Seven patients were managed with palliative chemotherapy only. Six patients received no treatment, while information regarding antineoplastic management is lacking in three cases.

Data on patient outcome were available in 22 cases. As expected, given the diagnosis of lung cancer at advanced stages (IIIB/IV in 84%), median survival was 4.5 months (range 1–42 months). The woman surviving for 42 months after diagnosis had a stage II squamous lung carcinoma at the third trimester and underwent pneumonectomy after delivery of a healthy infant. Data on foetal outcome were available in 23 cases. All 23 infants were born healthy and were doing well at a median follow-up of 14 months (range 2–60 months). Three of them were born premature. Of note, two infants presented malignant scalp deposits which were curatively resected: Both of them are alive and free from disease 5 years later. One infant born to a mother with small cell lung cancer presented visceral metastases, received intravenous cytotoxic chemotherapy and was in complete remission 1 year later.

Table 13.5 Characteristics of 25 reported cases of gestational lung carcinoma

N = 25	
Median age (range)	36 years (28–46)
Median gestational week (range)	29 (16–37)
Smoking history	
Yes	14
No	4
Histology	
NSCLC	18
SCLC	7
Stage	
I-II	4
III/IV	21
Therapy	
During pregnancy	2
Post-partum	14
No therapy	6
Chemotherapy	9
Radiotherapy	6
Surgery	3
Distant metastases	
Patient	16
Placenta	9
Foetus	3
Delivery of healthy infant	
Yes	25
No	0
Median survival (range)	4.5 months (1–42)

Placental involvement was present in 10 of 18 cases in which the placenta was examined at pathology. Lung cancer is the third most common gestational tumour spreading to the placenta, after melanomas and haematologic malignancies. The placenta should always be sent for pathologic evaluation after delivery and if it is found to be infiltrated by malignant cells, the infant should be screened and followed up for the possible development of metastases.

Overall, the available evidence does not establish a distinct biologic behaviour of lung cancer during pregnancy. Most tumours are diagnosed at advanced stages, a fact attributable to the masking of symptoms/signs from pregnancy, the avoidance of imaging studies utilising ionising radiation, the postponement of invasive diagnostic procedures and the low level of suspicion of managing physicians. Of course, a contribution to late diagnosis by fulminant disease course because of the gestational hormonal, immunosuppressive and perfusional environment cannot be ruled out. However, the outcome of pregnant patients does not seem to be different from that of non-pregnant patients with stage-matched tumours. Moreover, therapy of pregnant women is often deferred until after delivery, the delay in instituting treatment further compromising patient outcome. The rare patients with stage I/II NSCLC diagnosed in the first half of pregnancy should undergo surgical resection of the tumour, while patients in the late second/third trimester may opt for deferral until after delivery [203]. Stage IIIA patients should be treated with induction chemotherapy after the first trimester with relative safety, followed by definitive surgery or radiotherapy. Continuation of pregnancy may not be advised if radiotherapy is planned, although women with supradiaphragmatic Hodgkin lymphomas have been treated with carefully planned, restricted radiotherapy fields with appropriate abdominal shielding after the 17th gestational week without untoward effects for the embryo [204]. Intravenous cytotoxic chemotherapy has been administered with safety in pregnant patients after the first trimester, but experience with platinum salts, vinca alkaloids and taxanes, the most commonly used drugs in lung cancer, is restricted to a few case reports [205]. These show that the drugs are probably safe beyond the period of organogenesis. If the pregnant woman with stage IIIB/IV lung cancer is not willing to accept the low risk of congenital malformations (3%–5%), abortion and growth retardation (5%–10%) associated with chemotherapy in the second and third trimesters of pregnancy, the pregnancy should be terminated or treatment deferred until after delivery. For small cell lung cancer, intravenous cisplatin/etoposide may be administered after the first trimester and radiotherapy post-partum [206].

References

1. Wingo PA, Tong T, Bolden S (1995) Cancer statistics. CA Cancer J Clin 45: 8–30
2. Jemal A, Thomas A, Murray T et al. (2002) Cancer statistics, 2002. CA Cancer J Clin 52: 23–47
3. Nesbitt JC, Moise KJ, Sawyers JL (1985) Colorectal carcinoma in pregnancy. Arch Surg 120: 636–640
4. Girard RM, Lamarche J, Baillot R (1981) Carcinoma of the colon associated with pregnancy: report of a case. Dis Colon Rectum 24: 473–475
5. Nomura A (1990) An international search for causative factors of colorectal cancer. J Natl Cancer Inst 82: 894–895
6. Bernstein MA, Madoff RD, Caushaj PF (1993) Colon and rectal cancer in pregnancy. Dis Colon Rectum 36: 172–178
7. Van Voorhis B, Cruikshank DP (1989) Colon carcinoma complicating pregnancy: report of two cases. J Reprod Med 34: 923–927
8. Griffin PM, Liff JM, Greenberg RS et al. (1991) Adenocarcinomas of the colon and rectum in persons under 40 years old: a population-based study. Gastroenterology 100: 1033–1040
9. Cappell MS (2003) Colon cancer during pregnancy. Clin North Am Gastroenterol 32: 341–385
10. Shushan A, Stemmer SM, Reubinoff BE et al. (1992) Carcinoma of the colon during pregnancy. Obstet Gynecol Surv 47: 222–225
11. Brent RL (1980) Radiation teratogenesis. Teratology 21: 281–298
12. Reece EA, Assimakopoulos E, Zheng XZ et al. (1990) The safety of obstetric ultrasonography: concern for the fetus. Obstet Gynecol 76: 139–146
13. Kanal E (1994) Pregnancy and the safety of magnetic resonance imaging. Magn Reson Imaging Clin N Am 2: 309–317
14. Cappell MS, Sidhom O, Colon V (1996) A study at ten medical centres of the safety and efficacy of 48 flexible sigmoidoscopies and eight colonoscopies during pregnancy with follow-up of fetal outcome and with comparison to control groups. Dig Dis Sci 41: 2353–2360

15. Lamerz R, Reuder IL (1976) Significance of CEA determination in patients with cancer of the colon-rectum and the mammary gland in comparison to physiological states in connection with pregnancy. Bull Cancer 63: 575–586
16. Recalde M, Holyoke ED, Elias EG (1974) Carcinoma of the colon, rectum and anal canal in young patients. Surg Gynecol Obstet 139: 909–913
17. Arbman G, Nilsson E, Storgren-Fordell V et al. (1996) A short diagnostic delay is more important for rectal than for colonic cancer. Eur J Surg 162: 899–904
18. Kort B, Katz VL, Watson WJ. (1993) The effect of non obstetric operation during pregnancy. Surg Gynecol Obstet 177: 371–376
19. Saunders P, Milton PJD (1993) Laparotomy during pregnancy: an assessment of diagnostic accuracy and fetal wastage. BMJ 3: 165–167
20. Skilling JS (1998) Colorectal cancer complicating pregnancy. Obstet Gynecol Clin North Am 25: 417–421
21. Fetus and Newborn Committee. (1994) Canadian Paediatric Society and Maternal-Fetal Medicine Committee, Society of Obstetricians and Gynaecologists of Canada. Management of the woman with threatened birth of an infant of extremely low gestational age. CMAJ 151: 547–553
22. Walsh C, Fazio VW (1998) Cancer of the colon, rectum and anus during pregnancy: the surgeon's perspective. Gastroenterol Clin North Am 27: 257–267
23. Pentheroudakis G, Pavlidis N (2006) Cancer and pregnancy: Poena Magna, not anymore. Eur J Cancer 42: 126–140
24. Song H, Wu P, Wang Y et al. (1988) Pregnancy outcomes after successful chemotherapy for choriocarcinoma and invasive mole: long term follow up. Am J Obstet Gynecol 158: 538–545
25. Cardonick E, Iacobucci A (2004) Use of chemotherapy during human pregnancy. Lancet Oncol 5: 283–291
26. Briggs GG, Freeman RK, Yaffe SJ (2002) Folic acid. Drugs in pregnancy and lactation: a reference guide to fetal and neonatal risk. Philadelphia, Lippincott Williams Wilkins pp. 583–597
27. Doll DC, Ringeberg S, Yarbro JW (1988) Management of cancer during pregnancy. Arch Intern Med 148: 2058–2064
28. Korenaga D, Orita H, Mackawa S et al. (1997) Relationship between hormone receptor levels and cell-kinetics in human colorectal cancer. Hepatogastroenterology 44: 78–83
29. Slattery ML, Samowitz WS, Holden JA (2000) Estrogen and progesterone receptors in colon tumors. Am J Clin Pathol 113: 364–368
30. Chute GG, Willett WC, Colditz GA et al. (1991) A prospective study of reproductive history and exogenous estrogens on the risk of colorectal cancer in women. Epidemiology 2: 201–207
31. Smith C, Butler JA (1989) Colorectal cancer in patients younger than 40 years of age. Dis Colon Rectum 32: 843–846
32. Chan YM, Ngai SW, Lao TT (1999) Colon cancer in pregnancy: a case report. J Reprod Med 44: 733–736
33. Matley PJ, Dent DM, Madden MV et al. (1988) Gastric carcinoma in young adults. Am Surg 208: 539–596
34. Haas FJ (1984) Pregnancy in association with a newly diagnosed cancer-a population based epidemiologic assessment. Int J Cancer 34: 229–235
35. Dupont JB, Lee JR, Burton GR et al. (1978) Adenocarcinoma of the stomach—a review of 1497 cases. Cancer 41: 941–947
36. Ueo H, Matsuoka H, Tamura S et al. (1991) Prognosis in gastric cancer associated with pregnancy. World J Surg 15: 293–298
37. Jaspers VKI, Gillessen A, Quakernack K (1999) Gastric cancer in pregnancy: do pregnancy, age or female sex alter the prognosis? Eur J Obstet Gynecol 87: 13–22
38. Maeta M, Yamashiro H, Oka A et al. (1995) Gastric cancer in the young, with special reference to 14 pregnancy-associated cases: analysis based on 2325 consecutive cases of gastric cancer. J Surg Oncol 58 :191–195
39. Tso PL, Bringaze WL, Dauterive AH et al. (1987) Gastric carcinoma in the young. Cancer 59: 1362–1365
40. Wu CW, Chang YF, Yeh TH et al. (1994) Steroid hormone receptors in three human gastric cancer cell lines. Dig Dis Sci 39: 2689–2694
41. Furukawa H, Iwanaga T, Hiratsuka M et al. (1994) Gastric cancer in young adults: growth accelerating effect of pregnancy and delivery. J Surg Oncol 55: 3–6

42. Cappell MS, Colon VJ, Sidhom OA (1996) A study of eight medical centres of the safety and clinical efficacy of esophagogastroduodenoscopy in 83 pregnant females with follow-up of fetal outcome with comparison control groups. Am J Gastroenterol 91: 348–354
43. Donegan WL (1991) Invited commentary. World J Surg 15: 298
44. Bender S (1950) Placental metastases in malignant disease complicated by pregnancy. Br Med J 30: 980–981
45. Blackbourne LH, Jones RS, Catalano CJ, Iezzoni JC, Bourgeois FJ (1997) Pancreatic adenocarcinoma in the pregnant patient: case report and review of the literature. Cancer 79: 1776–1779
46. Porcel JM, Ordi J, Castells L et al. (1992) Probable pancreatic cancer in a pre-eclamptic patient. Eur J Obstet Gynecol 44: 80–82
47. Targarona EM, Pons MD, Gonzalez G et al. (1991) Is exocrine pancreatic cancer a hormone-dependent tumor? A study of the existence of sex hormone receptors in normal and neoplastic pancreas. Hepatogastroenterol 38(2): 16516–9
48. Teras LR, Patel AV, Rodriguez C et al. (2005) Parity, other reproductive factors, and risk of pancreatic cancer mortality in a large cohort of US women. Cancer Causes Control 16(9): 1035–1040
49. Pejovic T, Mari G, Schwartz PE (1991) Rare tumors in pregnancy. In: Lishner M, et al. Cancer and Pregnancy. Lippincott, Philadelphia
50. Lopez-Tomasetti Fernandez EM, Martin MA, Arteaga GI et al. (2005) Mucinous cystic neoplasm of the pancreas during pregnancy: the importance of proper management. J Hepatobiliary Pancreat Surg 12: 494–497
51. Kato M, Kubota K, Kita J et al. (2005) Huge mucinous cystadenoma of the pancreas developing during pregnancy: a case report. Pancreas 30: 186–188
52. Su LL, Biswas A, Wee A, Sufyan W (2006) Placental metastases from pancreatic adenocarcinoma in pregnancy. Acta Obstet Gynecol Scand 85: 626–627
53. British National Formulary (2000) Appendix 4: Pregnancy. British Medical Association and The Royal Pharmaceutical Society of Great Britain, BNF 40th edition, London, pp. 644–657
54. Lau WY, Leung WT, Ho S et al. (1995) Hepatocellular carcinoma during pregnancy and its comparison with other pregnancy-associated malignancies. Cancer 75: 2669–2676
55. Au WY, Lie AK, Liang R et al. (2002) Aggressive hepatocellular carcinoma complicating pregnancy after autologous bone marrow transplantation for non Hodgkin`s lymphoma. Bone Marrow Transplant 29: 177–179
56. Johnson PJ, Krashner N, Portmann B et al. (1978) Hepatocellular carcinoma in Great Britain: influence of age, sex, HbsAg status and etiology of underlying cirrhosis. Gut 19: 1022–1026
57. Jeng L, Lee W, Wang C et al. (1995) Hepatocellular carcinoma in a pregnant woman detected by routine screening of maternal alpha-fetoprotein. Am J Obstet Gynecol 172: 219–220
58. Kroll D, Mazor M, Zirkin H et al. (1991) Fibrolamellar carcinoma of the liver in pregnancy: a case report. J Reprod Med 36(11): 823–827
59. Cobey FC, Salem RR (2004) A review of liver masses in pregnancy and a proposed algorithm for their diagnosis and management. Am J Surg 187: 181–191
60. Jabbour N, Brenner M, Gagandeep S et al. (2005) Major hepatobiliary surgery during pregnancy: safety and timing. Am Surg 71: 354–358
61. La Vecchia C, Negri E, Franseschi S et al. (1992) Reproductive factors and the risk of hepatocellular carcinoma in women. Int J Cancer;52(3): 351–354
62. Mucci LA, Kupper HE, Tamimi R et al. (2001) Age at menarche and age at menopause in relation to hepatocellular carcinoma in women. BJOG 108: 291–294
63. Lambe M, Trichopoulos D, Hsieh CC et al. (1993) Parity and hepatocellular carcinoma. A population-based study in Sweden. Int J Cancer 55(5): 745–747
64. Rembriese R, Ptak W, Budak M (1974) The immuno-suppressive effect of mouse placental steroids. Experientia 30: 82–83
65. Moore JL, Martin JN (1992) Cancer and pregnancy. Obstet Gynecol Clin North Am 19: 815–827
66. Nowak AK, Stockler MR, Chow PK, Findlay M (2005) Use of tamoxifen in advanced stage hepatocellular carcinoma. A systematic review. Cancer 103: 1408–1414

67. Entezami M, Becker A, Ebert A et al. (1996) Hepatocellular carcinoma as a rare cause of an excessive increase in AFP during pregnancy. Gynecol Oncol 62: 405–407
68. Wingo AP, Tong T, Bolden S (1995) Cancer Statistics 1995. CA Cancer J Clin 45 :8–30
69. Landis SH, Murray T, Bolden S, Wingo PA (1999) Cancer statistics 1999 CA Cancer J Clin 49: 8–31
70. Chow WH, Devesa SS, WarRen JL, Fraumeni JF Jr. (1999) Rising incidence of Renal cancer in the United States. JAMA 281: 1628–1631
71. Kreiger N, Marrett LD, Dodds L, Hilditch S, Darlington GA (1993) Risk factors for renal cell carcinoma: results of a population-based case-control study. Cancer Causes Control 4(2): 101–110
72. Kamat AM, Shock RP, Naya Y, Rosser CJ, Slaton JW, Pisters LL (2004) Prognostic value of body mass index in patients undergoing nephrectomy for localized renal tumors. Urology 63(1): 46–50
73. Mellemgaard A, Engholm G, McLaughlin JK, Olsen JH (1994) Risk factors for renal-cell carcinoma in Denmark. III. Role of weight, physical activity and reproductive factors. Int J Cancer 56(1): 66–71
74. Lambe M, Lindblad P, Wuu J, Remler R, Hsieh CC (2002) Pregnancy and risk of renal cell cancer: a population-based study in Sweden. Br J Cancer 86(9): 1425–1429
75. Mundy A. Low-Stage RCC in pregnancy: Immunohistochemical evaluation. Personal communication
76. Loughlin KR (1995) The management of urological malignancies during pregnancy. Br J Urol 76(5): 639–644
77. Jennings SB, Gnarra JR, Walter MM, Zbar B, Linehan WM (1995) Renal cell carcinoma: Molecular genetics and clinical implications. Surg Oncol Clin N Am 4: 219–229
78. Latif F, Tory K, Gnarra J, Yao M, Duh FM, Orcutt ML, Stackhouse T, Kuzmin I, Modi W, Geil L et al. (1993) Identification of the von Hippel-Lindau disease tumor suppressor gene. Science 260(5112): 1317–1320
79. Gnarra JR, Zhou S, Merrill MJ, Wagner JR, Krumm A, Papavassiliou E, Oldfield EH, Klausner RD, Linehan WM (1996) Post-transcriptional regulation of vascular endothelial growth factor mRNA by the product of the VHL tumor suppressor gene. Proc Natl Acad Sci USA 93(20): 10589–10594
80. Walker JL, Knight EL (1986) Renal cell carcinoma in pregnancy. Cancer 58(10): 2343–2347
81. Cozzoli A, Teppa A, Gregorini G (2003) Spontaneous renal hemorrhage occurring during pregnancy. J Nephrol 16(4): 595
82. Schneider-Monteiro ED, Lucon AM, de Figueiredo AA, Rodrigues Junior AJ, Arap S (2003) Bilateral giant renal angiomyolipoma associated with hepatic lipoma in a patient with tuberous sclerosis. Rev Hosp Clin Fac Med Sao Paulo 58(2): 103–108
83. Herndon CD, Cain MP (2003) Antenatal hydroureteronephrosis presenting as an apparent solid renal mass. Urology 62(1): 144
84. Gnessin E, Dekel Y, Baniel J (2002) Renal cell carcinoma in pregnancy. Urology 60(6): 1111
85. Mydlo JH, Chawla S, Dorn S, Volpe MA, Shah S, Imperato PJ (2002) Renal cancer and pregnancy in two different female cohorts. Can J Urol 9(5): 1634–1636
86. Durrani OH, Ng L, Bihrle W 3rd. (2002) Chromophobe renal cell carcinoma in a patient with the Birt-Hogg-Dube syndrome. J Urol 168(4 Pt 1): 1484–1485
87. Qureshi F, Gabr A, Eltayeb AA (2002) Renal cell carcinoma (chromophobe type) in the first trimester of pregnancy. Scand J Urol Nephrol 36(3): 228–230
88. Ganzera S, Nguyen HN, Wiemann H, Schneider J, Jakubowski HD (2002) Retroperitoneal giant angiomyolipoma diagnosed post-partum with lymph node involvement. Dtsch Med Wochenschr 127(27): 1463–1466
89. Shiroyanagi Y, Kondo T, Tomita E, Onitsuka S, Ryoji O, Ito F, Nakazawa H, Toma H (2002) Nephron-sparing tumorectomy for a large benign renal mass: a case of massive bilateral renal angiomyolipomas associated with tuberous sclerosis. Int J Urol 9(2): 117–119
90. Gladman MA, MacDonald D, Webster JJ, Cook T, Williams G (2002) Renal cell carcinoma in pregnancy. J R Soc Med 95(4): 199–201
91. Dakir M, Aboutaieb R, Dahami Z, Meziane F, Ghazli M, Benjelloun S (2001) Kidney cancer and pregnancy Prog Urol 11(6): 1269–1273
92. Hatakeyama S, Habuchi T, Ichimura Y, Akihama S, Terai Y, Kakinuma H, Akao T, Sato S, Kato T (2002) Rapidly growing renal angiomyolipoma during pregnancy with tumor thrombus into the inferior vena cava: a case report. Nippon Hinyokika Gakkai Zasshi 93(1): 48–51

93. Henderson NL, Mason RC (2001) Juxtaglomerular cell tumor in pregnancy. Obstet Gynecol (5 Pt 2): 943–945
94. Tanaka M, Kyo S, Inoue M, Kojima T (2001) Conservative management and vaginal delivery following ruptured renal angiomyolipoma. Obstet Gynecol 98(5 Pt 2): 932–933
95. Mancuso A, Macri A, Palmara V, Scuderi G, Grosso M, Famulari C (2001) Chromophobe renal cell carcinoma in pregnancy: case report and review of the literature. Acta Obstet Gynecol Scand 80(10): 967–969
96. Khaitan A, Hemal AK, Seth A, Gupta NP, Gulati MS, Dogra PN (2001) Management of renal angiomyolipoma in complex clinical situations. Urol Int 67(1): 28–33
97. Mascarenhas R, McLaughlin P (2001) Haemorrhage from angiomyolipoma of kidney during pregnancy—a diagnostic dilemma. Ir Med J 94(3): 83–84
98. Kobayashi T, Fukuzawa S, Miura K, Matsui Y, Fujikawa K, Oka H, Takeuchi H (2000) A case of renal cell carcinoma during pregnancy: simultaneous cesarean section and radical nephrectomy. J Urol 163(5): 1515–1516
99. Shah J, Jones J, Miller MA, Patel U, Anson KM (1999) Selective embolization of bleeding renal angiomyolipoma in pregnancy. J R Soc Med 92(8): 414–415
100. Oka D, Mizutani S, Takao T, Inoue H, Nishimura K, Miyoshi S (1999) Spontaneous rupture of a renal angiomyolipoma in pregnancy: a case report. Hinyokika Kiyo 45(6): 423–425
101. Usta IM, Chammas M, Khalil AM (1998) Renal cell carcinoma with hypercalcemia complicating a pregnancy: case report and review of the literature. Eur J Gynaecol Oncol 19(6): 584–587
102. Lesourd B, Siquier J, Haillot O, Lanson Y (1997) Nephrectomy for cancer in pregnant women. Apropos of a case J Urol (Paris) 103(1–2): 59–61
103. Lesourd B, Peyrat L, Haillot O, Lanson Y (1998) Discovery of a renal chromophobe cell carcinoma in a pregnant woman. Apropos of a case. Ann Urol (Paris) 32(3):133–137
104. Forsnes EV, Eggleston MK, Burtman M (1996) Placental abruption and spontaneous rupture of renal angiomyolipoma in a pregnant woman with tuberous sclerosis. Obstet Gynecol 88 (4 Pt 2): 725
105. Pobil Moreno JL, Martinez Rodriguez J, Maestro Duran JL, Morales Lopez A (1996) Renal incidentaloma and pregnancy. Arch Esp Urol 49(7): 755–757
106. Yanai H, Sasagawa I, Kubota Y, Ishigooka M, Hashimoto T, Kaneko H, Nakada T (1996) Spontaneous hemorrhage during pregnancy secondary to renal angiomyolipoma. Urol Int 56(3): 188–191
107. Wolff JM, Jung PK, Adam G, Jakse G (1995) Nontraumatic rupture of the urinary tract during pregnancy. Br J Urol 76(5): 645–648
108. Farina LA (1995) Rapidly growing renal angiomyolipoma associated with pregnancy. Actas Urol Esp 19(5): 425–427
109. Monga M, Benson GS, Parisi VM (1995) Renal cell carcinoma presenting as hemolytic anemia in pregnancy. Am J Perinatol 12(2): 84–86
110. Gross AJ, Zoller G, Hermanns M, Ringert RH (1995) Renal cell carcinoma during pregnancy. Br J Urol 75(2): 254–255
111. Ponsot Y, Blouin D, Carmel M (1994) Hemorrhagic rupture of an angiomyolipoma during pregnancy. Review of the literature apropos of a case. Prog Urol 4(4): 578–581
112. Fernandez Arjona M, Minguez R, Serrano P, Sanz J, Teba F, Peinado F, Nieto S, Pereira I (1994) Rapidly-growing renal angiomyolipoma associated with pregnancy. Actas Urol Esp 18(7): 755–757
113. Smith DP, Goldman SM, Beggs DS, Lanigan PJ (1994) Renal cell carcinoma in pregnancy: report of three cases and review of the literature. Obstet Gynecol 83(5 Pt 2): 818–820
114. Thomas D, Henriet J, Schellinck P, Engelholm L, Corbusier A, Larsimont D (1994) Kidney cancer: fortuitous discovery of a para-uterine mass at the beginning of pregnancy. J Gynecol Obstet Biol Reprod (Paris) 23(2): 188–192
115. Bartha Rasero JL, Bedoya Bergua C, Diaz Cano S, Sanchez Ramos J (1993) Renal-cell adenocarcinoma and massive retroperitoneal hemorrhage during pregnancy. Arch Esp Urol 46(5): 421–423
116. Morrison JJ, Robinson RE (1992) Renal cell carcinoma: an unusual cause of second trimester hypertension. Br J Obstet Gynaecol 99(9): 775–776
117. Sheil O, Redman CW, Pugh C (1991) Renal failure in pregnancy due to primary renal lymphoma. Case report. Br J Obstet Gynaecol 98(2): 216–217

118. Gutierrez Banos JL, Portillo Martin JA, Martin Garcia B, Hernandez Rodriguez R (1990) Adenocarcinoma of the kidney in pregnancy. Presentation of a case. Arch Esp Urol 43(3): 296–297
119. Fraser WD, Auger M, Onerheim RM (1989) Renal oncocytoma in pregnancy: a case report. Can J Surg 32(2): 124–126
120. Meredith WT, Levine E, Ahlstrom NG, Grantham JJ (1988) Exacerbation of familial renal lymphangiomatosis during pregnancy. AJR Am J Roentgenol 151(5): 965–966
121. Ozmen M, Deren O, Akata D, Akhan O, Ozen H, Durukan T (2001) Renal lymphangiomatosis during pregnancy: management with percutaneous drainage. Eur Radiol 11(1): 37–40
122. Czerkwinski J, Marianowski L, Szymanowski J, Ulanowska D (1988) A case of spontaneous rupture of simple renal angioma in pregnancy. Wiad Lek 41(19): 1318–1321
123. Selli C, Bartolozzi C, Amorosi A, Carini M (1988) Incidental finding of renal cell carcinoma with histological regressive aspects in a pregnant woman. Eur Urol 15(3–4): 287–289
124. Lipman JC, Loughlin K, Tumeh SS (1987) Bilateral renal masses in a pregnant patient with tuberous sclerosis. Invest Radiol 22(11): 912–915
125. Atalla A, Page IJ, Young KR, Payne MJ, Elwood JS (1987) Rupture of angiomyolipoma of the kidney presenting as puerperal collapse. J R Army Med Corps 133(3): 166–168
126. Steiner H, Kullnig P, Petritsch P, Stenzel A, Ratschek M (1987) Renal cell carcinoma in a 19-year-old female manifested during pregnancy. ROFO Fortschr Geb Rontgenstr Nuklearmed 147(4): 457–459
127. Podluzhnyi GA, Braganets AM (1987) Spontaneous rupture of nephrocarcinoma in full-term pregnancy. Akush Ginekol (Mosk) (6): 67–68
128. Klein VR, Laifer S, Timoll EA, Repke JT (1987) Renal cell carcinoma in pregnancy. Obstet Gynecol 69(3 Pt 2): 531–533
129. Wiltschova M, Janku K, Uhlir M (1987) Grawitz tumor in pregnancy. Zentralbl Gynakol 109(16): 1042–1045
130. Ohba S, Moriguchi H, Tanaka S, Kobayashi Y, Ishiyama S, Gotoh K, Tozuka K, Tokue A, Yonese Y (1986) A case of renal cell carcinoma during pregnancy. Hinyokika Kiyo 32(5): 751–756
131. Malone MJ, Johnson PR, Jumper BM, Howard PJ, Hopkins TB, Libertino JA (1986) Renal angiomyolipoma: 6 case reports and literature review. J Urol 135(2): 349–353
132. Lewis EL, Palmer JM (1985) Renal angiomyolipoma and massive retroperitoneal hemorrhage during pregnancy. West J Med 143(5): 675–676
133. Snoddy WM, Nelson RP, Nyberg LM Jr, Turner WR Jr, Curry N, Betsill W Jr, Rous SN (1985) Symptomatic renal mass in a patient with a positive pregnancy test. J Urol 133(6): 1015–1018
134. Shinoda I, Takeuchi T, Fujimoto Y, Kuriyama M, Ban Y, Nishiura T, Setsuda O, Shinoda T (1985) A case of postpartum spontaneous rupture of an angiomyolipoma. Hinyokika Kiyo 31(6): 1027–1036
135. Pozzi V, Cappa F, De Bernardinis G, Ventura T, Mascaretti G (1985) A case of renal angiomyolipoma in pregnancy Minerva Ginecol 37(4): 147–152
136. Le Guillou M, Ferriere JM, Barthaburu D, Nony P, Piechaud T, Gaston R (1985) Renal cancer in the pregnant woman. Ann Urol (Paris) 19(1): 69–70
137. Steiner E, Devaud G, Etienne P, Colombeau P (1984) Isolated arterial hypertension during pregnancy disclosing a malignant tumor of the kidney. Apropos of a case. J Chir (Paris) 121(2): 123–125
138. Bozeman G, Bissada NK, Abboud MR, Laver J (1995) Adult Wilms' tumor: prognostic and management considerations. Urology 45(6): 1055–1058
139. Swierz J, Stawarz B (1994) Wilms' tumor in a 22-year old woman during pregnancy. Pol Tyg Lek 49(8–9): 198–199
140. Davis LW (1987) Wilms' tumor complicating pregnancy: report of a case. J Am Osteopath Assoc 87(4): 306–309
141. Karavasilis V, Briasoulis E, Mauri D, Zioga A, Pavlidis N (2003) Coexistence of renal cell carcinoma and pregnancy. A report of a case. F Clin Oncol 2(1): 68–71
142. Dumas JP, Colombeau P, Steiner E, Jouvie J (1984) Tumors of the kidney and pregnancy. Ann Urol (Paris) 18(5): 339–341
143. Harvey EB, Boice JD Jr, Honeyman M, Flannery JT (1985) Prenatal x-ray exposure and childhood cancer in twins. N Engl J Med 312(9):541–545
144. Pentheroudakis G, Pavlidis N (2006) Cancer and pregnancy: Poena Magna, not anymore. Eur J Cancer 42:126–140

145. Levine D, Barnes PD, Edelman RR (1999) Obstetric MR imaging. Radiology 211:609–617
146. Nagayama M, Watanabe Y, Okumura A, Amoh Y, Nakashita S, Dodo Y (2002) Fast MR imaging in obstetrics. Radiographics 22(3): 563–80; discussion 580–582
147. Shellock FG, Kanal E (1999) Safety of magnetic resonance imaging contrast agents. J Magn Reson Imaging 10: 477–484
148. Hendry WF (1997) Management of urological tumours in pregnancy. Br J Urol 80 (Suppl 1): 24–28
149. Rosen MA (1999) Management of anesthesia for the pregnant surgical patient. Anesthesiology 91(4): 1159–1163
150. Hiratsuka M, Minakami H, Koshizuka S, Sato I (2000) Administration of interferon-alpha during pregnancy: effects on fetus. J Perinat Med 28(5): 372–376
151. Ozaslan E, Yilmaz R, Simsek H, Tatar G (2002) Interferon therapy for acute hepatitis C during pregnancy. Ann Pharmacother 36(11): 1715–1718
152. Shiraishi H, Hayakawa S, Satoh K (1996) Murine experimental abortion by IL-2 administration is caused by activation of cytotoxic T lymphocytes and placental apoptosis. J Clin Lab Immunol 48(3): 93–108
153. Rezaei A, Dabbagh A (2002) T-helper-1 cytokines increase during early pregnancy in women with a history of recurrent spontaneous abortion. Med Sci Monit 8: CR607–CR610
154. Cutuli BF, Methlin A, Teissier E, Schumacher C, Jung GM (1990) Radiation therapy in the treatment of metastatic renal-cell carcinoma. Prog Clin Biol Res 348:179–186
155. Wax JR, Pinette MG, Blackstone J et al. (2002) Non-bilharzial bladder carcinoma complicating pregnancy: review of the literature. Obstet Gynecol Surv 57: 236–244
156. Castrillo HA, Villanueva Pena A, de Rodriguez E et al. (2005) Hematuria during pregnancy caused by a bladder tumour. Report of 2 cases. Actas Urol Esp 29:981–984
157. Spahn M, Bader P, Westermann D et al. (2005) Bladder carcinoma during pregnancy. Urol Int 74: 153–159
158. Mitra S, Williamson JG, Bullock KN et al. (2003) Bladder cancer in pregnancy. J Obstet Gynaecol 23: 440–442
159. Wax JR, Ross J, Marotto L et al. (2002) Nonbilharzial bladder carcinoma complicating pregnancy-treatment with BCG. Am J Obstet Gynecol 187: 239–240
160. Choate JW, Thiede A, Miller HC (1964) Carcinoma of the bladder in pregnancy- report of three cases. Am J Obstet Gynecol 90: 526–530
161. Dogra PN, Wadhwa SN, Gupta R (1991) Primary bladder carcinoma presenting during pregnancy-a report of two cases. Indian J Urol 8: 51–52
162. Hendry WF (1997) Management of urological tumours in pregnancy. Br J Urol (suppl 1)80: 24–28
163. Deneffe G, Lacquet LM, Verbeken E, Vermaut G (1988) Surgical treatment of bronchogenic carcinoma: a retrospective study of 720 thoracotomies. Ann Thorac Surg. 45(4): 380–383
164. Antkowiak JG, Regal AM, Takita H (1989) Bronchogenic carcinoma in patients under age 40. Ann Thorac Surg 47(3): 391-393
165. McDuffie HH, Klaassen DJ, Dosman JA (1989) Characteristics of patients with primary lung cancer diagnosed at age of 50 years or younger. Chest 96(6):1298–1301
166. Radzikowska E, Roszkowski K, Glaz P (2001) Lung cancer in patients under 50 years old. Lung Cancer 33(2–3): 203–211
167. Ramalingam S, Pawlish K, Gadgeel S, Demers R, Kalemkerian GP (1998) Lung cancer in young patients: analysis of a Surveillance, Epidemiology, and End Results database. J Clin Oncol 16(2): 651–657
168. Whooley BP, Urschel JD, Antkowiak JG, Takita H (1999) Bronchogenic carcinoma in young patients. J Surg Oncol 71(1): 29–31
169. Maruyama R, Yoshino I, Yohena T, Uehara T, Kanematsu T, Kitajima M, Teruya T, Ichinose Y (2001) Lung cancer in patients younger than 40 years of age. J Surg Oncol 77(3): 208–212
170. Green LS, Fortoul TI, Ponciano G, Robles C, Rivero O (1993) Bronchogenic cancer in patients under 40 years old. The experience of a Latin American country. Chest 104(5): 1477–1481
171. Bourke W, Milstein D, Giura R, Donghi M, Luisetti M, Rubin AH, Smith LJ (1992) Lung cancer in young adults. Chest 102(6): 1723–1729
172. Roviaro GC, Varoli F, Zannini P, Fascianella A, Pezzuoli G (1985) Lung cancer in the young. Chest 87(4): 456–459
173. Allen HH, Nisker JA (1986) Cancer in Pregnancy. Futura Publishing Company, Mt. Kisco, New York, p. 3

174. Doll DC, Ringenberg QS, Yarbro JW (1988) Management of cancer during pregnancy. Arch Intern Med 148(9): 2058–2064
175. Sutcliffe SB (1985) Treatment of neoplastic disease during pregnancy: maternal and fetal effects. Clin Invest Med 8(4): 333–338
176. Reynoso EE, Shepherd FA, Messner HA, Farquharson HA, Garvey MB, Baker MA (1987) Acute leukemia during pregnancy: the Toronto Leukemia Study Group experience with long-term follow-up of children exposed in utero to chemotherapeutic agents. J Clin Oncol 5(7):1098–1106
177. Pawelec D, Madey B (1976) Adenocarcinoma of the lung with metastasis in a 39-year-old pregnant woman. Pneumonol Pol 44(3): 283
178. Read EJ Jr, Platzer PB (1981) Placental metastasis from maternal carcinoma of the lung. Obstet Gynecol 58(3): 387–391
179. Reiter AA, Carpenter RJ, Dudrick SJ, Hinkley CM (1985) Pregnancy associated with advanced adenocarcinoma of the lung. Int J Gynaecol Obstet 23(1): 75–78
180. Stark P, Greene RE, Morgan G, Hildebrandt-Stark HE (1985) Lung cancer and pregnancy. Radiologe 25(1): 30–32
181. Suda R, Repke JT, Steer R, Niebyl JR (1986) Metastatic adenocarcinoma of the lung complicating pregnancy. A case report. J Reprod Med 31(12): 1113–1116
182. Dildy GA 3rd, Moise KJ Jr, Carpenter RJ Jr, Klima T (1989) Maternal malignancy metastatic to the products of conception: a review. Obstet Gynecol Surv 44 (7): 535–540
183. Bruhwiler H, Wild A, Luscher KP (1988) Bronchus cancer and pregnancy. Geburtshilfe Frauenheilkd 48(9): 654–655
184. Delerive C, Locquet F, Mallart A, Janin A, Gosselin B (1989) Placental metastasis from maternal bronchial oat cell carcinoma. Arch Pathol Lab Med 113(5): 556–558
185. Harpold TL, Wang MY, McComb JG, Monforte HL, Levy ML, Reinisch JF (2001) Maternal lung adenocarcinoma metastatic to the scalp of a fetus. Case report. Pediatr Neurosurg 35(1): 39–42
186. Janne PA, Rodriguez-Thompson D, Metcalf DR, Swanson SJ, Greisman HA, Wilkins-Haug L, Johnson BE (2001) Chemotherapy for a patient with advanced non-small-cell lung cancer during pregnancy: a case report and a review of chemotherapy treatment during pregnancy. Oncology 61(3): 175–183
187. Jackisch C, Louwen F, Schwenkhagen A, Karbowski B, Schmid KW, Schneider HP, Holzgreve W (2003) Lung cancer during pregnancy involving the products of conception and a review of the literature. Arch Gynecol Obstet 268(2): 69–77
188. Tolar J, Coad JE, Neglia JP (2002) Transplacental transfer of small-cell carcinoma of the lung. N Engl J Med 346(19): 1501–1502
189. Kochman AT, Rabczynski JK, Baranowski W, Palczynski B, Kowalski P (2001) Metastases to the products of conception from a maternal bronchial carcinoma. A case report and review of literature. Pol J Pathol 52(3): 137–140
190. Mujaibel K, Benjamin A, Delisle MF, Williams K (2001) Lung cancer in pregnancy: case reports and review of the literature. J Matern Fetal Med 10(6): 426–432
191. Walker JW, Reinisch JF, Monforte HL (2002) Maternal pulmonary adenocarcinoma metastatic to the fetus: first recorded case report and literature review. Pediatr Pathol Mol Med 21(1): 57–69
192. Wong CM, Lim KH, Liam CK (2003) Metastatic lung cancer in pregnancy. Respirology 8(1): 107–109
193. Stewart A, Kneale GW (1970) Radiation dose effects in relation to obstetric x-rays and childhood cancers. Lancet 1(7658): 1185–1188
194. Bithell JF, Stiller CA (1988) A new calculation of the carcinogenic risk of obstetric X-raying. Stat Med 7(8): 857–864
195. Yoshimoto Y (1990) Cancer risk among children of atomic bomb survivors. A review of RERF epidemiologic studies. Radiation Effects Research Foundation. JAMA 264(5): 596–600
196. Jemal A, Thomas A, Murray T, Thun M (2002) Cancer statistics, 2002. CA Cancer J Clin 52(1): 23–47
197. Barr J.S (1953) Placental metastases from a bronchial carcinoma. J Obstet Gynaecol Br Emp 60: 895–897
198. Hesketh J (1962) A case of carcinoma of the lung with secondary deposits in the placenta. J Obstet Gynaecol Br Comm 69: 514
199. Jones EM (1969) Placental metastases from bronchial carcinoma. Br Med J 2 (655): 491–492
200. Penha DS, Salge AK, Tironi F et al. (2006) Bronchogenic carcinoma of squamous cells in a young pregnant woman. Ann Diagn Pathol 10: 235–238

201. Folk JJ, Curioca J, Nosovitch JT, Silverman RK (2004) Poorly differentiated large cell adenocarcinoma of the lung metastatic to the placenta: a case report. J Reprod Med 49: 395–397
202. Bahhady IJ, Ernst A (2004) Risks of and recommendations for flexible bronchoscopy in pregnancy. Chest 126: 1974–1981
203. Bains MS, Beattie EJ Jr. (1974) Thoracic surgery in pregnancy. In: HRK Barber, EA Gaber (eds). Surgical disease in pregnancy. WB Saunders, Philadelphia, pp. 62–76
204. Redman JR, Bajorunas DR, Lacher MJ (1990) Hodgkin's disease: pregnancy and progeny. In: Lacher MJ, Redman JR (eds). Hodgkin's disease, The Consequence of survival. Lea & Febiger, Philadelphia, pp. 244–266
205. Potluri V, Lewis D, Burton GV (2006) Chemotherapy with taxanes in breast cancer during pregnancy: case report and review of the literature. Clin Breast Cancer 7:167–170
206. Leslie KK, Koil C, Rayburn WF (2005) Chemotherapeutic drugs in pregnancy. Obstet Gynecol Clin North Am 32: 627–640

14 Melanoma During Pregnancy: Epidemiology, Diagnosis, Staging, Clinical Picture

M. Lens

Recent Results in Cancer Research, Vol. 178

14.1 Introduction

Since the incidence of cutaneous melanoma is continuing to increase among all fair-skinned populations, the coexistence of melanoma and pregnancy or desire to conceive is increasing as well. Cutaneous melanoma may be the most frequently encountered malignancy during pregnancy. The influence of pregnancy on the development and prognosis of melanoma has been a matter of intense research for years. For many years, there has been controversy in the medical community regarding the correlation of female reproductive factors and hormones with the development and outcome of malignant melanoma.

This paper addresses epidemiological aspects of melanoma during pregnancy and the current evidence on the effect of hormonal and reproductive factors on incidence and prognosis of melanoma. Results from epidemiological studies assessing effect of pregnancy on melanoma have been analysed in detail. Diagnostic aspects of cutaneous melanoma during pregnancy are evaluated. Staging and clinical presentation of cutaneous melanoma during pregnancy are discussed.

14.2 Epidemiology

Cutaneous melanoma (CM) represents a significant and growing public health burden since the number of melanoma cases worldwide is increasing faster than any other cancer. During the past several decades, there has been a steady increase in the incidence of cutaneous melanoma among all fair-skinned populations [1]. The annual increase in incidence rate varies between populations, but in general has been on the order of 3%–7% per year for fair-skinned populations [2].

CM is now the fourth most common cancer in Australia and New Zealand, the seventh most common in the USA and Canada, and the tenth most common in Scandinavia [3]. In the UK, melanoma is the 11th most common cancer in women and the 12th most common cancer in men [4].

Most of the increased incidence is owed to increased numbers of superficial spreading melanoma. Many epidemiologists are attributing the increase of melanoma incidence to improved surveillance techniques with early diagnosis and changes in lifestyle in terms of excessive exposure to sunlight [5].

In the US general population, the age-adjusted incidence rates of melanoma are higher in males than females [6]. However, melanoma incidence rates are higher for females than males during the reproductive years (first four decades of life except childhood). In Western and Northern Europe the incidence of melanoma is higher in women at all ages (Fig. 14.1).

In the United Kingdom around a third of all cases occur in people aged less than 50 years and in the age group of 20–39 years cutaneous melanoma is the second most common cancer [7]. About 30%–35% of all CM in women occur during their childbearing years. Thus, the coexistence of melanoma and pregnancy or desire to conceive is increasing and melanoma may be the most frequently encountered malignancy during pregnancy. The real incidence of malignant melanoma during pregnancy is unknown. Smith and Randall, in 1969, reported an incidence of 2.8 per 1,000 deliveries [8]. The estimated incidence of melanoma in pregnancy is from 2.8 to 5 cases

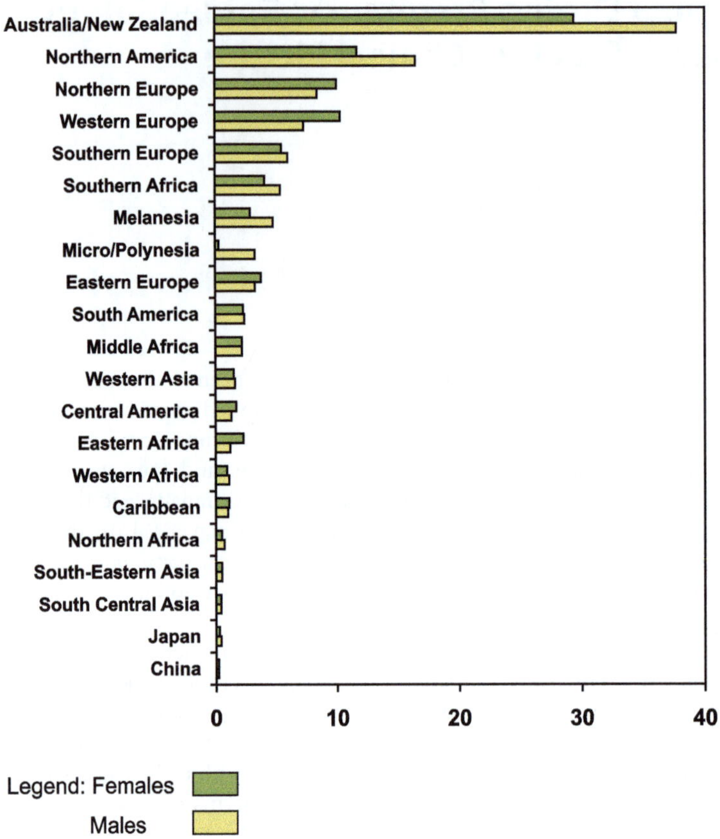

Fig. 14.1 World age-standardised incidence rates, malignant melanoma, by sex, 2002 estimates (rate per 100,000 population)

per 100,000 pregnancies [9]. The Registry of the German Dermatological Society revealed that 1% of female melanoma patients were pregnant and 40.5% were found to be in premenopausal status [10].

In Sweden, in the period 1973–1984, melanoma was the most common cancer type appearing during pregnancy, and it accounted for 24.5% of all cases of malignancies in pregnant women [11]. Data from the largest cohort study examining the association between pregnancy and melanoma using the data from the Swedish National and Regional Registries showed that among all women ($n=19{,}337$) diagnosed with primary cutaneous melanoma in the period from 1958 until December 1999, 28.6% were diagnosed with melanoma during childbearing age, while 0.9% were diagnosed with melanoma during pregnancy [12].

Melanoma mortality rates have been rising in most fair-skinned populations throughout the world in the past few decades [13]. Although there were contrasting trends in melanoma mortality between different countries, an increase in mortality rate from melanoma has been on the order of 2% annually [14]. The lower increase in melanoma mortality compared with the increase in melanoma incidence has been explained by improvements in early diagnosis and management of cutaneous melanoma. However, recent statistics from many countries show that mortality appears to be levelling off, indicating that secondary prevention has been more effective [15]. Data from the WHO database show that in Western Europe, mortality rates have recently levelled off [estimated annual percentage change (EAPC) from −13.6% (n.s.) to 3.3%], whereas in Eastern and Southern Europe mortality rates are still increasing [EAPC −1.8% (n.s.) to 7.2%] [16].

Despite the rising melanoma incidence, fortunately, there has been a marked concomitant improvement in survival [17]. Recent data demonstrating a strong trend towards prognostically more favourable CM are most likely due to earlier diagnosis. Some epidemiologists consider that survival is on the rise also because of the change in the behaviour of CM: It tends to be thinner, less aggressive and more curable than in the past [18].

Although the long-term survival rate for patients with metastatic melanoma is only 5%, early detection of CM carries in general an excellent prognosis [19]. However, survival is strongly associated with Breslow thickness of the melanoma. Five-year relative survival varies from over 90% for patients with thin tumours to about 40% for those with thick tumours [15].

The influence of pregnancy on the development and prognosis of melanoma has been a matter of intense research for years. Over the past 50 years, the data from epidemiological studies evaluating the influence of pregnancy on the prognosis in women with melanoma have been conflicting. Since 1951, when Pack and Scharnagel reported that women diagnosed with melanoma during pregnancy have extremely poor prognosis because of the rapid development of metastases [20], several other studies have suggested that melanoma diagnosed during pregnancy is associated with a high risk of disease progression and increased mortality risk [21, 22]. Other studies failed to document an adverse effect of pregnancy on melanoma prognosis [23]. However, the majority of these studies were case reports and uncontrolled studies. There are five controlled studies which have examined the effect of pregnancy on outcome in women with melanoma [24–28], and all of them fail to demonstrate a statistically significant difference in survival rate when comparing women diagnosed with melanoma (AJCC stage I and II) during pregnancy with women of the same age diagnosed with melanoma while non-pregnant. However, these studies contained considerable methodological flaws, and thus their results should be interpreted with caution.

Recent large population-based studies showed that pregnancy does not appear to have an adverse effect on survival in women with clinically localised melanoma [12, 29]. The results from the population-based study of 412 women with malignant melanoma diagnosed during or within 1 year after pregnancy in California from 1991 to 1999 found no data to support a more advanced stage, thicker tumors, increased metastases to lymph nodes, or a worsened survival in women with localised melanoma associated with pregnancy [29].

Analysis of survival data from the Swedish cohort study showed that among 5,535 women diagnosed with melanoma during childbearing age in the period between 1958 and 1999 the overall survival rate from cutaneous melanoma was 82.1% [12]. The incidence mortality rate in pregnant and non-pregnant women was 1,315/100,000 person-years and 1,102/100,000 person-years of follow-up, respectively.

At the end of follow-up (median follow-up 11.5 years), the survival of pregnant women with melanoma was not worse than the survival of non-pregnant women with melanoma (85% and 82%, respectively). Log rank test did not detect a statistically significant difference in overall survival in women with melanoma diagnosed during pregnancy when compared with women with melanoma diagnosed while non-pregnant ($\chi 2 = 0.84$, df = 1, $p = 0.36$) (Fig. 14.2).

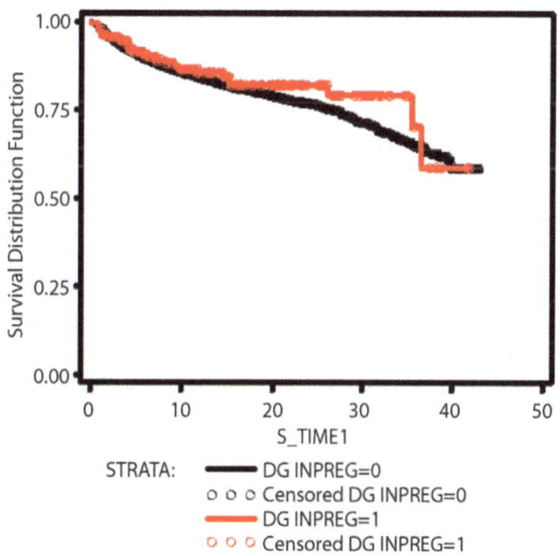

Fig. 14.2 Kaplan-Meier curves of the probability of survival for women with pregnancy-associated melanoma compared with women with non-pregnancy associated melanoma (Swedish cohort study). *Red line*, women with melanoma diagnosed during pregnancy. *Black line*, women with melanoma diagnosed while non-pregnant. *S_time1*, survival time in years

After adjustment for potential confounders (Breslow thickness, tumour site, Clark level and age) in a multivariable Cox model in 2,101 women, pregnancy status at the time of diagnosis of melanoma was not related to survival (hazard ratio for death in the pregnant group was 1.08; 95% CI: 0.60–1.93). However, Breslow thickness and tumour site were highly significant independent prognostic factors of overall survival in these female melanoma patients. Women with a higher Breslow tumour thickness category had a significantly higher risk of death than those with a lower Breslow category (HR = 2.16, 95% CI: 1.80–2.58). Also, women with axial tumours (head and neck and trunk melanomas) had a poorer prognosis than those with tumours localised on the extremities (HR = 2.51, 95% CI: 1.78–3.56).

Some other studies confirmed that the prognosis for women with melanoma during pregnancy is dependent on tumour thickness, which is the major single determinant of overall survival [30].

Sun exposure, particularly recreational or intermittent sun exposure, is the major known etiologic factor for melanoma, and it may interact with other important risk factors [31]. Intensive efforts were devoted to identify other risk factors for melanoma in addition to the well-known cutaneous factors and those variables related to UV exposure.

The roles of endogenous sex hormones, exogenous sex hormones and reproductive factors in the causation of cutaneous melanoma of the skin in women were extensively examined and debated in several studies with inconsistent findings. Many studies showed that neither reproductive factors nor exogenous and endogenous hormones contribute significantly to an increased risk of melanoma [32, 33]. Results from the Nurses' Health Study showed that the risk of pre-menopausal melanoma may be increased among women who are current oral contraceptive users, particularly among those with longer durations of use [34].

Currently there is no evidence that exogenous oestrogens, either oral contraceptives or hormone replacement therapy, have a role in the aetiology of melanoma.

A pooled analysis of 10 case-control studies examining the effect of oral contraceptive use on women's risk of melanoma indicated a lack of effect of oral contraceptives on cutaneous melanoma risk in women [35]. The pooled odds ratio (pOR) for the association between oral contraceptive use for 1 year or longer compared to no use at any time or use for less than 1 year was 0.86 (95% CI: 0.74–1.01). A systematic review of 18 case-control studies revealed no evidence for an aetiological role of oral contraceptives in the development of cutaneous melanoma [36]. The summary ORs estimated from both fixed-effects and random-effects models were each 0.95; the 95% CI were 0.87–1.04 and 0.87–1.05, respectively, indicating no association.

The use of hormone replacement therapy in post-menopausal women who had melanoma was seriously criticised in the past. At present, there appears to be no justification for withholding this potentially beneficial therapy from menopausal women who have undergone treatment for melanoma [37].

There are insufficient data to understand the role of hormones in outcome from melanoma. Results from epidemiological studies demonstrated that women have more favourable prognosis than men [38]. This sex-specific difference in prognosis of cutaneous melanoma may be explained by the hypothesis that oestrogens may be responsible for the inhibition of melanoma growth.

Several studies suggested that endogenous 17-β-estradiol metabolite 2-methoxyoestradiol (2-ME) formed by granulosa cells inhibits angiogenesis and suppresses tumour growth in many malignant tumours [39]. Although various molecular targets have been proposed for 2-ME, the actual mechanism of its anti-proliferative and apoptotic activities is still undefined.

Some studies suggested that pregnancy after melanoma might have a protective role. The results from the Swedish cohort study showed that parity status after diagnosis of primary melanoma is not an important prognostic factor in the multivariate analysis: There was no statistically significant difference in overall survival in women with no pregnancies subsequent to the diagnosis of primary melanoma when compared with women who had pregnancies after the diagnosis and treatment of the primary cutaneous melanoma (hazard ratio for death in women who had pregnancy subsequent to the diagnosis of melanoma was 0.58; 95% CI: 0.32–1.05) [12]. However, this issue needs further research.

For many years epidemiologists also tried to address the question of whether a previous pregnancy is associated with a more favourable outcome for women subsequently diagnosed with melanoma. Some studies found that women with pregnancies before the development of melanoma had a better five-year survival rate from melanoma than women without previous pregnancies (77% and 68%, respectively) [40]. In contrast, some other studies found no difference for nulliparous versus parous women in five-year melanoma survival rates (63% vs. 61%) [41].

However, there is clinical evidence that pregnancy history may play a role in risk of cutaneous melanoma in women. The results from a collaborative analysis of original data from 10 completed case-control studies including 2,391 cases and 3,199 controls found a reduced risk of melanoma among women with higher parity (≥5 vs. no live births pOR 0.76, 95% CI 0.49–1.18, each live birth pOR 0.95, 95% CI 0.91–0.99, p trend = 0.05) [42].

Another important epidemiological aspect of melanoma during the pregnancy is the possibility of transplacental metastases. Although metastases to the foetus via the placenta are rare, melanoma is the most common culprit [43]. With placental involvement, foetal risk of melanoma metastasis is approximately 22%. Maternally derived melanoma metastasis in the infant is almost invariably fatal.

14.3 Diagnosis

The diagnosis of melanoma is always made by clinical examination, tumour excision and pathological examination. Classically, the "ABCD" mnemonic method developed by the American Cancer Society in 1985 to facilitate evaluation of pigmented lesions and improve early diagnosis of malignant melanoma is used to describe the most common characteristics of a melanoma [44]. The ABCD mnemonic analyses four clinical features: A = asymmetry; B = border irregularity; C = colour variegation; D = diameter greater than 6 mm. Recently, in light of recent data regarding the existence of small-diameter (≤6 mm) melanomas, it has been suggested that the ABCD criteria for the gross inspection of pigmented skin lesions and early diagnosis of cutaneous melanoma should be expanded to ABCDE (to include "evolving") [45].

Differential diagnosis includes seborrhoic keratosis, traumatised or irritated naevus, lentigo, hemangioma, pigmented basal cell carcinoma, pigmented actinic keratosis, angiokeratoma, dermatofibroma and blue naevus.

The final diagnosis of melanoma is made on the basis of an excisional biopsy and histological examination. Any lesion suspected of being a melanoma should be removed entirely with free margins. The pathologist should be given all clinical information regarding the patient and specimen, including any personal or family history of melanoma, the site and size of the lesion and its morphologic characteristics. A complete histopathology report should include type of melanoma (superficial spreading, nodular, etc.), dimensions, margin status, tumour thickness according to Breslow, the level of invasion (Clark's level), presence or absence of ulceration, mitotic index, presence or absence of vascular and lymphatic invasion, lymphocytic infiltration (tumour-infiltrating lymphocyte host response), growth phase (radial or vertical) and presence or absence of regression.

Several studies have suggested that women diagnosed with melanoma during pregnancy are more likely to have thicker tumours because of delays in diagnosis or hormonal or growth factor stimulation [12]. Although it is known that naevi change during pregnancy (become darker and larger) and that the increased pigmentation occurs during pregnancy together with general physiological changes, physicians caring for pregnant women must be always alert to the potential of melanoma and not routinely dismiss these changes as being secondary effects of pregnancy. Thus, careful examination of naevi is required during pregnancy.

It is often stated that naevi may darken and enlarge during pregnancy and that the increased pigmentation during pregnancy combined with the general physiological changes which take place in pregnancy could make the detection of a slight change in a mole more difficult, or the woman less concerned than she would be otherwise [17].

In the diagnosis of cutaneous melanoma, various stage-dependent diagnostic procedures are widely performed. However, the situation becomes more complicated in pregnant women because of the potential hazardous side effects to the foetus. Thus, the diagnosis of melanoma during pregnancy presents some unique and difficult challenges for both patients and providers. One of the open questions is whether or not to perform lymphatic mapping and sentinel lymph node biopsy in pregnant women. Lymphatic mapping and sentinel lymph node biopsy are an essential part of the diagnosis and staging of patients with melanoma. This technique provides important prognostic data in patients with early-stage melanoma and identifies patients with nodal metastases whose survival can be prolonged by immediate lymphadenectomy. Sentinel node mapping has been adopted as a standard staging procedure in many melanoma units. However, currently there are no data on the safety of sentinel node mapping in pregnant patients. Although there is limited experience that lymphatic mapping and sentinel node biopsy are feasible in pregnant women, there is still no general endorsement of such procedures during pregnancy [46]. It is suggested that potential risks of radioactive tracers used during the procedure should be clearly explained to the patient and well balanced against the risk of omitting nodal staging by sentinel biopsy. Furthermore, in pregnant women other staging imaging tests should be limited to those associated with the lowest exposure to ionising radiation. Abdominal plain films, isotope scans and computerised tomography should be avoided [47].

Another important aspect of diagnosis of melanoma during pregnancy is a careful gross and histological examination of the placenta by pathologists in women with known or suspected metastatic melanoma.

14.4 Staging

Accurate stratification of patients into prognostic categories and meaningful comparisons across patient populations are achieved by means of a standardised and uniformly accepted cancer staging system.

Currently the staging of disease in melanoma patients is carried out based upon Union Internationale Contre le Cancer/American Joint Committee on Cancer staging (UICC/AJCC) system. Upon critical review of the accuracy of the previous AJCC staging system for cutaneous melanoma, a more useful staging system was proposed. Changes were suggested after retrospective evaluation of the published data as well as a reanalysis of the University of Alabama and Sydney Melanoma Unit databases ($n=4,568$) for patients with primary melanoma using an overlay graphic technique to compare the Kaplan-Meier survival curves of patients with melanoma and examine the impact of powerful prognostic factors (level of invasion, presence of ulceration, local recurrences, satellite metastases, in-transit metastases and extent of nodal metastasis) on survival [48] This final version of the new melanoma AJCC staging system became official with publication of the sixth edition of the AJCC Cancer Staging Manual on January 1, 2003 [49, 50] (Table 14.1). Results from the prognostic factors analysis from the pooled data from 13 prospective databases were used to validate the proposed staging system [51]).

To improve the accuracy of the previous AJCC staging system the following modifications were made in the new staging system:

1. Clark's level of invasion was eliminated from the T category (except for T1 melanomas), since it adds little to prognosis and tends to be less accurate and less reproducible than tumour thickness (Breslow).
2. Tumour thickness stratification cut-offs were changed to 1, 2 and 4 mm since these numbers provided a better prediction of prognosis and were easier to use than the previously used cutoffs of 0.75, 1.5 and 4 mm.
3. Ulceration as an independent prognostic pathologic feature was incorporated into the T category.
4. All patients with stage I, II and III disease are staged up when a primary melanoma is ulcerated.
5. The number of metastatic lymph nodes and the delineation of microscopic versus macroscopic lymph node metastases are used in the N classification.

Table 14.1 The new AJCC staging system

Stage	Primary tumour (pT)	Lymph node (N)	Distant metastases (M)
0	In situ tumours	No nodes	None
IA	<1.0 mm, no ulceration	No nodes	None
IB	<1.0 mm with ulceration	No nodes	None
	1.01–2.0 mm, no ulceration	No nodes	None
IIA	1.01–2.0 mm with ulceration	No nodes	None
	2.01–4.0 mm, no ulceration	No nodes	None
IIB	2.01–4.0 mm with ulceration	No nodes	None
	>4.0 mm, no ulceration	No nodes	None
IIC	>4.0 mm with ulceration	No nodes	None
IIIA	Any Breslow thickness, no ulceration	Micrometastases in nodes	None
IIIB	Any Breslow thickness, with ulceration	Micrometastases in nodes	None
	Any Breslow thickness, no ulceration	Up to three palpable nodes	None
	Any Breslow thickness ± ulceration	No nodes but in-transit metastases or satellites	None
IIIC	Any Breslow thickness with ulceration	Up to three palpable nodes	None
	Any Breslow thickness ± ulceration	Four or more palpable nodes or matted nodes or in-transit metastases with nodes	None
IV			M1: skin, subcutaneous or distant lymph nodes M2: lung M3: all other sites or any site with raised LDH

6. The site of distant metastases and the presence of elevated serum LDH are incorporated in the M category.
7. Satellite metastases around a primary melanoma and in-transit metastases are now grouped into a single staging entity and classified as stage III disease.
8. A new convention is added for defining clinical and pathologic staging so as to take into account the new staging information gained from intraoperative lymphatic mapping and sentinel lymph node biopsy.

14.5 Clinical Picture

Cutaneous melanoma has been classified, on the basis of distinctive clinical and histopathological characteristics, into four major types:

1. Superficial spreading melanoma;
2. Nodular melanoma;
3. Acral lentiginous melanoma;
4. Lentigo maligna melanoma.

14.5.1 Superficial Spreading Melanoma

Superficial spreading melanoma (SSM) is the most common type of cutaneous melanoma. It accounts for approximately 70% of all primary melanomas in Caucasian populations [52]. This type of melanoma has peak incidence in the fourth and fifth decades of life. Superficial spreading melanoma can be located on any anatomic site of the body, but the most common sites are the areas of the body intermittently exposed to the sun, such as the lower extremities in females and the back in males. This type of melanoma has a tendency for slow growth. SSM usually originates in a pre-existing naevus. The number and size of naevi are more strongly associated with the risk for superficial spreading melanoma [53].

14.5.2 Nodular Melanoma

Nodular melanoma (NM) is the second most widespread type of melanoma, comprising around 10%–15% of all melanomas. It has a peak incidence in middle age. The most frequent anatomic sites for the development of NM are the trunk, head and neck. It is thought that NM usually develops on normal skin and not from a pre-existing naevus. The main characteristic of NM is a rapid growth.

14.5.3 Lentigo Maligna Melanoma

Lentigo maligna melanoma (LMM) accounts for approximately 5%–10% of all melanomas. It is mostly seen in an older population, with a peak incidence in the seventh decade of life. Typical sites for the development of LMM are the face (particularly cheeks and nose) and the neck. The risk for the development of LMM is associated with a long-term cumulative sun exposure.

LMM has a prolonged intraepidermal radial growth phase that often lasts 10–20 years, known as lentigo maligna or Hutchinson freckle. Some authors have considered LMM to be a precursor of malignant melanoma, whereas others have considered it to be melanoma in situ [54]. Recently, a hypothesis has been proposed that lesions termed lentigo maligna represent a spectrum of lesions ranging from atypical melanocytic proliferation with a low risk of progression to melanoma to lesions that are already melanoma in situ [55].

14.5.4 Acral Lentiginous Melanoma

Acral lentiginous melanoma (ALM) represents approximately 2%–8% of all melanomas in caucasian populations. This variant of melanoma is the most common expression of melanoma among populations with a relatively low incidence of melanoma (African-Americans, Asians and Hispanics), where it may account for more than half of all melanomas [56]. ALM appears on the palms, soles and subungual sites, with a peak incidence in the seventh decade.

Two most common types of melanoma during pregnancy are superficial spreading melanoma and nodular melanoma. In the Swedish cohort study 68% of patients were diagnosed with SSM during pregnancy, while 15% had nodular melanoma. Similar results were achieved in other studies evaluating melanoma during pregnancy.

References

1. Parkin DM, Bray F, Ferlay J, Pisani P (2005) Global cancer statistics, 2002. CA Cancer J Clin 55(2): 74–108
2. Diepgen TL, Mahler V (2002) The epidemiology of skin cancer. Br J Dermatol146(Suppl. 61): 1–6
3. Marks R (2000) Epidemiology of melanoma. Clin Exp Dermatol 25: 459–463
4. Lens MB, Dawes M (2004) Global perspectives of contemporary epidemiological trends of cutaneous malignant melanoma. Br J Dermatol 150(2): 179–185
5. MacKie RM (1998) Incidence, risk factors and prevention of melanoma. Eur J Cancer 34 (suppl. 2): S3–S6
6. Anonymous (2003) Stat bite: incidence of and mortality from melanoma of the skin, 1975–2000. J Natl Cancer Inst 95(13): 933
7. Cancer Research UK (2006) Malignant melanoma factsheet May 2006. Available at: www. info.cancerresearchuk.org. Accessed November 9, 2006

8. Smith RS, Randall P (1969) Melanoma during pregnancy. Obstet Gynecol 34: 825–829
9. Dillman RO, Vandermolen LA, Barth NM, Bransford KJ (1996) Malignant melanoma and pregnancy. West J Med 164: 156–161
10. Garbe C (1993) [Pregnancy, hormone preparations and malignant melanoma]. Hautarzt 44: 347–352
11. Matthiasen L, Berg G (1989) Malignant melanoma, the most common cancer type, first appearing during pregnancy. Läkartidningen 86: 2845–2848
12. Lens MB, Rosdahl I, Ahlbom A, Farahmand BY, Synnerstad I, Boeryd B, Newton Bishop JA (2004) Effect of pregnancy on survival in women with cutaneous malignant melanoma. J Clin Oncol 22(21): 4369–4375
13. Brochez L, Naeyaert JM (2000) Understanding the trends in melanoma incidence and mortality: where do we stand? Eur J Dermatol10(1): 71–75
14. Severi G, Gilles GG, Robertson C et al. (2000) Mortality from cutaneous melanoma: evidence for contrasting trends between populations. Br J Cancer 82(11): 1887–1891
15. Downing A, Newton-Bishop JA, Forman D (2006) Recent trends in cutaneous malignant melanoma in the Yorkshire region of England; incidence, mortality and survival in relation to stage of disease, 1993–2003. Br J Cancer 95(1): 91–95
16. de Vries E, Bray FI, Coebergh JW, Parkin DM (2003) Changing epidemiology of malignant cutaneous melanoma in Europe 1953–1997: rising trends in incidence and mortality but recent stabilizations in western Europe and decreases in Scandinavia. Int J Cancer 107(1): 119–126
17. Rigel DS, Friedman RJ, Kopf AW et al. (1996) The incidence of malignant melanoma in the United States: Issues as we approach the 21st century. J Am Acad Dermatol 34: 839–847
18. Burton RC, Armstrong BK (1995) Current melanoma epidemic: a nonmetastasizing form of melanoma? World J Surg 19(3): 330–333
19. Cummins DL, Cummins JM, Pantle H, Silverman MA, Leonard AL, Chanmugam A (2006) Cutaneous malignant melanoma. Mayo Clin Proc 81(4): 500–507
20. Pack GT, Scharnagel IM (1951) Prognosis of malignant melanoma in pregnant women. Cancer 4: 324–334
21. Sutherland CM, Loutfi A, Mather FJ, Carter RD, Krementz ET (1983) Effect of pregnancy upon malignant melanoma. Surg Gynecol Obstet 157: 443–446
22. Trapeznikov NN, Khasanov SR, Iavorskii VV (1987) Melanoma of the skin and pregnancy. Voproxy Onkologii 33: 40–46
23. Holly EA (1986) Melanoma and pregnancy. Recent Results Cancer Res 102: 118–126
24. Reintgen DS, McCarty KS Jr, Vollmer R, Cox E, Seigler HF (1985) Malignant melanoma and pregnancy. Cancer 55: 1340–1344
25. McManamny DS, Moss ALH, Pocock PV, Briggs JC (1989) Melanoma and pregnancy: a long-term follow-up. Br J Obstet Gynaecol 96: 1419–1423
26. Wong JH, Sterns EE, Kopald KH, Nizze JA, Morton DL (1989) Prognostic significance of pregnancy in stage I melanoma. Arch Surg 124: 1227–1231
27. Slingluff CL Jr, Reintgen DS, Volmer RT, Seigler HF (1990) Malignant melanoma arising during pregnancy—a study of 100 patients. Ann Surg 211: 552–559
28. MacKie RM, Bufalino R, Morabito A, Sutherland C, Cascinelli N (1991) Lack of effect of pregnancy on outcome of melanoma—The World Health Organisation Melanoma Programme. Lancet 337: 653–655
29. O'Meara AT, Cress R, Xing G, Danielsen B, Smith LH (2005) Malignant melanoma in pregnancy. A population-based evaluation. Cancer 103(6): 1217–1226
30. Daryanani D, Plukker JT, De Hullu JA, Kuiper H, Nap RE, Hoekstra HJ (2003) Pregnancy and early-stage melanoma. Cancer 97(9): 2248–2253
31. Berwick M, Armstrong BK, Ben-Porat L, Fine J, Kricker A, Eberle C, Barnhill R (2005) Sun exposure and mortality from melanoma. J Natl Cancer Inst 97(3): 195–199
32. Osterlind A, Tucker MA, Stone BJ, Jensen OM (1988) The Danish case-control study of cutaneous malignant melanoma. III. Hormonal and reproductive factors in women. Int J Cancer 42(6): 821–824
33. Smith MA, Fine JA, Barnhill RL, Berwick M (1998) Hormonal and reproductive influences and risk of melanoma in women. Int J Epidemiol 27(5): 751–757
34. Feskanich D, Hunter DJ, Willett WC, Spiegelman D, Stampfer MJ, Speizer FE et al. (1999) Oral contraceptive use and risk of melanoma in premenopausal women. Br J Cancer 81(5): 918–923

35. Karagas MR, Stukel TA, Dykes J, Miglionico J, Greene MA, Carey M et al. (2002) A pooled analysis of 10 case-control studies of melanoma and oral contraceptive use. Br J Cancer 86(7): 1085–1092
36. Pfahlberg A, Hassan K, Wille L, Lausen B, Gefeller O (1997) Systematic review of case-control studies: oral contraceptives show no effect on melanoma risk. Publ Health Rev 25: 309–315
37. Durvasula R, Ahmed SM, Vashisht A, Studd JW (2002) Hormone replacement therapy and malignant melanoma: to prescribe or not to prescribe? Climacteric 5(2): 197–200
38. Thörn M, Adam HO, Ringborg U, Bergrström R, Krusemo UB (1987) Long-term survival in malignant melanoma with special reference to age and sex as prognostic factors. J Natl Cancer Inst 79: 969–974
39. Fotsis T, Zhang Y, Pepper MS, Adlercreutz H, Montesano R, Nawroth PP, Schweigerer L (1994) The endogenous oestrogen metabolite 2-methoxyoestradiol inhibits angiogenesis and suppresses tumour growth. Nature 368(6468): 237–239
40. Hersey P, Morgan G, Stone DE, McCarthy WH, Milton GW (1977) Previous pregnancy as a protective factor against death from melanoma. Lancet 1(8009): 451–452
41. Elwood JM, Coldman AJ (1978) Previous pregnancy and melanoma prognosis. Lancet 2(8097): 1000–1001
42. Karagas MR, Zens MS, Stukel TA, Swerdlow AJ, Rosso S, Osterlind A et al. (2006) Pregnancy history and incidence of melanoma in women: a pooled analysis. Cancer Causes Control 17(1): 11–19
43. Alexander A, Samlowski WE, Grossman D, Bruggers CS, Harris RM, Zone JJ et al. (2003) Metastatic melanoma in pregnancy: risk of transplacental metastases in the infant. J Clin Oncol 21(11): 2179–2186
44. Friedman RJ, Rigel DS, Kopf AW (1985) Early detection of malignant melanoma: the role of physician examination and self-examination of the skin. CA Cancer J Clin 35: 130–151
45. Abbasi NR, Shaw HM, Rigel DS, Friedman RJ, McCarthy WH, Osman I et al. (2004) Early diagnosis of cutaneous melanoma: revisiting the ABCD criteria. JAMA 292(22): 2771–2776
46. Mondi MM, Cuenca RE, Ollila DW, Iv JH, Levine EA (2007) Sentinel lymph node biopsy during pregnancy: initial clinical experience. Ann Surg Oncol 14: 218–221
47. Pavlidis NA (2002) Coexistence of pregnancy and malignancy. Oncologist 7(4): 279–287
48. Buzaid AC, Ross MI, Balch CM, Soong S, McCarthy WH, Benjamin RS et al. (1997) Critical analysis of the current American Joint Committee on Cancer staging system for cutaneous melanoma and proposal of a new staging system. J Clin Oncol 15: 1039–1051
49. Balch CM, Buzaid AC, Soong SJ, Atkins MB, Cascinelli N, Coit DG et al. (2001) Final version of the American Joint Committee on Cancer staging system for cutaneous melanoma. J Clin Oncol 19(16): 3635–3648
50. American Joint Committee on Cancer (2002) Melanoma of the skin. Greene FL, Page DL, Fleming ID, Fritz A, Balch CM, Haller DG, et al., eds. AJCC Cancer Staging Manual. 6th ed. New York: Springer Verlag
51. Balch CM, Soong SJ, Gershenwald JE, Thompson JF, Reintgen DS, Cascinelli N et al. (2001) Prognostic factors analysis of 17600 melanoma patients: validation of the American Joint Committee on Cancer melanoma staging system. J Clin Oncol 19(16): 3622–3634
52. MacKie RM (2000) Malignant melanoma: clinical variants and prognostic indicators. Clin Dermatol 25: 471–475
53. Holly EA, Kelly JW, Shpall SN, Chiu SH (1987) Number of melanocytic nevi as a risk factor for malignant melanoma. J Am Acad Dermatol 17: 459–468
54. Cohen LM (1995) Lentigo maligna and lentigo maligna melanoma. J Am Acad Dermatol 33: 923
55. Crowson AN, Magro CM, Sanchez-Carpintero I, Mihm MC Jr. (2002) The precursors of malignant melanoma. Recent Results Cancer Res 160: 75–84
56. Halder RM, Ara CJ (2003) Skin cancer and photoaging in ethnic skin. Dermatol Clin 21(4): 725–732

15 Melanoma During Pregnancy: Therapeutic Management and Outcome

H. J. Hoekstra

Recent Results in Cancer Research, Vol. 178

15.1 Introduction

The epidemiology, diagnosis, staging, and clinical picture of melanoma during pregnancy are described in Chap. 14. The real incidence of melanoma during pregnancy is still unknown. Pregnancy-related risk factors might play a role in melanoma as in breast cancer (Karagas et al. 2006). The prognosis of cutaneous melanoma is based on the Breslow thickness, the presence or absence of ulceration, and the mitotic rate of the tumor (Balch et al. 2001; Francken et al. 2004). In general the clinical outcome of solid cancer treatment, disease-free and overall survival, is based on the stage of the disease, that is, the lower the stage, the better the outcome. The behavior of melanoma is, unfortunately, unpredictable.

The influence of pregnancy on the prognosis of women with a history of melanoma or pregnant women in whom a melanoma is diagnosed has been controversial since the first publication of Pack and Scharnagel in 1951, in which they described 10 pregnant patients diagnosed with melanoma and a mortality rate of 50% (Pack and Scharnagel 1951). It has been hypothesized that hormonal, reproductive, and/or growth factors influence prognosis during pregnancy. There are no clear indications that exogenous hormonal stimulation or hormonal changes during pregnancy stimulate the growth of the primary tumor or of potential micrometastases, that is, affect disease outcome (Neifeld and Lippman 1980; Flowers et al. 1987; Lecavalier et al. 1990). Furthermore, there is also no relation between the use of oral contraceptives and prognosis (Pfahlberg et al. 1997; Grin et al. 1998; Gefeller et al. 1998). As yet, there is no conclusive evidence that the timing of melanoma during or near the time of pregnancy adversely affects the clinical course or prognosis of the disease (George et al. 1960; Reintgen et al. 1985; Slingluff et al. 1990; MacKie et al. 1991; Antonelli et al. 1996; Teplitzky et al. 1998; Pavlidis 2002; Daryanani et al. 2003). In vitro fertilization in a woman previously diagnosed with melanoma also does not affect survival (Venn et al. 1995).

When a skin lesion becomes suspicious during pregnancy and the diagnosis of melanoma is considered, an excisional biopsy should be performed, followed by appropriate staging and treatment. Several well-controlled studies showed that the survival in pregnant woman with stage I and II melanoma did not show any overall and disease-free survival difference if they were adequately treated (George et al. 1960; Reintgen et al. 1985; Slingluff et al. 1990; MacKie et al. 1991; Antonelli et al.1996; Teplitzky et al. 1998; Pavlidis 2002; Daryanani et al. 2003). Recent studies indicated that melanomas detected during pregnancy were in general thicker than those in nonpregnant women (George et al. 1960; Reintgen et al. 1985; Slingluff et al. 1990; MacKie et al. 1991; Travers et al. 1995; Antonelli et al. 1996; Teplitzky et al. 1998; Pavlidis 2002; Daryanani et al. 2003). The prognosis is therefore related to the tumor thickness and not related to the pregnancy. Presumably diagnosis of melanoma is delayed during pregnancy and therefore thicker lesions are diagnosed (Wrone et al. 1999). Two recent population-based studies did not support a more advanced stage, thicker tumors, increased lymphatic metastatic disease, or worsened survival (Lens et al. 2004; O'Meara et al. 2005).

When a recurrence of a previously treated melanoma or an unknown primary melanoma is encountered during pregnancy, appropriate treatment is indicated after optimal staging.

In both described situations, recurrent melanoma or melanoma first diagnosed during pregnancy, the specific (surgical) treatment is extensively discussed by the surgical oncologist, dermatologist, and/or obstetrician with the patient and her partner. Consultation with a radiation oncologist and/or medical oncologist may sometimes be indicated. In certain circumstances there might be even an indication for termination of the pregnancy.

This chapter focuses on the diagnostic and therapeutic management of primary and recurrent melanoma during pregnancy.

15.2 Diagnostic Biopsy

Only a small proportion of nevi (6%) show a change during pregnancy (Pennoyer et al. 1997). When a suspicious skin lesion is encountered, digital dermatoscopy has the potential to increase the diagnostic accuracy for such a lesion (Kittler et al. 2002). A suspicious lesion with change in size, shape, or color, or one that itches, diagnosed during pregnancy should always be excised, and this should not be deferred until after delivery (MacKie 1999). The excisional biopsy involves complete removal of skin with a 1- to 2-mm clinical margin and a deep margin in the subcutaneous fat underneath all epithelial appendant structures and can be safely performed during pregnancy. A narrow diagnostic excision preserves the normal lymphatic flow and will lead to a minimal scar in case the lesion turns out to be benign. When an excisional biopsy is not possible, a full-thickness, incisional biopsy should be obtained. The prognosis of melanoma patients may be worse after incisional biopsy (Rampen et al. 1980). The diagnostic excision or incision can be safely performed under local anesthesia. It is important to inform the pathologist with respect to the pregnancy when a mole is excised, since pregnancy-related changes might lead to a misinterpretation of the microscopic picture of the mole (MacKie 1999).

15.3 Local Excision

The reason for a wide local excision of a melanoma is based on the fact that a melanoma might be surrounded by "centripetal lymphatic spread." The risk of the presence of satellites is increased with the Breslow thickness of the melanoma. Five completed prospective randomized trials addressed the surgical excision margin for primary melanoma of the skin as summarized in Table 15.1 (Veronesi and Cascinelli 1991; Cohn-Cedermark et al. 2000; Balch et al. 2001; Khayat et al. 2003; Thomas et al. 2004). For melanoma in situ an excision margin of 0.5 cm is adequate. The currently advised resection margins for melanoma Breslow thickness ≤2.0 mm is 1 cm, for Breslow thickness 2.0–4 mm is 2 cm, and for >4 mm is at least 2 cm, as summarized in Table 15.2. Reexcision is preferably performed under general or regional anesthesia with primary closure of the skin. When this is impossible a split skin graft might be used. Tissue transfers are generally not recommended, since they might preclude the early detection of a local recurrence. Small excisions can also be performed under local anesthesia. If excision needs to be performed under general anesthesia, fetal heart rate monitoring can be performed, if indicated.

Table 15.1 Prospective randomized surgical excision trials in cutaneous melanoma

Author	Year	N	Tumor thickness (mm)	Randomized surgical arms (cm)
Veronesi	1991	612	≤2	1 vs. 3
Balch	2001	486	1–4	2 vs. 4
Cohn-Cedermark	2002	989	≤2	2 vs. 5
Khayat	2003	362	≤2	2 vs. 5
Thomas	2004	900	>2	1 vs. 3

Table 15.2 Recommended excision margin in cutaneous melanoma

Tumor thickness (mm)	Excision margin (cm)
In situ	0.5–1
0–1	1
1–2	1
2–4	2
>4	At least 2

15.4 Lymphatic Mapping

In most patients with localized melanoma of less than 4-mm Breslow thickness, wide local excision is a curative treatment, although 15%–20% will develop locoregional disease. Various prospective and retrospective studies have not shown any benefit of an elective lymph node dissection (ELND) in improving the disease and/or overall survival of melanoma patients (Sim et al. 1986; Balch et al. 1996; Cascinelli et al. 1998). Therefore, Morton developed the technique of sentinel lymph node biopsy (SLNB) in the early nineties in order to achieve a better staging of patients with clinical stage I and II melanoma (Morton et al. 1992). SLNB is one of the most significant advances in the treatment of melanoma during the last decade. Research has shown that SLNB does indeed lead to better staging and is the most powerful prognostic factor related to recurrence and survival for localized melanoma (Gershenwald et al. 1999; de Vries et al. 2005). When metastases are found in the sentinel lymph node, completion lymph node dissection (CLND) is recommended. The technique of the SLNB is well defined. Lymphoscintigraphy with ^{99m}technetium-labeled colloids is used in combination with intraoperative blue dye. The SLNB in itself seems to be a minimally invasive procedure, although there is a minimal treatment-related short- and long-term morbidity after CLND, wound infection and slight edema (Morton et al. 2005; de Vries et al. 2005, 2006). Whether SLNB and CLND influence survival is being investigated in the multicenter selective lymphadenectomy trial (MSLT I). It will take a number of years before the final results of the MSLT I become available. A recent interim analysis reported that for intermediate thickness (1.2–3.5 mm) the results of sentinel node biopsy showed that the 5-year survival rate was higher among those who underwent immediate lymphadenectomy than among those in whom lymphadenectomy was delayed (72.3 ± 4.6% vs. 52.4 ± 5.9% with a p value of .004) (Morton et al. 2006).

The use of sentinel node mapping in melanoma during pregnancy is controversial for two reasons. The rate of allergic reactions to blue dye is as high as 2%. The incidence of life-threatening anaphylactic reaction requiring resuscitation is ±1% (Cimmino et al. 2001; Albo et al. 2001). Lymphoscintigraphy cannot be combined with blue dye, since vital blue dye is contraindicated in pregnant patients. Radioactive colloid alone can be used in the SLN mapping, since the lymphoscintigraphy leads to a negligible dose to the fetus of 0.014 mGy or less, a radiation dose not increasing the incidence of fetal malformation. This is much less than the National Council on Radiation Protection and Measurements limit for a pregnant woman (Pandit-Taskar et al. 2006). Although lymphoscintigraphy without blue dye does not harm the fetus, we do not recommend SLNB with lymphoscintigraphy in pregnant women, since the MSLT I trial still has not proven any benefit in overall survival, the primary endpoint of the trial (Morton et al. 2006).

If a lymphatic mapping is considered it is advised that no more than 10 MBq be injected and that surgical excision of the lesion site be performed within 6 h. The fetus will then be receiving approximately 33 μSv, equivalent to 6 days' natural background radiation. For women who are in the middle or end stage of pregnancy and had undergone a diagnostic excision with uninvolved margins, the definitive treatment, wide local excision and SLNB, might be postponed until delivery.

15.5 Therapeutic Lymph Node Dissection

When a patient is diagnosed with clinical palpable lymph nodes of a melanoma there is an indication for an optimal staging for further disseminated disease. Whole body positron emission tomography (PET), computer tomography (CT), and even magnetic resonance imaging (MRI) are widely used in the staging of stage III melanoma. In general PET will lead to staging up in 20%–25% of clinical stage III patients (Bastiaannet et al. 2006). Staging procedures in pregnant women must avoid ionizing radiation. The exposure of the fetus to lymphoscintigraphy or CT scan does not significantly increase the risk of prenatal death or malformation when performed correctly. The use of CT scanning is based on the duration of the gestation period. PET, however, is contraindicated during pregnancy. Pregnant women should not undergo MRI in the first 3 months of pregnancy, unless the only reasonable alternative imaging involves the use of X-ray procedures (Campbell and Campbell 2006).

The majority of these patients still require a therapeutic lymph node dissection (TLND). When there are no contraindications for a surgical intervention, the TLND should not be delayed because the woman is pregnant. It is known that pregnancy in women with occult metastases may promote earlier appearance of metastatic disease. Since the doubling time of metastatic disease is unknown, delay might result in a more advanced disease.

The surgical techniques for TLND for melanoma are well described (Coit 1992). Lateral or posterolateral neck dissection, axillary dissection including level III, and superficial groin dissection can easily be performed during pregnancy. In contrast, the deep part of the groin dissection might be difficult during pregnancy. However, in late stages of pregnancy it might be advisable to delay surgery to allow the pregnancy to be completed or to initiate early delivery to allow the surgical procedure.

Extensive nodal disease, extranodal disease, angioinvasion, and/or microscopic involvement of the resection margins might be an indication for adjuvant radiation treatment (Bastiaannet et al. 2005). The radiation treatment is postponed until the end of the pregnancy.

15.6 Local Recurrence and/or In-Transit Metastases and Disseminated Disease

The treatment of local recurrence and/or in-transit metastases is primarily a curative local treatment that might consist of surgical resection, cryosurgery, or laser ablation. The techniques of hyperthermic isolated limb perfusion or isolated limb infusion with melphalan for local disease confined to the limbs are contraindicated during pregnancy.

In case of disseminated disease during pregnancy, the available treatment options are limited. Since no proven effective chemotherapy regimen for melanoma is yet available, it is recommended that pregnant woman who have systemic disease should not be offered any chemotherapy. Vaccine therapy is also excluded in pregnant woman. In case of disseminated disease with regional disease, a therapeutic lymph node dissection is seldom indicated and palliative resection of the involved node(s) is sufficient. In-transit metastases can easily be treated by cryosurgery or laser ablation, which can be performed on an outpatient basis. If the recurrences are too large for local treatment, palliative surgical resections can be performed under general, regional, or even local anesthesia. Surgery is the only curative treatment option for disseminated disease. If surgery can render a nonpregnant patient NED, 5-year survival rates up to 20%–39% can be achieved (Hsueh et al. 2002). Therefore, an aggressive surgical approach seems also warranted in pregnant women.

In pregnant patients with disseminated disease termination of the pregnancy will not alter the prognosis of the mother. In women with stage III and IV during pregnancy it is important to examine the placenta histologically for evidence of metastatic disease. Placental and fetal metastasis from maternal melanoma is exceptionally rare (Altman et al. 2003; Alexander et al. 2003). Melanoma is the most common type of cancer to metastasize to the placenta and the fetus. If metastases are found in the placenta, there is a 20% risk of metastatic disease to the fetus. The baby should be carefully monitored for metastatic disease during the first year.

15.7 Pregnancy and Melanoma History

The incidence of melanoma is increasing also in women of childbearing age. Those women may desire to become pregnant. There are no data that pregnancy or hormone use adversely affects prognosis (George et al. 1960; Reintgen et al. 1985; Slingluff et al. 1990; MacKie et al. 1991; Antonelli et al. 1996; Pfahlberg et al. 1997; Grin et al. 1998; Gefeller et al. 1998; Teplitzky et al. 1998; Pavlidis 2002; Daryanani et al. 2003). The risk of recurrence of a melanoma increases with Breslow thickness, and the majority of the patients will develop a recurrence within 24 months (Francken et al. 2005). Therefore, pregnancy is not advisable for at least 2 years in patients with melanoma >1.5 mm and at least 5 years in women with stage III melanoma. The idea behind this advice is to avoid the tragedy that a healthy newborn loses his mother (Merkus and Teepen 1998). If recurrences develop during pregnancy it is disastrous for the patient, not only emotionally but also medically. Beside the options for surgical treatment, radiation and chemotherapy treatment might harm the fetus. Although the risk for placental and fetal metastasis is minimal, they may develop. The placentas of women with known or suspected melanoma should be carefully examined by the pathologist. When placenta involvement occurs, the fetal risk of melanoma metastasis is approximately 22%.

15.8 Conclusion

Pregnancy or hormone use has no adverse, long-term effect on survival in patients with clinically localized melanoma. An alternative to oral contraceptives is nonhormonal contraception. Pregnant patients may present with thicker melanoma. The surgical resection margins in women with melanoma diagnosed during pregnancy are well defined, and customized sentinel node biopsy procedure in stage I and II patients might be discussed. The indication for therapeutic lymph node dissection in stage III is not different from that in nonpregnant patients, although systemic or vaccine treatment is contraindicated. The treatment of recurrences diagnosed during pregnancy is "tailored" to the type of recurrence and the pregnancy. The prognosis of women with primary or recurrent melanoma diagnosed during pregnancy, overall and disease-free survival, is related to tumor thickness, ulceration, and stage of disease. Pregnant patients should therefore be counseled regarding these factors. The surgical principles of melanoma treatment during pregnancy are summarized in Table 15.3.

Table 15.3 Surgical principles of melanoma treatment during pregnancy

Suspicious skin lesion
Suspicious lesions should be examined with digital dermatoscopy
Diagnostic excision of a suspicious lesion under local anesthesia with 5-mm margin
Melanoma stage I and II
Staging of melanoma stage I and II: chest X-ray and no sentinel lymph node biopsy
Treatment of stage I and II melanoma: Breslow 0–2 mm, excision under with 1-cm margin, Breslow 2–4 mm with 2-cm margin, and Breslow>4 mm with at least 2-cm margin
Melanoma stage III
Staging of melanoma stage III: chest X-ray, no further staging with PET, CT, or MRI
Treatment of stage III nodal disease: therapeutic lymph node dissection
Treatment of stage III disease: in-transit metastases or satellitosis, tailored to the extent of the disease, excision, cryosurgery, laser ablation
Melanoma stage IV
Staging of stage IV disease: tailored to the gestation period
Treatment of stage IV disease: tailored to the patient, gestation period, and extent of the disease; local treatment (surgery, cryosurgery, laser ablation, radiation treatment) or systemic treatment. Termination of pregnancy based on the extent of the disease and/or gestation period. Inspection of the placenta and histopathology of the placenta after delivery

References

Albo D, Wayne JD, Hunt KK et al. (2001) Anaphylactic reactions to isosulfan blue dye during sentinel lymph node biopsy for breast cancer. Am J Surg 182: 393–398

Alexander A, Samlowski WE, Grossman D et al. (2003) Metastatic melanoma in pregnancy: risk of transplacental metastases in the infant. J Clin Oncol 21: 2179–2186

Altman JF, Lowe L, Redman B et al. (2003) Placental metastasis of maternal melanoma. Am Acad Dermatol 49: 1150–1154

Antonelli NM, Dotters DJ, Katz VL et al. (1996) Cancer in pregnancy: a review of the literature. Part I and II. Obstet Gynecol Surv 51: 125–134

Balch CM, Soong SJ, Gershenwald JE et al. (2001) Prognostic factors analysis of 17,600 melanoma patients: validation of the American Joint Committee on Cancer melanoma staging system. J Clin Oncol 19: 3622–3634

Balch CM, Soong SJ, Smith T et al. (2001) Investigators from the Intergroup Melanoma Surgical Trial. Long-term results of a prospective surgical trial comparing 2 cm vs. 4 cm excision margins for 740 patients with 1–4 mm melanomas. Ann Surg Oncol 8: 101–108

Balch CM, Soong SJ, Bartolucci AA et al. (1996) Efficacy of an elective regional lymph node dissection of 1 to 4 mm thick melanomas for patients 60 years of age and younger. Ann Surg 224: 255–263

Bastiaannet E, Beukema JC, Hoekstra HJ (2005) Radiation therapy following lymph node dissection in melanoma patients: treatment, outcome and complications. Cancer Treat Rev 31: 18–26

Bastiaannet E, Oyen WJ, Meijer S et al. (2006) Impact of [18F]fluorodeoxyglucose positron emission tomography on surgical management of melanoma patients. Br J Surg 93: 243–249

Campbell FA, Campbell C (2006) Comment on: Magnetic resonance imaging for stage IV melanoma during pregnancy. Arch Dermatol 142: 393

Cascinelli N, Morabito A, Santinami M et al. (1998) Immediate or delayed dissection of regional nodes in patients with melanoma of the trunk: a randomised trial. WHO Melanoma Programme. Lancet 351: 793–796

Cimmino VM, Brown AC, Szocik JF et al. (2001) Allergic reactions to isosulfan blue during sentinel node biopsy—a common event. Surgery 130: 439–442

Cohn-Cedermark G, Rutqvist LE, Andersson R et al. (2000) Long term results of a randomized study by the Swedish Melanoma Study Group on 2-cm versus 5-cm resection margins for patients with cutaneous melanoma with a tumor thickness of 0.8–2.0 mm. Cancer 89: 1495–1501

Coit DG (1992) Lymph node dissection in malignant melanoma. Surg Oncol Clin North Am 1: 157–335

Daryanani D, Plukker JT, De Hullu JA et al. (2003) Pregnancy and early stage melanoma. Cancer 97: 2248–2253

Flowers JL, Seigler HF, McCarty KS Sr et al. (1987) Absence of estrogen receptor in human melanoma as evaluated by a monoclonal antiestrogen receptor antibody. Arch Dermatol 123: 764–765

Francken AB, Shaw HM, Thompson JF et al. (2004) The prognostic importance of tumor mitotic rate confirmed in 1317 patients with primary cutaneous melanoma and long follow-up. Ann Surg Oncol 11: 426–433

Francken AB, Bastiaannet E, Hoekstra HJ (2005) Follow-up in patients with localised primary cutaneous melanoma. Lancet Oncol 6: 608–621

Gefeller O, Hassan K, Wille L (1998) Cutaneous malignant melanoma in women and the role of oral contraceptives. Br J Dermatol 138: 122–124

George PA, Fortner JG, Pack GT (1960) Melanoma with pregnancy. A report of 115 cases. Cancer 13: 854–859

Gershenwald JE, Thompson W, Mansfield PF et al. (1999) Multi-institutional melanoma lymphatic mapping experience: the prognostic value of sentinel lymph node status in 612 stage I or II melanoma patients. J Clin Oncol 17: 976–983

Grin CM, Driscoll MS, Grant-Kels JM (1998) The relationship of pregnancy, hormones, and melanoma Semin Cutan Med Surg 17: 167–171

Hsueh EC, Essner R, Foshag LJ et al. (2002) Prolonged survival after complete resection of disseminated melanoma and active immunotherapy with a therapeutic cancer vaccine. J Clin Oncol 20: 4549–4554

Karagas MR, Zens MS, Stukel TA et al. (2006) Pregnancy history and incidence of melanoma in women: a pooled analysis. Cancer Causes Control 17: 11–19

Khayat D, Rixe O, Martin G et al. (2003) Surgical margins in cutaneous melanoma (2 cm versus 5 cm for lesions measuring less than 2.1-mm thick). Cancer 97: 1941–1946

Kittler H, Pehamberger H, Wolff K et al. (2002) Diagnostic accuracy of dermoscopy. Lancet Oncol 3: 159–165

Lecavalier MA, From L, Gaid N (1990) Absence of estrogen receptors in dysplastic nevi and malignant melanoma. J Am Acad Dermatol 23 :242–246

Lens MB, Rosdahl I, Ahlbom A et al. (2004) Effect of pregnancy on survival in women with cutaneous malignant melanoma. J Clin Oncol 22: 4369–4375

MacKie RM, Bufalino R, Morabito A et al. (1991) Lack of effect of pregnancy on outcome of melanoma. For The World Health Organisation Melanoma Programme. Lancet 337: 653–655

MacKie RM (1999) Pregnancy and exogenous hormones in patients with cutaneous malignant melanoma. Curr Opin Oncol 11: 129–131

Merkus JM, Teepen JL (1998) The indispensable anamnesis: in-vitro fertilization in a woman under treatment for melanoma. Ned Tijdschr Geneeskd 142: 2073–2075

Morton DL, Wen DR, Wong JH et al. (1992) Technical details of intraoperative lymphatic mapping for early stage melanoma. Arch Surg 127: 392–399

Morton DL, Cochran AJ, Thompson JF et al. (2005) Sentinel node biopsy for early-stage melanoma: accuracy and morbidity in MSLT-I, an international multicenter trial. Ann Surg 242: 302–311

Morton DL, Thompson JF, Cochran AJ et al. (2006) Sentinel-node biopsy or nodal observation in melanoma. N Engl J Med 355: 1307–1317

Neifeld JP, Lippman ME (1980) Steroid hormone receptors and melanoma. J Invest Dermatol 74: 379–381

O'Meara AT, Cress R, Xing G et al. (2005) Malignant melanoma in pregnancy. A population-based evaluation. Cancer 103: 1217–1226

Pack GT, Scharnagel IM (1951) The prognosis for malignant melanoma in the pregnant woman. Cancer 4: 324–334

Pandit-Taskar N, Dauer LT, Montgomery L et al. (2006) Organ and fetal absorbed dose estimates from 99mTc-sulfur colloid lymphoscintigraphy and sentinel node localization in breast cancer patients. J Nucl Med 47: 1202–1208

Pavlidis NA (2002) Coexistence of pregnancy and malignancy. Oncologist 7: 279–287. Erratum: Oncologist 7: 585, 2002.

Pennoyer JW, Grin CM, Driscoll MS et al. (1997) Changes in size of melanocytic nevi during pregnancy. Am Acad Dermatol 36: 378–382

Pfahlberg A, Hassan K, Wille L et al. (1997) Systematic review of case-control studies: oral contraceptives show no effect on melanoma risk. Public Health Rev 25: 309–315

Rampen FHJ, Van Houten WA, Hop WCJ (1980) Incisional procedures and prognosis in malignant melanoma. Clin Exp Dermatol 5: 313–420

Reintgen DS, McCarty KS Jr, Vollmer R et al. (1985) Malignant melanoma and pregnancy. Cancer 55: 1340–1344

Sim FH, Taylor WF, Pritchard DJ et al. (1986) Lymphadenectomy in the management of stage I malignant melanoma: a prospective randomized study. Mayo Clin Proc 61: 697–705

Slingluff CL Jr, Reintgen DS, Vollmer RT et al. (1990) Malignant melanoma arising during pregnancy. A study of 100 patients. Ann Surg 211: 552–557

Teplitzky S, Sabates B, Yu K et al. (1998) Melanoma during pregnancy: a case report and review of the literature. J La State Med Soc 150: 539–543

Thomas JM, Newton-Bishop J, A'Hern R et al. (2004) Excision margins in high-risk malignant melanoma. N Engl J Med 350: 757–766

Travers RL, Sober AJ, Berwick M et al. (1995) Increased thickness of pregnancy-associated melanoma. Br J Dermatol 132: 876–883

Venn A, Watson L, Lumley J et al. (1995) Breast and ovarian cancer incidence after infertility and in vitro fertilisation. Lancet 346: 995–1000

Veronesi U, Adamus J, Bandiera DC et al. (1982) Delayed regional lymph node dissection in stage I melanoma of the skin of the lower extremities. Cancer 49: 2420–2430

Veronesi U, Cascinelli N (1991) Narrow excision (1-cm margin). A safe procedure for thin cutaneous melanoma. Arch Surg 126: 438–441

Vries M de, Vonkeman WG, van Ginkel RJ et al. (2005) Morbidity after axillary sentinel lymph node biopsy in patients with cutaneous melanoma. Eur J Surg Oncol 31: 778–783

Vries M de, Jager PL, Suurmeijer AJ et al. (2005) Sentinel lymph node biopsy for melanoma: prognostic value and disadvantages in 300 patients. Ned Tijdschr Geneeskd 149: 1845–1851

Vries M de, Vonkeman WG, van Ginkel RJ et al. (2006) Morbidity after inguinal sentinel lymph node biopsy and completion lymph node dissection in patients with cutaneous melanoma. Eur J Surg Oncol 32: 785–789

Wrone DA, Duncan LM, Sober AJ (1999) Melanoma and pregnancy: eight questions with discussion. J Gend Specif Med 2: 52–54

16 Metastatic Involvement of Placenta and Foetus in Pregnant Women with Cancer

N. Pavlidis, G. Pentheroudakis

Recent Results in Cancer Research, Vol. 178

16.1 Introduction

The coexistence of cancer with pregnancy is a rare event. The estimated frequency is around 1 case of cancer every 1,000 gestations. During the last decades and especially in developed countries the incidence is probably increasing because of delay of pregnancy into the late reproductive years [1, 2].

The management of these patients is unique since it involves two persons: the mother and the foetus. Because of the absence of strict diagnostic or therapeutic guidelines, both gynaecologists and oncologists should try to benefit the mother's life, to treat curable cancers, to protect the foetus from toxic treatments and to retain the mother's reproductive system intact. Every decision should always be taken after a thorough discussion among the doctor, the pregnant mother and her partner.

The most common malignant tumours arising in pregnancy are breast cancer, cervical cancer, haematological malignancies and melanoma, followed by lung cancer, thyroid cancer, gastrointestinal and gynecological cancer as well as by sarcomas [1].

The diagnosis and staging work-up of pregnant mothers with cancer should always be limited to those associated with the smallest hazardous effect on the mother and the foetus. Radiation therapy should be avoided, whereas chemotherapy can safely be provided during the second or third trimester of pregnancy [2].

16.2 Incidence

Reliable epidemiological data on metastatic involvement of the products of conception are lacking since: (a) routine histological examination of the placenta is not always performed, (b) most newborns do not have a proper follow-up, (c) cancer could be expected to induce abortion and eliminate the possibility of such metastasis or (d) many pregnant women have only localised disease without metastatic spread.

During the last decades four reviews have appeared in the medical literature, in which approximately 100 cases were reported (Table 16.1). The first review was published in 1970 with 24 cases and the second in 1989 with 52 patients, and in 2003 two reports with 62 and 87 cases have seen the light of publication [3–6].

Although placental invasion is a rare phenomenon, it seems that foetal involvement is even more uncommon accounting for the one fourth of those cases with affected placentas [1].

Metastatic transmission to placenta or foetus is most frequently seen in melanoma (30%), leukemias and lymphomas (15%), breast cancer (14%) and lung cancer (13%), followed by bone or soft tissue sarcomas, gynaecological malignancies, gastric cancer or other tumours [1, 2, 5, 6].

16.3 Histopathological Findings

Maternal blood circulation in the placenta drains into the intervillous space, where the anchoring villous projections are located. Foetal trophoblasts consisting of the syncytiotrophoblasts (outer layer) and the cytotrophoblasts (inner layer of Langhans) line the villous projections. Maternal and foetal circulation are separated by three components: the trophoblast, the villous connective tissue and the capillary wall [7, 8] (Fig. 16.1).

Table 16.1 Metastatic involvement of products of conception

Tumor type	No. of cases	Involvement		Reference
		Placenta	Foetus	
Melanoma	28	25/28	6/28	17–43
Breast cancer	14	14/14	0/14	49–61
Lung cancer	13	11/13	3/13	5, 16, 63–78
Leukaemias	10	7/10	3/10	89–97
Lymphomas	7	7/7	3/7	83–88
Gastrointestinal cancer	9	9/9	1/9	13, 57, 102–108
Sarcomas	8	8/8	0/8	17, 109–115
Head-neck cancer	3	3/3	1/3	101, 114, 115
Ovarian cancer	2	2/2	0/2	47, 48
CUP	2	2/2	0/2	106, 118
Cervical cancer	1	1/1	0/1	12
Adrenal cancer	1	1/1	0/1	119
Total	98	90/98	17/98	

CUP, carcinoma of unknown primary

Probably the trophoblast plays the role of a physical barrier in recognising and rejecting foreign maternal antigens expressed by the cancer cells. Phagocytosis of maternal cells by the syncytiotrophoblast is a normal function during the implantation phase [9]. However, phagocytosis and destruction of tumour cells by the villous syncytiotrophoblasts and the villous trophoblasts have also been reported [10, 11].

Vertical transmission of cancer cells to placenta or foetus is exceptionally uncommon. Most malignant tumours involving the products of conception metastasise through the haematogenous route, whereas lymphatic dissemination or contiguous invasion are less common metastatic pathways [5]. Lymphatic spread has been mostly observed in cervical cancer associated with pregnancy [12].

Histologically, tumour cell sequestration in the intervillous spaces intermixed with the maternal blood has been observed in all cases of placental metastatic deposits suggesting haematogenous spread of tumour [13] (Fig. 16.2). On the other hand, foetal metastases are always preceded by invasion of the chorionic villous by cancer cells [3, 7, 13].

16.4 Review by Tumour Type

16.4.1 Melanoma

It is important to note that the incidence of melanoma has been increasing lately, representing the main cause of cancer death in women of childbearing age.

Melanoma constitutes 8% of all cancers occurring with pregnancy, with an estimated incidence of 0.1 to 2.8 per 1,000 pregnancies [14, 15]. Despite the fact that melanoma is not the most common cancer during pregnancy, it is most likely to metastasise to the products of conception. Melanoma accounts for 58% of all gestational cancer affecting the embryo. The likelihood of embryonal metastasis in a pregnant patient with melanoma has been estimated to be about 17% [6, 16].

Several explanations have been postulated for this "melanoma tropism" to trophoblastic tissue, such as (a) placental overexpression of melanocytes, (b) release of adhesion molecules, growth factors such as PGF and HGF or angiogenic molecules such as VEGF by melanoma cells favouring placental seeding or (c) inad-

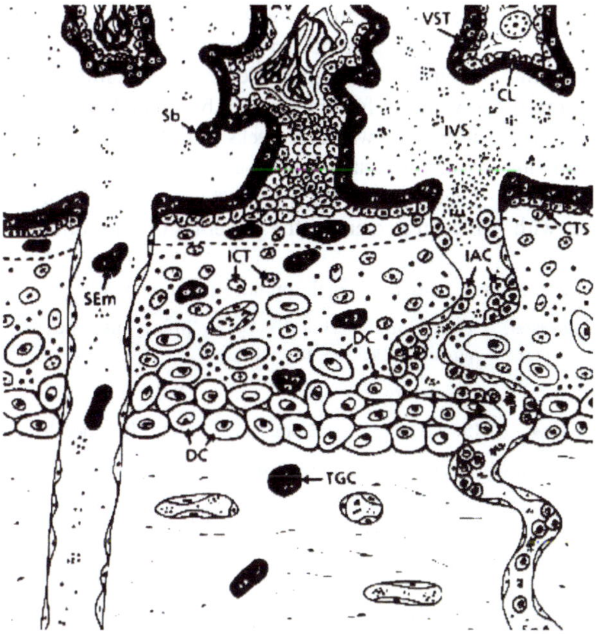

Fig. 16.1 Uterine insertion of the human placenta. *AV*, anchoring villi; *CCC*, cytotrophoblast cell column; *CL*, villous cytotrophoblast, Langhans layer; *CTS*, cytotrophoblast shell; *DC*, cells of the maternal decidua basalis; *IAC*, intra-arterial trophoblast cell in the walls and lumen of the maternal spiral artery; *ICT*, interstitial cytotrophoblast at the insertion of the basal plate; *IVS*, intervillous space; *Sb*, syncytiotrophoblast bud; *SEm*, syncytiotrophoblast embolus carried by the venous blood returning from the placenta to the maternal circulation; *SpA*, maternal uteroplacental spiral artery; *TGC*, trophoblast multinucleate giant cell; *UVL*, uterine vein lumen; *VST*, syncytiotrophoblast of the chorionic villous tissue. (Reprinted from [5] with permission)

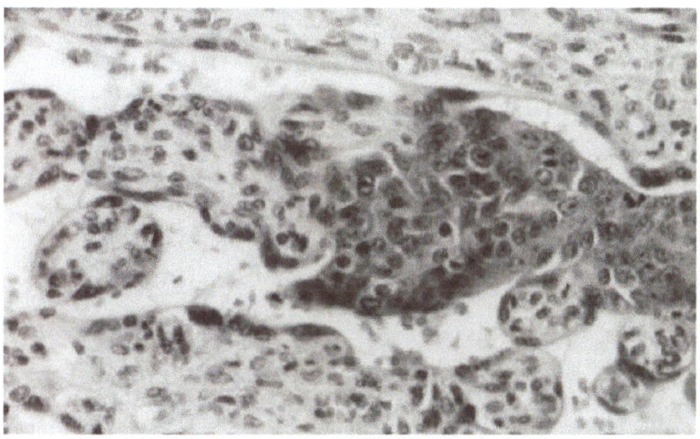

Fig. 16.2 The tumour cells in the intervillous space with discrete infiltration of chorionic villi. (Reprinted from [5] with permission)

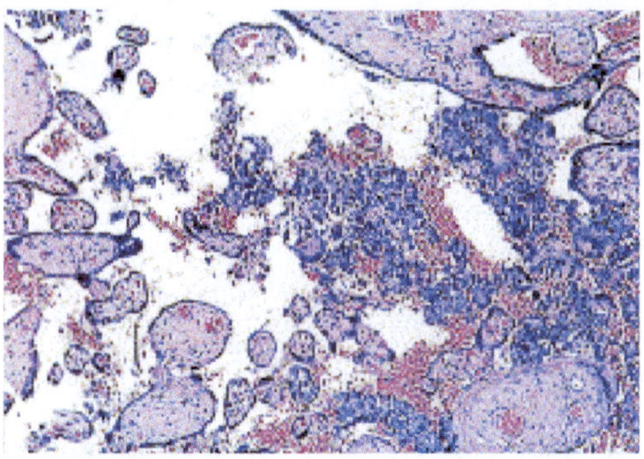

Fig. 16.3 Sections of placenta show multiple aggregates of atypical epithelioid cells in the intervillous space. (H&E; original magnification ×100). (Reprinted from [43] with permission)

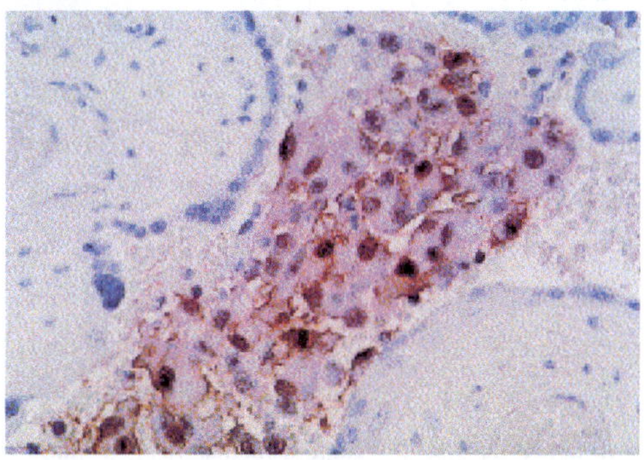

Fig. 16.4 Atypical epithelioid cells show nuclear and cytoplasmic staining with S100 protein, a finding consistent with metastatic melanoma. (S100 stain; original magnification ×400). (Reprinted from [43] with permission)

equate immune response due to immaturity [6] (Figs. 16.3, 16.4).

During the period 1918 to 2006, 28 pregnant patients with melanoma have been reported (MEDLINE database after 1966) (Table 16.2). After microscopic evaluation 25 of these patients had placental involvement, and in six foetal metastases were found. In another three cases with foetal invasion, there was no report on corresponding placental involvement [6, 17–43].

From the extensive review of Alexander et al. several useful findings can be elicited. Mean age at delivery was 29.5 weeks (range 18–43) and the melanoma stages were as follows: stage I 23%, stage II 18%, stage III 18% and stage IV 41%. Eleven percent of the placentas did not undergo

Table 16.2. Maternal and foetal characteristics of 28 melanoma cases involving the products of conception

Reference/year	Site of presentation or metastatic sites	Maternal survival	Gestational age at birth	Foetal metastasis	Infant outcome
Markus 1918 [17]	Brain	5 h	Premature	-	Death 12 hours
Weber 1930 [18]	Left thigh	55 days	38 weeks	In 5 organs	Death 10.5 months
Gottron 1940 [19]	Right back	2 months	Term	Presumed	Death 5 months
Dargeon 1950 [20]	Right leg	4 days	8 months	In 8 organs	Death 10.5 months
Byrd 1954 [21]	Left thigh	3 weeks	3rd trimester	-	Death 24 hours
Reynolds 1955 [22]	Right foot	38 days	Term	-	NED 10 months
Freedman 1960 [23]	Right chest wall	42 days	36 weeks	Skin (resolved)	NED 2 years
Aronsson 1963 [24]	Diffuse at autopsy	4 days	34 weeks	Soft tissue, lung (resolved)	NED 2 years
Brodsky 1965 [25]	Mid-interscapular	17 days	38 weeks	In 13 organs	Death 48 days
Stephenson 1971 [26]	Back	3 months	Term		NED 2 years
Holcomb 1975 [27]	Left scapula	18 days	6 months		NED 47 days
Sokol 1976 [28]	Mid-back	54 days	31 weeks		Death 2 days
Smythe 1976 [29]	Left breast	20 days	8 months	-	NED 9 months
Gillis 1976 [30]	Right arm	7.5 months	32 weeks	-	NED 2 years
Russel 1977 [31]	Back	2 weeks	36 weeks	-	NED 5 months
Looi 1979 [32]	Right shoulder	6 weeks	33 weeks	-	NED 1 month
Moller 1986 [33]	Right calf	1 month	31 weeks	-	NED 6 months
Anderson 1989 [34]	Left scapula	6 months	38 weeks	-	NED 1 year
Brossard 1994 [35]	Right buttock	4 days	34 weeks	-	NED 1 year
Marsh 1996 [36]	Choroid	3 weeks	36 weeks	-	NED ?
Dillman 1996 [37]	Brain, liver, lung	5 months	34 weeks	-	NED ?
Baergen 1997 [38]	Right shoulder	7 days	31 weeks	-	NED 7 months
Dipaola 1997 [39]	Left shoulder	1 month	30 weeks	-	NED 17 months
Johnston 1998 [40]	Back	4 days	31 weeks	-	NED 1 year
Ferreira 1998 [41]	Left shoulder	2 days	28 weeks	Skin	Stillborn
Merkus 1998 [42]	Right medial thigh	8 weeks	35 weeks	-	NED 4 years
Alexander 2003 [6]	Right labia majora	56 days	38 weeks	-	NED 10 months
Altman 2003 [43]	Left arm	19 months	31 weeks	-	NED 19 months

M, male; F, female; NED, no evidence of disease

Table modified from [6]

microscopic examination, 55% showed microscopic metastases and 33% showed both gross and microscopic metastatic sites. Concerning foetal characteristics, 55% were males and 45% females, with a mean birth weight of 2.240 g, while 50% of them were delivered by a caesarean section. The clinical manifestations of foetal metastases in the newborn were mainly characterised by skin lesions (brown nodules) or abdominal swelling. The mean follow-up was 14.2 months. Survival data indicated that 26% of the foetuses died with disease in a median duration of 48 days, 70% were alive without disease with a median follow-up of 12 months and only 4% were stillbirths [6].

The clinical course of pregnant patients with advanced melanoma is often followed by serious complications, with prematurity the most common complication especially if the placenta is involved. The mean gestational age is estimated to be 34 weeks [6].

Infant disease-free survival up to 1 year may be translated to an absence of risk of metastatic involvement. There is no report of development of metastasis after 11 months of age [34]. Two of the six cases reported with skin and/or lung metastases had spontaneous resolution of the metastatic lesions and are alive without evidence of disease at 2 years [22, 23].

Various maternal or foetal prognostic factors have been implicated such as maternal age, primiparity, disease onset, number of maternal metastatic sites, primary site or foetal age at birth. From the results of Alexander et al., however, none of these factors were related to prognosis except one, that of foetal gender. Males comprised 80% of all infants with metastatic melanoma and 75% with metastasis of all cancers [6].

16.4.2 Breast and Gynaecological Cancers

Breast cancer and cervical cancer are the most frequent malignant tumours associated with pregnancy. The incidence is approximately 1:2,000–1:10,000 pregnancies [44, 45]. Ovarian cancer is much more rare, with 40% being germ cell tumours [46].

Despite the fact that cervical cancer is a common tumour in pregnancy, only one case with placental involvement has been reported [12]. Also, two other cases with ovarian cancer were found to have placental invasion [47, 48]. However, in none of these three cases have metastases to the foetuses been described.

In addition, 14 cases of pregnant women with breast cancer have been diagnosed with metastatic spread to the placenta but none to the foetuses [49–61].

16.4.3 Lung Cancer

Lung cancer is not a common pregnancy-associated tumour, ranking far beyond breast cancer, cervical cancer, leukaemias and lymphomas as well as melanoma.

Smoking during the female reproductive age is the main cause of cancer death. Almost 30% of young women smoke, and 20%–30% of this population continue to smoke during pregnancy [62].

Since 1953 almost 20 cases of lung cancer associated with pregnancy have been published. Thirteen of these cases showed involvement of the products of conception. Eleven had placental and three had foetal metastatic spread, while no information on placental status was available in two patients with foetal involvement.

Maternal characteristics of the entire population of pregnant mothers with lung cancer showed a mean age of 35 years and a positive smoking history in 60%. The most common histologic type was non-small-cell lung cancer (60%–70%), the rest being small-cell lung cancer. Maternal distant metastases in visceral organs at the time of diagnosis were found in half of the patients. In most cases systemic chemotherapy was postponed to the postpartum period. Prognosis was poor, with a mean survival of 8 months [5]. All three reported infants with metastatic involvement showed skin lesions to the scalp with intracranial metastases [69, 71, 73].

16.4.4 Leukaemias and Lymphomas

The incidence of the coexistence of lymphomas and leukaemias with pregnancy is 1:1,000–1:6,000 and 1:75,000–1:100,000, respectively. Hodgkin lymphoma is more common than non-Hodgkin lymphomas [1, 2].

Hodgkin lymphoma is predominantly presented at earlier stages I–II (70%), while non-Hodgkin lymphomas at more advanced stages III–IV (70%–80%) [79]. From a review of 37 cases of lymphomas during pregnancy, a site predilection for mediastinum and a tendency to involve breast, ovary and uterus were observed [80]. The most common histologic types are nodular sclerosis for Hodgkin lymphoma and high-grade B-cell lymphomas for non-Hodgkin lymphomas. Acute leukaemias and especially myelomonocytic leukaemias are more frequently associated with pregnancy, whereas chronic leukaemias are rarely seen since they occur at older ages [81].

Among all malignancies affecting the placenta and foetus, leukaemias and lymphomas represent 15% of all tumours [5].

The first report of a lymphosarcoma involving the product of conception was in 1900 [82]. Since then, 7 cases of lymphomas [83–88] and 10 cases of leukemias [89–97] have been described, 6 of which had also foetal involvement. There is only one, not well-documented case of Hodgkin lymphoma in 1926 affecting both the placenta and the foetus [83]. All the rest were aggressive non-Hodgkin lymphomas. In most cases of non-Hodgkin lymphomas with placental involvement the tumour invasion was grossly visible, while microscopic tumour cells were found in the intervillous space (Figs. 16.5, 16.6).

Transmission of maternal leukaemic cells to the infants is very rare. Only three cases have been reported. In two cases mothers were suffering from acute lymphocytic leukaemias and both infants died in the first year of life [98]. In the third case, the mother was diagnosed with acute monocytic leukaemia and her infant was also diagnosed with an identical type of leukaemia at 20 months of age [97].

16.4.5 Gastrointestinal Cancers

Cancers of the gastrointestinal tract associated with pregnancy are rare tumours, since the population affected by these diseases are seen after the fifth decade of life. So far 300 cases of colorectal cancers, 131 cases of gastric cancer, 40 cases of hepatoma and 5 cases of pancreatic cancers have been described during gestation [2, 99–101].

There are four cases of gastric carcinoma with

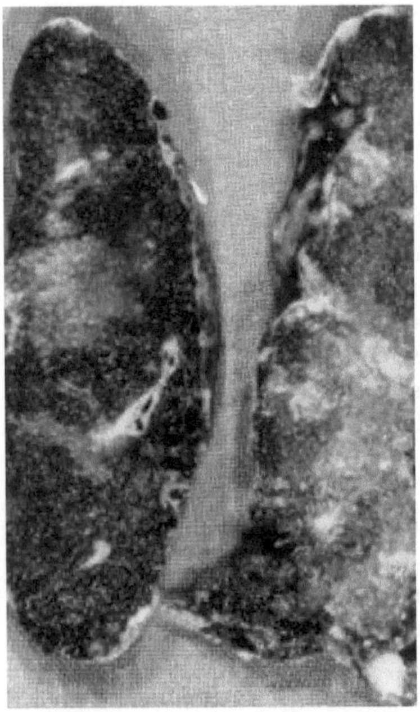

Fig. 16.5 Sections of the placenta showing numerous whitish lymphoma nodules of various size. (Reprinted from [86] with permission)

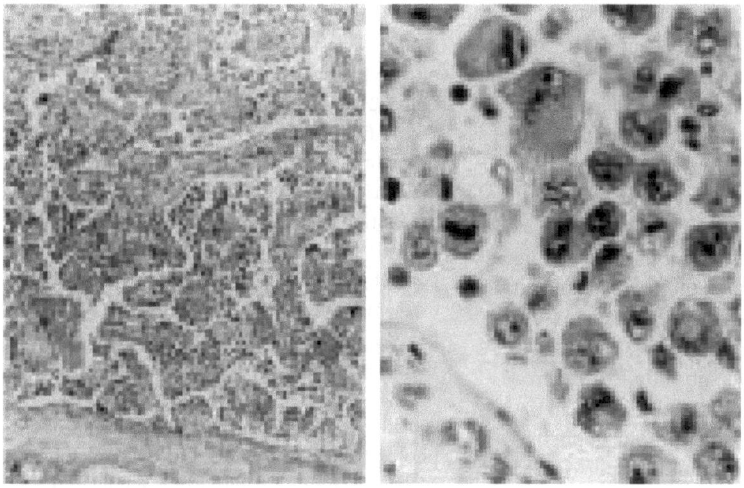

Fig. 16.6 a Low-power view showing the intervillous space massively infiltrated by anaplastic large cell lymphoma cells. The villous stroma is not involved. b Morphologic characteristics of malignant cells which are of varying size and show a striking nuclear pleomorphism with binucleated cells and some crown-like nuclei. The cytoplasm is abundant with some tiny vacuoles. (Reprinted from [86] with permission)

placental metastases without foetal involvement in one, no information in two and detection of tumour cells in the amniotic fluid in the last with no evidence of foetal metastases [102–105]. Also, three cases of pancreatic cancer involving the placenta are available in the literature. None of these cases had foetal involvement [57, 106, 107]. In addition, there is one reported case of hepatoma metastatic to the foetus and one case of rectal cancer with placental metastases [13, 108].

16.4.6 Other Tumours

Other malignant tumours have also been sporadically reported to involve the products of conception.

Although sarcomas are extremely rare tumours in association with pregnancy, there are eight reported cases of sarcomas metastatic to the products of conception [17,109–115]. None of these invaded the foetuses. Almost all were soft-tissue sarcomas (myxoid sarcoma, angiosarcoma, myeloblastoma or PNET tumours), and only one was skeletal Ewing sarcoma.

Other rare cancers such as squamous head and neck tumours (3 cases reported) [103, 116, 117], carcinomas of unknown primary site (2 cases) [106, 118] and adrenal adenocarcinoma (1 case) [119] with placental involvement have also been published.

16.5 Patient Registrations and Doctor Recommendations

Since the first report in 1866 [108] of metastatic involvement of the products of conception, there are in total no more than 100 cases reported in the literature. Therefore, both the real incidence as well as the biological properties of this phenomenon are still poorly understood. More extensive and accurate data are desperately needed in order to clarify them further.

It has been suggested that all identifiable cases of metastatic disease to the placenta or foetus should be included in Cancer Registry Data as well as reported in the literature. In the United States there are two registries available, one for "Pregnancies Exposed to Cancer Chemotherapy" at the University of Oklahoma Medical Center Section of Genetics (940 NE 13th Street, Room B2418, Oklahoma City, OK 73104, USA; telephone: 405-271-8697; e-mail: john.mulvihill@ouhsc.edu) [120] and one for "Long-term Follow-up of High-Risk Infantile Melanoma Population" at the University of Utah within the Tom C. Mathews, Jr Familial Melanoma Research Clinic at Huntsman Cancer Institute.

Another source is the Consortium of Cancer in Pregnancy Evidence (CCoPE) and the development of the On-line Cancer in Pregnancy Consultative Forum, which has been in operation since 2000, providing clinicians with access to expert guidance. In addition, it serves as a data collection centre. The Forum can be visited at www.motherisk.org/cforum.

A number of recommendations concerning the safety of the mother and the foetus directed to both obstetricians and the pediatricians are important to be followed: [2, 3, 6, 34, 38, 44]:

1. The placenta should be submitted to macroscopic and histopathologic examination in order to rule out microscopic tumour deposits.
2. Cytologic examination should be performed in both maternal and umbilical cord blood. "Buffy coat" preparations are also advised.
3. If metastases are found in both the placenta and the embryo, especially in melanomas, further immunohistochemical, karyotypic and cytogenetic studies as well as HLA typing contribute to the accurate identification of the malignant clone.
4. Neonates should be clinically examined for palpable skin lesions, organomegaly or other masses. If no metastases are present, a close follow-up of the healthy baby every 6 months for 2 years with physical examination, chest X-ray and liver function tests (including lactate dehydrogenase) is recommended.

References

1. Pavlidis N (2002) Coexistence of pregnancy and malignancy. Oncologist 7: 279–287
2. Pentheroudakis G, Pavlidis N (2006) Cancer and pregnancy: poena magna, not anymore. Eur J Cancer 42(2): 126–140
3. Potter JF, Schoeneman M (1970) Metastasis of maternal cancer to the placenta and fetus. Cancer 25: 380–388
4. Dildy GA, Moise KJ, Carpenter RJ, Kilma T (1989) Maternal malignancy metastatic to the products of conception: a review. Obstet Gynecol Surv 44: 535–540
5. Jackisch C, Louwen F, Schwenkagen A, et al. (2003) Lung cancer during pregnancy involving the products of conception and a review of the literature. Arch Gynecol Obstet 268: 69–77
6. Alexander A, Samlowski WE, Grossman D, et al. (2003) Metastatic melanoma in pregnancy: risk of transplacental metastases in the infant. J Clin Oncol 21: 2179–2186
7. Fox H (1987) Non-trophoblastic tumours of the placenta. In: Haines H, Taylor CW, Fox H (eds). Obstetrical and gynaecological pathology, vol II, 3rd edition. Churchill Livingstone, Edinburgh, pp 1030–1044
8. Panigel M (1993) The origin and structure of the extraembryonic tissue. In: Redman CWG, Sargent IL, Starkey PM (eds). The human placenta. Blackwell Scientific Publications, Cambridge, pp 3–32
9. Gardner R (1975) Origins and properties of trophoblast. In: Edwards RG, Howe CWS, Johnson MH (eds). Immunobiology of trophoblast. Cambridge University Press, Cambridge, pp 43–65
10. Wang T, Hamann W, Hartge R (1983) Structural aspects of a placenta from a case of maternal acute lymphatic leukemia. Placenta 4: 185–196
11. Harpold TL, Wang MY, McComb J, et al. (2001) Maternal lung adenocarcinoma metastatic to the scalp of a fetus. Pediatr Neurosurg 35: 39–42
12. Cailliez D, Moirot MH, Fessard C, Hemet J, Philipe E (1980) Localisation placentaire d' un carcinoma du col uterine. J Gynecol Obstet Biol Reprod (Paris) 9: 461–463
13. Rothman LA, Cohen CJ, Astarloa J (1973) Placental and fetal involvement by maternal malignancy: a report of rectal carcinoma and review of the literature. Am J Obstet Gynecol 116: 1023–1034
14. Villani GM, Goldberg GL (2000) Nongenital malignancies, in Cohen W (ed): Cherry and Merkatz's Complications of Pregnancy. Philadelphia, PA, Lippincott Williams and Wilkins, pp 624–627
15. O'Reily S, Chakravarthy A (1999) Other cancers in pregnancy, in Trimble E, Trimble C (eds): Cancer Obstetrics and Gynecology. Philadelphia, Lippincott Williams and Wilkins, pp 249–259
16. Dildy GA, Moise KJ, Carpenter RJ, et al. (1989) Maternal malignancy metastatic to the products of conception: A review. Obstet Gynecol Surv 44: 535–540
17. Markus N (1918) Gleichzeitige entwicklung melanosarcoma ovarii und carcinoma hepder schwangerschaft, eklampsie, placentarmetastazen. Arch F Gynakol 92: 659–678
18. Weber FP, Schwarz E, Hellenchmied R (1930) Spontaneous inoculation of melanotic sarcoma from mother to foetus. Br Med J 1: 537–539

19. Gottron H, Gertler W (1940) Zur frage des ubertritts von melanogen der mutter au den saugling uber die muttermilch. Arch Dermatol Syph 181: 91–98
20. Dargeon HW, Eversole JW, Del Duca V (1950) Malignant melanoma in an infant. Cancer 3: 299–306
21. Byrd BF, McGanity WJ (1954) The effect of pregnancy on the clinical course of malignant melanoma. South Med J 47: 196–200
22. Reynolds AG (1955) Placental metastasis from malignant melanoma: Report of a case. Obstet Gynecol 6: 205–209
23. Freedman WL, McMahon FJ (1960) Placental metastasis: review of the literature and report of a case of malignant melanoma. Obstet Gynecol 16: 550–560
24. Aronsson S (1963) A case of transplacental tumor metastasis. Acta Pediatr Scand 52: 123–134
25. Brodsky I, Baren M, Kahn SB, et al. (1965) Metastasis melanoma malignant from mother to fetus. Cancer 18: 1048–1054
26. Stephenson HE Jr, Terry CW, Lukens JN, et al. (1971) Immunologic factors in human melanoma „metastatic" to products of gestation (with exchange transfusion of infant to mother). Surgery 69: 515–522
27. Holcomb BW, Thigpen JT, Puckett JF, et al. (1975) Generalized melanosis complicating disseminated malignant melanoma in pregnancy: a case report. Cancer 35: 1459–1464
28. Sokol RJ, Hutchison P, Cowan D, et al. (1976) Amelanotic melanoma metastatic to the placenta. Am J Obstet Gynecol 124: 431–432
29. Smythe AR, Underwood PB Jr, Kreutner A Jr. (1976) Metastatic placental tumors: report of three cases. Am J Obstet Gynecol 125: 1149–1151
30. Gillis H II, Mortel R, McGavran MH (1976) Maternal malignant melanomametastatic to the products of conception: Report of a case. Gynecol Oncol 4: 38–42
31. Russell P, Laverty CR (1977) Malignant melanoma metastases in the placenta: a case report. Pathology 9: 251–255
32. Looi LM, Wang F (1979) Malignant melanoma metastases in chorionic villi: a case report. Malays J Pathol 2: 73–75
33. Moller D, Ipsen L, Asschenfeldt P (1986) Fatal course of malignant melanoma during pregnancy with dissemination to the products of conception. Acta Obstet Gynecol Scand 65: 501–502
34. Anderson JF, Kent S, Machin GA (1989) Maternal malignant melanoma with placental metastasis: a case report with literature review. Pediatr Pathol 9: 35–42
35. Brossard J, Abish S, Bernstein ML, et al. (1994) Maternal malignancy involving the products of conception: a report of malignant melanoma and medulloblastoma. Am J Pediatr Hematol Oncol 16: 380–383
36. Marsh RD, Chu NM (1996) Placental metastasis from primary ocular melanoma: A case report. Am J Obstet Gynecol 174: 1654–1655
37. Dillman RO, Vandermolen LA, Barth NM, et al. (1996) Malignant melanoma and pregnancy: ten questions. West J Med 164: 156–161
38. Baergen RN, Johnson D, Moore T, et al. (1997) Maternal melanoma metastatic to the placenta: A case report and review of the literature. Arch Pathol Lab Med 121: 508–511
39. Dipaola RS, Goodin S, Ratzell M, et al. (1997) Chemotherapy for metastatic melanoma during pregnancy. Gynecol Oncol 66: 526–530
40. Johnston SR, Broadley K, Henson G, et al. (1998) Management of metastasis melanoma during pregnancy. Br Med J 316: 848–849
41. Ferreira CM, Maceira JM, Coelho JM (1998) Melanoma and pregnancy with placental metastases: Report of a case. Am J Dermatopathol 20: 403–407
42. Merkus JM, Teepen JL (1998) The indispensable anamnesis: In-vitro fertilization in a woman under treatment for melanoma. Ned Tijdschr Geneeskd 142: 2073–2075
43. Altman JF, Lower L, Redman B, et al. (2003) Placental metastasis of maternal melanoma. J Am Acad Dermatol 49: 1150–1154
44. Smith LH, Dalrymple JL, Leiserowitz GS, et al. (2001) Obstetrical deliveries associated with maternal malignancy in California, 1992 through 1997. Am J Obstet Gynecol 184(7): 1504–1512
45. Nevin J, Soeters R, Dehaeck K, et al. (1995) Cervical carcinoma associated with pregnancy. Obstet Gynecol Surv 50: 228–239
46. Jolles CJ (1989) Gynecologic cancer associated with pregnancy. Semin Oncol 176: 417–424
47. Horner EN (1960) Placental metastasis. Case report: maternal death from ovarian cancer. Obstet Gynecol 15: 566–572
48. Patsner B, Mann WJ Jr, Chumas J (1989) Primary invasive ovarian adenocarcinoma with brain and placental metastases: a case report. Gynec Oncology 33:112–115

49. Cross RG, O'Connor MH, Hooland PDJ (1951) Placental metastasis of breast carcinoma. J Obstet Gynaecol Br Emp 58: 810–811
50. Rosemond GP (1964) Management of patients with carcinoma of the breast in pregnancy. Ann NY Acad Sci 114: 851–856
51. Pisarki T, Mrozewski A (1964) Przerzut raka sutka do lozyska (The mammary gland cancer to the placenta). Ginekol Pol 35: 277–286
52. Rewell RE, Whitehouse WL (1966) Malignant metastasis to the placenta from carcinoma of the breast. J Pathol Bacteriol 91: 225–256
53. Benirschke K, Driscoll SG (1967) The pathology of the human placenta. Springer, Berlin Heidelberg New York
54. Metler S, Werner B, Mayer J (1970) Prerzuty raka sutka do lozyska (mammary cancer metastases to the placenta). Ginekol Pol 41: 301–307
55. Angate AY, Loubiere R, Battesti F, Coulibaly AO, Fretillere M (1975) Metastase placentaire secondaire a un cancer du sein avec survie de trente et un mois de l'enfant. Chirurgie 101: 121–128
56. Salamon MA, Sherer DM, Saller DN Jr, Metlay LA, Sickel JZ (1994) Placental metastases in patients with recurrent breast carcinoma. Am J Obstet Gynecol 171(2): 573–574
57. Eltorky M, Khare VK, Osborne, P, Shanklin DR (1995) Placental metastasis from maternal carcinoma. A report of three cases. J Reprod Med 40(5): 399–403
58. Ackerman J, Gilbert-Barness E (1997) Malignancy metastatic to the products of conception: A case report with literature review. Pediatr Pathol Lab Med 17: 577–586
59. Dunn JS Jr, Anderson CD, Brost BC (1999) Breast carcinoma metastatic to the placenta. Obstet Gynecol 94:846
60. Ben Brahim E, Mrad K, Driss M, et al. (2001) Placental metastasis of breast cancer. Gynecol Obstet Fertil 29: 545–548
61. Lehner R, Strohmer H, Jirecek S (2001) Placental insufficiency and maternal death caused by advanced stage of breast cancer in third trimester. Eur J Obstet Gynecol Reprod Biol 99: 272–273
62. Roth LK, Taylor HS (2001) Risk of smoking to reproductive health: assessment of women's knowledge. Am J Obstet Gynecol 1849: 934–939
63. Barr JS (1953) Placental metastasis from a bronchial carcinoma. J Obstet Gynaecol Br Emp 60: 895–897
64. Hesketh J (1962) A case of carcinoma of the lung with secondary deposits in the placenta. J Obstet Gynaecol Br Emp 69: 514
65. Jones EM (1969) Placental metastasis from bronchial carcinoma. Br Med J 2: 491–492
66. Read EJ, Platzer RB (1981) Placental metastasis from maternal carcinoma of the lung. Obstet Gynecol 58: 387–391
67. Suda R, Repke JT, Steer R, Niebly JR (1986) Metastatic adenocarcinoma of the lung complicating pregnancy: a case report. J Reprod Med 31: 1113–1116
68. Delerive C, Locquet F, Mallart A, Janin A, Gosselin B (1989) Placental metastasis from maternal bronchial oat cell carcinoma. Arch Pathol Lab Med 113: 556–558
69. Harpold TL, Wang MY, McComb J, et al. (2001) Maternal lung adenocarcinoma metastatic to the scalp of a fetus. Pediatr Neurosurg 35: 39–42
70. Kochman AT, Radczynski JK, Baranowski W, et al. (2001) Metastases to the products of conception from a maternal bronchial carcinoma. A case report and review of literature. Pol J Pathol 52(3): 137–140
71. Walker JW, Reinisch JF, Monforte HL (2002) Maternal pulmonary adenocarcinoma metastatic to the fetus: first recorded case report and literature review. Pediatr Pathol Mol Med 21: 57–69
72. Tolar J, Coad JE, Neglia JP (2002) Transplacental transfer of small-cell carcinoma of the lung. N Engl J Med 346: 1501–1502
73. Teksam M, McKinney A, Short J, et al. (2004) Intracranial metastasis via transplacental (vertical) transmission of maternal small cell lung cancer to fetus: CT and MRI findings. Acta Radiol 45(5): 577–579
74. Reiter AA, Carpenter RJ, Dudrick AJ, Hinkley C (1985) Pregnancy associated with advanced adenocarcinoma of the lung. Int J Gynaecol Obstet 23: 78–85
75. Stark P, Green RE, Morgan G, Hildebrandt–Stark HE (1985) Lung cancer and pregnancy. Radiologe 25: 30–32
76. Brühwiler H, Wild A, Lüscher KP (1988) Lung cancer and pregnancy. Geburtshilfe Frauenheilkd 45: 654–655
77. Jaenne PA, Rodriguez-Thompsen D, Metcalf DR, et al. (2001) Chemotherapy for a patient with advanced non-small cell lung cancer during pregnancy: a case report and a review of chemotherapy treatment during pregnancy. Oncology 63: 175–183

78. Pawelec D (1976) Adenocarcinoma of the lung with metastasis in a 39-year-old pregnant woman. Pneumonol Pol 44: 283
79. Lishner M, Zemlickis P, Degendorfer P, et al. (1992) Maternal and foetal outcome following Hodgkin's disease in pregnancy. Br J Cancer 65: 114–117
80. Pohlman B, Lyons JA, Macklis RM (1999) Lymphoma in pregnancy. In: Trimble EL, Trimble CL, (eds). Cancer Obstetrics and Gynaecology. Philadelphia, Pa: Lippincott Williams and Wilkins, pp 209–238
81. Peleg D, Ben Ami M (1998) Lymphoma and leukemia complicating pregnancy. Obstet Gynecol Clin North Am 25: 365–383
82. Berghinz G (1900) Linfosarcoma acuta della madre; metastasi milari nel fegato del feto. Gazetta degli Ospedali di Milano 21:606 (abstract in J Am Med Assoc 34: 1558)
83. Priesel A, Winkelbauer A (1926) Placentare Übertragung des Lymphogranuloms. Virchows Arch (Patho Anat) 262: 749
84. Tsujimura T, Matsumoto K, Aozasa K (1993) Placental involvement by maternal non-Hodgkin's lymphoma. Arch Pathol Lab Med 117: 325–327
85. Pollack RN, Sklarin NT, Rao S, Divon MY (1993) Metastasis placental lymphoma with maternal human immunodeficiency virus infection. Obstet Gynecol 81: 856–857
86. Meguerian-Bedoyan Z, Lamant L, Hopfner C, et al. (1997) Anaplastic large cell lymphoma of maternal origin involving the placenta: case report and literature survey. Am J Surg Pathol 21: 1236–1241
87. Catlin EA, Roberts JD Jr, Erana R, et al. (1999) Transplacental transmission of natural-killer-cell lymphoma. N Engl J Med 341: 85–91
88. Nishi Y, Suzuki S, Otsubo Y, et al. (2000) B-cell-type malignant lymphoma with placental involvement. J Obstet Gynaecol Res 26: 39–43
89. Biermann HR, Aggeler PM, Thelander H, Kely KH, Cordes L (1956) Leukemia in pregnancy: a problem in transmission in man. JAMA 161: 220–223
90. Gramblett HG, Friedmann JL, Najjar S (1958) Leukemia in an infant born of a mother with leukaemia. N. Engl J Med 259: 727–729
91. Diamandopoulos GT, Hertig AT (1963) Transmission of leukaemia and allied diseases from mother to fetus. Obstet Gynecol 21: 150–154
92. Rigby PG, Hanson TA, Smith RS (1964) Passage of leukaemia cells across the placenta. N Engl J Med 271: 124–127
93. Bernard J, Jacquillat C, Chavelet F (1964) Leucémie aigue d'ume enfant de 5 mois née d'une mére attainte de leucémie aiguë au moment de l'accouchement. Nouv Rev Fr Hematol 4: 140–146
94. Las Heras J, Leal G, Haust MD (1986) Congenital leukaemia with placental involvement. Report of a case with ultrastructural study. Cancer 58: 2278–2281
95. Honore LH, Brown LB (1990) Intervillous placental metastasis with maternal myeloid leukaemia. Arch Pathol Lab Med 114: 450.
96. Sheikh SS, Khallifa MA, Marley EF, Bagg A, Lage JM (1996) Acute monocytic leukemia (FAB MS) involving the placenta associated with delivery of a healthy infant: case report and discussion. Int J Gynecol Pathol 15(4): 363–366
97. Osada S, Horibe K, Oiwa K, et al. (1990) A case of infantile acute monocytic leukaemia caused by vertical transmission of the mother's leukaemia cells. Cancer 65: 1146–1149
98. Catanzarite VA, Ferguson JE II (1984) Acute leukemia and pregnancy: A review of management and outcome, 1973–1982. Obstet Gynecol Surv 39: 663–678
99. Cappell MS. Colon cancer during pregnancy. Clin North Am Gastroenterol 2003; 32:341–85.
100. Ueo H, Matsuoka H, Tamura S, et al. (1991) Prognosis in gastric cancer associated with pregnancy. World J Surg 15: 293–298
101. Jaspers VKI, Gillessen A, Quakernack K (1999) Gastric cancer in pregnancy: Do pregnancy, age or female sex alter the prognosis? Eur J Obstet Gynecol 87: 13–22
102. Senge J (1912) Sekundäre carcinosis der Plazenta bei primären Magenkarzinom. Beitz Pathol 53:532–549
103. Bender S (1950) Placental metastasis in malignant disease complicated by pregnancy: with a report of two cases. Br Med J 1: 980–981
104. Almanza-Marquer R, Jurado-Jurado MB, Steta-Mondragon J, et al. (2002) Pregnancy complicated by acute lymphangitic adenomatosis, metastasis and disseminated intravascular coagulation: a case report. J Reprod Med 47: 421–423

105. Khatib F, Shaya M, Samueloff A (2003) Gastric carcinoma with metastasis to the placenta and amniotic fluid: case report and review of the literature. Eur J Obstet Gyne Reprod Biol 107: 208–209
106. Smythe AR, Underwood PB Jr, Kreutner AR (1976) Metastatic placental tumors: Report of three cases. Am J Obstet Gynecol 125: 1149–1151
107. Su LL, Biswas A, Wee A, Sufyan W (2006) Placental metastases from pancreatic adenocarcinoma in pregnancy. Acta Obstet Gynecol Scand 85(5): 626–627
108. Friedreich N (1866) Beitrag zur Pathologie das Krebses. Virchows Arch (Pathol Anat) 36: 465
109. Walz K (1906) Über Plazentatumoren. Verh Dtsch Ges Pathol 10: 279–284
110. Hill K, Stolte H (1970) Metastasen eines retrothekalen Sarkoms der Lunge im intevillösen Raun der Plazenta. Verch Dtsch Ges Path 54: 665
111. Frick R, Rummel H, Heberling D, Schmidt WO (1977) Placental metastases from a maternal angioblastic sarcoma of the vagina. Geburtshife Frauenheilkd 37: 216–220
112. Greenberg P, Collins JD, Voet RL, Jariwala L (1982) Ewing's sarcoma metastatic to placenta and ovary. Placenta 3: 191–197
113. Sedgely MG, Ostor AG, Fortune DW (1985) Angiosarcoma of breast metastasis to the ovary and placenta. Aust NZJ Obstet Gynaecol 25: 299–302
114. Pollack RN, Pollack M, Rochon L (1993) Pregnancy complicated by medulloblastoma with metastases to the placenta. Obstet Gynecol 81: 858–859
115. Sakurai H. Mitsuhashi N, Ibuki Y, et al. (1998) Placental metastasis from maternal primitive neuroectodermal tumor. Am J Clin Oncol 21: 39–41
116. Orr Jr, Grizzle WE, Huddleston JF (1982) Squamous cell carcinoma metastasis to placenta and ovary. Obstet Gynecol 59(suppl): 81S–83S
117. Dessable L, Dalmon C, Roche B, et al. (2005) Placental metastases from a maternal squamous cell tumor of the maxillary. Eur J Obst Gyne Repr Biology 123: 117–118
118. Gourley C, Monqghan HM, Beattiee G, Court S, et al. (2002) Intrauterine death resulting from placental metastases in adenocarcinoma of unknown primary. Clin Oncol (R Coll Radiol) 14(3): 213–216
119. Gray J, Kenny M, Sharpey-Schafer EP (1939) Metastasis of maternal tumor to products of gestation. J Obstet Gynaecol Br Emp 46: 8–14
120. Randall T (1993) National registry seeks scare data on pregnancy outcomes during chemotherapy. JAMA 269: 323

17 The Obstetric Care of the Pregnant Woman with Cancer

M. K. Dhanjal, S. Mitrou

Recent Results in Cancer Research, Vol. 178

17.1 Introduction

The care of the pregnant woman with cancer represents an immense challenge for doctors and other health professionals because of the complex ethical and therapeutic dilemmas raised. Appropriate and timely investigation and treatment may be lifesaving for the mother, but may have devastating effects on the developing fetus. Cancer occurs rarely in pregnancy, complicating approximately 1 in 1,000 live births. As women delay their first pregnancy to their third and fourth decades, the number of women suffering malignancy in pregnancy is expected to rise. Women with malignancy should be managed by a specialist multidisciplinary team including obstetricians, medical and surgical oncologists, radiologists, oncology nurses and midwives.

This chapter covers the physiological changes in pregnancy, the obstetric care of a pregnant woman affected by cancer, fetal consequences of maternal disease and treatment, and timing and mode of delivery.

17.2 Physiological Changes in Pregnancy

Pregnancy does not usually affect the natural history of cancer, but the physiological changes of pregnancy can simulate symptoms suggestive of spread of disease, alter drug metabolism and increase risks of thromboses and infection.

17.2.1 Cardiovascular System

Peripheral vascular resistance falls by up to 40% in pregnancy because of relaxation of arterial smooth muscle. This results in a 5- to 15-mmHg fall in the diastolic blood pressure by the end of the first trimester, which then returns to pre-pregnancy levels. Heart rate, stroke volume and myocardial contractility increase, resulting in a 50% rise in the cardiac output by 24 weeks of gestation which is sustained until term, except in the supine position, when the gravid uterus causes aorto-caval compression. Cardiac output increases by a further 30%–50% during labour. After delivery there is an autotransfusion of up to 1 l of blood, which further increases cardiac output. Cardiac output returns to pre-pregnancy levels within 2 weeks of delivery.

17.2.2 Respiratory System

Pregnant women often complain of a sensation of breathlessness, which in cancer patients may raise concern of lung metastases. However, in pregnancy there is a progressive increase in oxygen demands. Progesterone increases the sensitivity of the respiratory centres to CO_2, resulting in an increased tidal volume and respiratory alkalosis. The respiratory rate, PEFR, FEV1 and vital capacity (VC) remain unchanged and the residual volume (RV) decreases by 20%.

17.2.3 Urinary System

In pregnancy the kidneys increase by 1 cm in size and the ureters become physiologically dilated because of the muscle-relaxing effects of progesterone and the pressure effect of the growing uterus. An increase in renal blood flow and glomerular filtration results in lower urea and creatinine levels.

17.2.4 Haematology

Anaemia is not uncommon in pregnancy and is partly dilutional because of a greater rise in plasma volume compared to red blood cell mass and partly related to iron deficiency. Iron absorption from the gut, total serum iron-binding capacity and transferrin increase because of the increased demand; however, serum iron and ferritin still tend to decrease. Haemoglobin over 10.5 g/dl does not require further investigations in pregnancy. The reticulocyte and white cell count increase whilst a gestational thrombocytopenia may result in platelet levels as low as 100×10^9/l.

17.2.5 Drug Metabolism During Pregnancy

Changes occurring in pregnancy influence the therapeutic effectiveness of chemotherapeutic agents. Gastric motility and small bowel transit are slowed, especially in the third trimester, which may alter absorption and bioavailability of oral drugs. By 32 weeks of gestation, there is a 40% increase in plasma volume which can result in drug dilution. Albumin levels fall substantially as pregnancy advances, increasing the bioavailability of protein-bound drugs. Clearance of drugs excreted by the kidney increases as renal blood flow increases in pregnancy, resulting in a 50% rise in glomerular filtration rate. The activity of some hepatic metabolic pathways is enhanced, which may reduce the plasma concentration of some drugs cleared by the liver.

17.2.6 Increased Thrombotic Risk During Pregnancy

Pregnancy is a hypercoagulable state with a significantly increased risk of thromboembolism up to 6 weeks postnatally. The concentration of clotting factors is increased and there is reduced fibrinolysis. Obstruction of venous return by the enlarging uterus results in venous stasis which affects the left leg more than the right. Delivery may cause trauma to the pelvic veins, further increasing the thrombotic risk.

As malignancy itself is prothrombotic, serious consideration should be given to thromboprophylaxis in pregnancy. Additional risk factors such as a maternal age over 35 years, increased body mass index (BMI), thrombophilia and grandmultiparity may warrant thromboprophylaxis with low-molecular-weight heparin antenatally and in the puerperium. Temporary risk factors including dehydration from hyperemesis, surgery, long-haul air travel and infection may require thromboprophylaxis for the duration of the risk factor.

17.3 Antenatal Care

17.3.1 Maternal Issues

Pregnant women with co-existing malignancy should be looked after by a multidisciplinary team of specialists and mothers-to-be should actively take part in the decision making process at all times. Although the current trend is to reduce the antenatal visits of pregnant women, the need for closer surveillance of cancer patients is a sine qua non. Despite the lack of evidence-based guidance regarding the antenatal management of cancer patients or survivors, a senior obstetrician should be involved in their care in collaboration with oncologists and other health professionals [1].

The diagnosis of cancer makes a woman re-evaluate her life and it is unusual for women with a current malignancy to wish to conceive before treatment is complete. Chemotherapeutic agents and pelvic radiotherapy can render a woman infertile. She may therefore request freezing of eggs or in vitro fertilisation and freezing of embryos before such treatment. Those with a previous hormonally responsive tumour such as breast cancer or melanoma are advised to wait at least 2 years after treatment before conceiving [2]. These women should be provided with effective contraception. If an unexpected pregnancy occurs in a woman who is undergoing treatment, or who has been advised to delay pregnancy, she should be carefully counselled regarding the maternal and fetal risks of continuing with the pregnancy. Termination of pregnancy should be offered if appropriate.

Most cases of malignancy in pregnancy present as a de novo diagnosis. Diagnosis is often delayed because of non-specific symptoms which may occur in malignancy and in pregnancy. It is imperative to institute appropriate investigations of suspicious symptoms or biopsy lesions so that an early diagnosis can be made. Fetal risks of treatment may make health professionals reluctant to treat the mother aggressively at the time of diagnosis. The mother's decision may also be to put the unborn fetus first and delay treatment. Unfortunately, this could result in the mother not surviving the disease. Careful in-depth counselling should occur and informed decisions should be respected. Social workers may need to be involved if the mother is not expected to survive after the birth of her child.

17.3.1.1 First Trimester

The booking visit at the antenatal clinic allows a detailed history to be taken and a full general examination to be performed. In addition to routine booking blood tests, blood should be taken for renal, liver and bone studies. Depending on the site of the malignancy further tests may be necessary, such as ultrasound scanning, echocardiography, and lung function tests [1]. Folic acid 400 mcg daily reduces the incidence of neural tube defects if taken from pre-conception to 12 weeks of gestation [3]. Risk factors for thrombosis can be assessed and thromboprophylaxis commenced if appropriate. An ultrasound scan will confirm fetal viability and stage of gestation and inform regarding multiple pregnancy. Fetal screening tests for chromosomal abnormalities should be offered. Plans should be made for further multidisciplinary care. Women who have had a malignancy in the past and who are in remission should be treated as normal and should have regular follow-up visits with their oncologist. If they present with symptoms of a recurrence, this should be investigated urgently.

17.3.1.2 Second and Third Trimesters

Abdominal examination of the uterus is performed routinely at every visit. Further physical examination should be guided by presenting symptoms. Although breast and pelvic examinations are not carried out routinely in an otherwise uncomplicated pregnancy, this may be required in women with previous breast or gynaecological cancer. Tumour markers in pregnancy are often elevated and should be interpreted with caution [4].

Imaging techniques using ultrasound are safe at any stage of gestation. Magnetic resonance imaging (MRI) can be performed safely in the second and third trimesters. There are few safety data on the use of MRI in the first trimester, although there have been no reports of adverse effects. MRI should not be withheld in the first trimester if clinically necessary. X-rays can be performed safely with appropriate shielding. CT of chest and V/Q scan carry negligible radiation risk when shielding is used; hence they are commonly used for the diagnosis of pulmonary embolism. However, multiple testing with such scans in pregnancy may reach the total dose of 1 cGy, which is the threshold for safe fetal exposure [5].

17.3.1.3 Symptom Control

Analgesics

Paracetamol is safe in pregnancy and is a first-line analgesic. Non-steroidal anti-inflammatory drugs (NSAIDs) are generally avoided because of premature closure of the ductus arteriosus via their inhibition of prostaglandin E_2 production. However, ductal flow impairment is rare before 27 weeks and resolves within 24 hours of NSAID discontinuation, and indomethacin (used in the short term at later stages of gestation for the arrest of pre-term labour) appears to be safe. NSAIDs also affect the fetal kidney, causing reversible oligohydramnios. There have been recent concerns over the use of aspirin and NSAIDs before pregnancy and in the first trimester. Analgesic doses of NSAIDs have been associated with miscarriage, and some data are emerging of an association between NSAIDs, cardiac defects and orofacial clefts [6]. Opiates are suitable for more severe pain. If used close to delivery, they can result in neonatal withdrawal effects. Paediatricians should be warned so that they can arrange to wean the neonates off the medication.

Nausea and Vomiting

Nausea and vomiting may result from the pregnancy in the first trimester, the malignancy or the use of chemotherapy. First-line agents are metoclopromide, cyclizine, promethazine, prochlorperazine and domperidone, which may be used in combination. These have all been used widely in hyperemesis gravidarum and have not been found to be teratogenic. Ondansetron is widely used in patients on chemotherapy. Its use in pregnancy has been limited to those with severe hyperemesis gravidarum as a second-line agent; however, reassuring safety profiles are emerging. Prednisolone is an alternative effective second-line agent. It should only be used after failure of combination first-line agents as there is a weak association between oral cleft in the newborn and maternal first trimester corticosteroid use.

Constipation

Bulk-forming laxatives, lactulose and senna can be used safely in the management of constipation.

Infections

Pregnancy results in an increased susceptibility to infections normally dealt with by the cell-mediated immune system. Infections combated mainly by the humoral immune system are not increased. Infections in immunosuppressed cancer patients can be aggressive and need early effective treatment. Clinicians should have a very low threshold in prescribing antibiotics if an infection is suspected. Asymptomatic bacteriuria and urinary tract infections are common in pregnancy and can lead to pyelonephritis, septicaemia and pre-term labour. They should both be actively sought at each antenatal visit and treated. Premature rupture of membranes can lead to chorioamnionitis, which can cause life-threatening maternal and foetal infection. The altered drug metabolism in pregnancy often lowers the maternal serum levels of drugs such as antibiotics and may lead to subtherapeutic levels, particularly if lower doses are used.

Penicillins freely cross the placenta, but with no harmful effects to the fetus. During pregnancy, their dose needs to be increased. The combination of amoxicillin and clavulanic acid (Augmentin) is an effective agent against aerobic and anaerobic infections but is used with some caution in pregnancy as it has been shown to be associated with an increased rate of necrotising enterocolitis in the newborn. Cephalosporins and metronidazole are safe in pregnancy and are commonly used as broad-spectrum agents in combination. The macrolide erythromycin is safe and commonly used in penicillin allergy and community-acquired pneumonia and as prophylaxis in preterm pre-labour rupture of membranes. Clarithromycin appears to be safe and has fewer maternal gastric side effects than erythromycin [7]. Nitrofurantoin can be safely used in urinary infections, but may cause neonatal haemolysis if used at term. Trimethoprim should be avoided in the first trimester as it is a folate antagonist. Gentamicin can be used in gram-negative sepsis or as prophylaxis against infective endocarditis, but maintenance of gentamicin levels is essential as subtherapeutic levels occur with standard doses in pregnancy. Aminoglycosides can cause damage to the fetal eighth cranial nerve, but this risk is mainly with streptomycin rather than gentamicin or tobramycin. Imipenem and meropenem have been used in pregnancy, but few safety data are available. Quinolones such as ciprofloxacin have been found to cause congenital arthropathy in animal studies and are therefore avoided in pregnancy. Tetracyclines are contraindicated in pregnancy as high parenteral doses can be hepatotoxic to the mother and cause tooth discoloration and inhibition of fetal bone growth [8].

17.3.2 Fetal Issues

17.3.2.1 Fetal Malformations

The detection of structural abnormalities is important particularly if a fetus has been exposed to radiation or chemotherapy in the first trimester. Second-trimester biochemical screening alone is used to identify chromosomal abnormalities but has poor sensitivities. Interpretation could be difficult in the presence of an AFP- or HCG-producing tumour. Nuchal translucency is more sensitive and can also give an indication of fetal cardiac abnormalities. Definitive tests for chromosomal abnormalities (chorionic villus sampling or amniocentesis) should be carried out only if indicated. First-trimester ultrasound (transabdominal and transvaginal combined) may be able to pick up gross abnormalities such as neural tube defects, gastroschisis and multi-dysplastic kidneys. Most malformations can be detected by ultrasound scanning between 18 and 20 weeks and fetal echocardiography at 23 weeks can be employed if cardiac defects are suspected. Fetal MRI scanning is available in some tertiary centres, allowing more detailed studies of foetal anatomy [1, 9, 10].

Any patient requiring chemotherapy in pregnancy should have regular fetal growth ultrasound scans, with assessment of liquor volume and umbilical Doppler studies which will confirm fetal well-being [1].

17.4 Delivery

One of the milestones in the management of pregnant women with cancer is the decision to deliver in order to introduce or continue cancer treatment.

17.4.1 Timing of Delivery

The decision to end the pregnancy and deliver the fetus depends mainly on the urgency of the requirement to treat the mother with potentially fetotoxic agents. If maternal outcome or survival is reduced by delaying treatment, serious consideration should be given to either terminating the pregnancy or delivering a pre-term baby, depending on gestational age.

The lower limit of fetal viability is generally agreed to be 24 weeks of gestation or a fetal weight of 500 g. Survival figures from the UK EPICure study in 1995 showed that 39% of babies delivered before 26 weeks of gestation survived to discharge. Gestation specific survival rates were 11%, 26% and 44% at 23, 24 and 25 weeks, respectively. Of the survivors, by 6 years of age, between 25% and 46% (depending on addition of cognitive measures to physical disability) were not functioning within the normal range, or had a disability which would prevent them from being independent [11, 12]. More current population-based data suggest that survival is increasing at these very pre-term stages of gestation. In a recent report from Belgium, survival increased from 49% at 24 weeks to 72% at 26 weeks. However, it is as yet unknown whether the proportion of these surviving children with disability is also improving. In the Belgian study, those without neurological sequelae and specific intensive care complications at the time of discharge from hospital were only 7% if delivered at 25 weeks and 28% if delivered at 26 weeks of gestation [13].

If urgent treatment (surgery, chemotherapy or radiotherapy) is necessary, the options are to:

- Terminate the pregnancy if less than 24 weeks gestation and then continue with the treatment or
- Deliver the baby and continue with the treatment or
- Commence treatment without delivery, after considering the risks of the treatment to the fetus. In this instance, if surgery is required, this is best performed after the first trimester to minimise fetal risk. If chemo- or radiotherapy is subsequently required, it may be possible to delay this until after a viable gestational age is reached. Alternatively, if urgent chemotherapy is necessary, it may be possible to administer this before the foetus reaches an appropriate gestational age for delivery, if it is considered that the chemotherapy risk for the foetus is minimal

If the fetus is less than 30 weeks gestation and the treatment can be safely delayed for a few weeks, this may be appropriate to optimise outcome. This is particularly relevant between 24 and 26 weeks of gestation, when fetal survival increases by 3% with each extra day in utero.

17.4.2 Antenatal Steroids

Antenatal corticosteroid administration reduces neonatal complications and improves outcome with pre-term deliveries. Forty to fifty percent of babies born before 32 weeks will develop respiratory distress syndrome (RDS), which is a significant contributing factor to the mortality and morbidity of prematurity. Antenatal steroids reduce the risk of neonatal RDS, intraventricular haemorrhage and death in babies delivered before 34 weeks of gestation, primarily by enhancing fetal lung maturation. They also reduce the cost and duration of neonatal intensive care. They have a very good safety profile and their administration as a single course of two doses carries minimal risks for the mother and the baby.

If contemplating delivery between 24 and 34 weeks of gestation, betamethasone 12 mg intramuscularly in two doses 24 h apart should be administered to the mother. Betamethasone should be given at least 24 h to 7 days before delivery to achieve optimal effect. Dexamethasone has been used with the same efficacy, but is associated with an increased risk of periventricular leukoplakia compared to betamethasone. Repeated courses of steroids are not indicated as there is lack of evidence to support the benefits and there are serious concerns of multiple courses of steroids and neurological development [14].

17.4.3 Mode of Delivery

The mode of delivery depends on the gestational age, fetal presentation, previous obstetric history and presence of a pelvic mass. A vaginal delivery is preferable to a caesarean section unless there is an obstetric indication for surgery, an obstructing pelvic mass or a gynaecological malignancy [4].

Caesarean section carries many risks which may be compounded by the malignancy itself, or by its treatment. The recovery time is also longer than that following a vaginal birth. There is a 20-fold increased risk of infection following caesarean section [15]. A patient requiring chemotherapy immediately after delivery is therefore at serious risk of wound infection and dehiscence from the additional effect of immunosuppression [16]. Thrombo-embolism is more common after a caesarean section. Malignancy increases this risk further, such that women should be given thromboprophylaxis with LMWH for up to 6 weeks postnatally. The risks of haemorrhage and hysterectomy are increased with a caesarean section and the overall mortality is five times greater than vaginal delivery. The neonnate is also at increased risk of transient tachypnoea of the newborn (TTN) with a caesarean section, which may necessitate admission to the special care baby unit [15].

17.5 Conclusion

Cancer complicating pregnancy is a rare life paradox and a multidisciplinary team approach in a tertiary setting would be appropriate. Medical, surgical, psychological and ethical issues should be dealt with by specialists and the pregnant woman should be given the best available evidence-based information in order to make informed decisions.

References

1. Antenatal care: Routine care for the healthy woman (2003). NICE Clinical Guideline CG 006
2. Pentheroudakis G, Pavlidis N (2006) Cancer and pregnancy: poena magna, not anymore. Eur J Cancer 42(2): 126–140
3. Periconceptional folic acid and food fortification in the prevention of neural tube defects (2003). RCOG Scientific advisory committee opinion paper 4
4. Leiserowitz GS (2006) Managing ovarian masses in pregnancy. Obstet Gynecol Surv 61(7): 463–470
5. Fattibene P, Mazzei F, Nuccetelli C, Risica S (1999) Prenatal exposure to ionising radiation: sources, effects and regulatory aspects. Acta Paediatr 88: 693–702
6. Koren G, Florescu A, Costei AM, Boskovic R, Moretti ME (2006) Nonsteroidal anti-inflammatory drugs during third trimester and the risk of premature closure of the ductus arteriosus: a meta-analysis. Ann Pharmacother 40(5): 824–829
7. Kenyon S, Boulvain M, Neilson J (2004) Antibiotics for preterm rupture of membranes: a systematic review. Obstet Gynecol 104(5 pt 1): 1051–1057
8. Nahum GG, Uhl K, Kennedy DL (2006) Antibiotic use in pregnancy and lactation: what is and is not known about teratogenic and toxic risks. Obstet Gynecol 107(5): 1120–1138

9. Mole RH (1987) Irradiation of the embryo and fetus. Br J Radiol 60: 17–31
10. Partridge AH, Garber JE (2000) Long-term outcomes of children exposed to anti-neoplastic agents in utero. Semin Oncol 27: 712–726
11. Wood NS, Marlow N, Costeloe K, Gibson AT, Wilkinson AR (2000) Neurologic and developmental disability after extremely preterm birth. EPICure Study Group. N Engl J Med 343: 378–384
12. Costeloe K (2006) EPICure: facts and figures: why preterm labour should be treated. BJOG 113 (Suppl 3): 10–12
13. Vanhaesebrouck P, Allegaert K, Bottu J, Debauche C, Devlieger H, Docx M et al. (2004) The EPIBEL study: outcomes to discharge from hospital for extremely pre-term infants in Belgium. Pediatrics 114: 663–675
14. Antenatal corticosteroids to prevent respiratory distress syndrome (2004) RCOG Green top guideline No. 7
15. Caesarean section (2004) National collaborating centre for women's and children's health. Clinical guideline
16. Reynosa E, Shepherd F, Messner H et al. (1987) Acute leukaemia in pregnancy: The Toronto Leukaemia Study Group experience with long-term follow-up of children exposed in utero to chemotherapeutic agents. J Clin Oncol 5: 1098–1106

18 Fertility Issues and Options in Young Women with Cancer

K. Oktay, M. Sönmezer

Recent Results in Cancer Research, Vol. 178

18.1 Introduction

Nearly 1,400,000 new cancer cases were expected in the year 2006, of which 679,450 would occur in women (Jemal et al. 2006). Around 8% of all female cancers occur under the age of 40 years, which corresponds to approximately 55,000 women in the United States (Oktay and Yih 2002). When all female cancers are considered, despite an increase in the cancer incidence by 0.3% per year from 1987 to 1999, the death rates for all cancers combined decreased by 0.6% per year from 1992 to 1999 as a result of improvements in current treatment modalities including surgical techniques, radiation therapy, multiagent chemotherapy, and hematopoietic stem cell transplantation (Reis et al. 1999; Jemal et al. 2004). The cure rates for certain malignancies now exceed 90%. As a result, more women survive cancer every year to face the challenging long-term complications of the treatment. These include but are not limited to growth disorders, cardiovascular problems, neurocognitive abnormalities, second malignant tumors, and reproductive failure, all of which substantially impair the quality of life of the cancer survivor (Leung et al. 2000; Shusterman and Meadows 2000; Bhatia 2002; Tauchmanova et al. 2002). Many chemotherapy regimens are gonadotoxic, mainly because of inclusion of alkylating agents (Brogan and Dillon 2000; Sonmezer and Oktay 2004). The risk of ovarian failure may increase up to ninefold in cancer survivors receiving cyclophosphamide-based combination chemotherapy (Byrne et al. 1992; Meirow and Nugent 2001), and ovarian failure is almost inevitable in patients undergoing preconditioning with chemoradiation before hematopoietic stem cell transplantation (Sanders et al. 1988). Even when these patients were not sterilized by high-dose chemo-/radiotherapy, there may be an increased risk for complications during pregnancy such as early pregnancy loss, premature labor, and low birth weight (Sanders et al. 1996; Chiarelli et al. 2000; Green et al. 2002a,b).

The picture is similar with pediatric cases. By the year 2010, as many as 1 in 250 patients will have survived *childhood* malignancies (Bleyer 1990). As the number of patients surviving childhood cancers and as the number reaching reproductive ages increases, pediatric patients and parents have begun to face some critical long-term cancer treatment-related issues. Among the concerns are whether chemo-/radiotherapy will cause any growth problems, or whether future reproductive function and childbearing will be affected. If in fact this child grows to have children, will the offspring be healthy?

This heightened awareness of the effects of various cancer treatments on fertility resulted in a surge in the number of patients seeking help to preserve their fertility (Oktay et al. 2003, 2005a). In response, a number of cryopreservation techniques have emerged to preserve fertility. The advent of in vitro fertilization (IVF) and its current worldwide utilization have resulted in the development of successful cryopreservation techniques for excess embryos. The cryopreservation techniques have further been applied to unfertilized mature and immature human oocytes (Porcu et al. 1997; Polak deFried et al. 1998) and ovarian tissue (Bahadur and Steele 1996; Oktay and Karlikaya 2000; Poirot et al. 2002; Oktay et al. 2004a). In this chapter, we review not only the underlying gonadal physiology and the mechanism of damage by cancer treatments, but also current as well as emerging techniques of fertility preservation.

18.2 Gonadal Damage Associated with Chemotherapy and Radiotherapy

18.2.1 Ovarian Physiology and the Impact of Chemotherapy on Ovarian Follicles

Multiagent chemotherapy constitutes the basis of the modern cancer treatment. Ovaries, which are stocked with irreplaceable follicles, are extremely sensitive to most cytotoxic drugs (Sonmezer and Oktay 2004; Oktay et al. 2001). The end result of the chemotherapy can range from damage to steroid-producing cells and/or oocytes of developing ovarian follicles (granulosa and theca cells), which can cause temporary amenorrhea, to apoptotic death of primordial follicles, that results in premature ovarian failure. Ultrastructurally, ovarian exposure to chemotherapeutics is associated with marked follicle loss (Familiari et al. 1993). Factors that can potentially modify the risk of chemotherapy-induced ovarian failure are summarized in Table 18.1.

In the neonatal period the first signs of ovarian differentiation are observed at 6–8 weeks of gestation, which is reflected by mitotic proliferation of germ cells reaching its maximum, 6–7 million oogonia, at 16–20 weeks (Speroff and Fritz 2005). After mitotic replication, oogonia enter the 1st meiotic division and are transformed to oocytes, which are arrested at diplotene. Over the next 20 weeks of gestation, the total number of germ cells falls to 1–2 million at birth as a result of a rapid and massive atresia of oocytes. In consequence of the continuing depletion, the number of germ cells is further reduced to 300,000–500,000 at puberty.

Table 18.1 Factors that can modify the risk of chemotherapy-related gonadal failure

Age of the patient
Type of chemotherapeutic agents
Cumulative dose of alkylating agent
Concomitant use of abdominopelvic radiation therapy
Ovarian reserve[a]
Schedule of implementation[b]

[a] If ovarian reserve was already compromised by a previous ovarian surgery or radiotherapy, the risk of ovarian failure is increased

[b] Whether schedule of implementation is an independent variable or related to cumulative dose of the implemented agent remains to be resolved

A minimum of 85 days is required for the full development of a primordial follicle that differentiates in to an antral follicle leading to ovulation. In adult ovary more than 90% of the ovarian reserve is made up of primordial follicles at resting stage that include an oocyte arrested at the prophase of 1st meiotic division. Even though the mechanism of primordial follicle growth initiation is still not understood, it is clearly an FSH-independent process; FSH receptors are not expressed until these follicles initiate growth and reach multilayer stages (Oktay et al. in press).

Some chemotherapeutic agents are more commonly associated with permanent and irreversible gonadal damage, such as cyclophosphamide, chlorambucil, melphalan, busulfan, nitrogen mustard, procarbazine, ifosphamide, and thiotepa (Sonmezer and Oktay 2004; Warne et al. 1973; Koyama et al. 1977; Fisher et al. 1979; Viviani et al. 1985; Mackie et al. 1996). Among the moderately gonadotoxic agents are cisplatin and adriamycin, while bleomycin, actinomycin D, vincristine, methotrexate, and 5-fluorouracil are associated with mild or no gonadotoxicity (Table 18.2). Although there is limited evidence, paclitaxel may also be gonadotoxic, but this remains to be verified (Oktay et al. 2005b). In a recent study the impact of breast cancer chemotherapy was investigated in patients receiving either adriamycin and cyclophosphamide (AC) or AC plus taxanes. Patients were assessed 6 months after chemotherapy, and a second assessment was done after a mean of 28.2 months after chemotherapy when patients were interviewed regarding menstruation and menopausal symptoms. Although the short-term incidence of amenorrhea was higher in patients who were treated with taxanes, no significant long-term impact of taxanes on ovarian function was demonstrated by day 2–3 FSH and estradiol evaluation (Reh et al. 2006).

Cyclophosphamide is the most recognized agent to cause damage to oocytes and granulosa cells. In a recent mouse study, cyclophosphamide-induced follicular damage occurred in a dose-dependent manner, even at low doses of

Table 18.2 The degree of gonadotoxicity of the chemotherapeutic agents

Risk is high	
	Cyclophosphamide
	Melphalan
	Procarbazine
	Busulfan
	Nitrogen mustard
	Chlorambucil
Risk is moderate	
	Adriamycin
	Cisplatin
	Paclitaxel*
	Risk is low
	Methotrexate
	Bleomycin
	Actinomycin D
	5-Fluorouracil
	Vincristine

*Needs to be verified in further studies

20 mg/kg (Meirow et al. 1999). Relative risk of premature ovarian failure was reported to be between 4 and 9.3 in patients receiving cyclophosphamide (Byrne et al. 1992; Meirow and Nugent 2001). Sanders and colleagues reported that the probability of having ovarian failure in patients receiving high-dose cyclophosphamide before hematopoietic stem cell transplantation (HSCT) was 0.35 by 7 years (Sanders et al. 1988).

During the last 10–15 years before the onset of menopause, primordial follicle loss is accelerated, which is reflected by a constant decrease in inhibin B levels and increase in FSH levels. As a consequence, a smaller number of follicles that are more prone to cell division errors begin to grow each cycle, until menopause occurs, when the number of follicles falls below 1,000. Because of this, older women with a low primordial follicle pool have a higher risk of developing ovarian failure compared with young women with higher primordial follicle numbers. Consistent with this biological fact, earlier studies demonstrated that a cumulative cyclophosphamide dose of 5.2 g caused amenorrhea in women in their forties, 9.3 g in women in their thirties, and 20.4 g in women in their twenties (Koyama et al. 1977).

One of the major weaknesses of the preexisting studies assessing the impact of chemotherapy on ovarian function is the utilization of *amenorrhea* as a surrogate marker for infertility. Although irregular menstrual pattern or amenorrhea is expected to occur in a significant number of patients during the courses of chemotherapy, or even last for some period of time after completion of the chemotherapy, many patients return to a cyclical menstrual pattern (Wallace et al. 1989a; Brewer et al. 1999; Tangir et al. 2003). Gonadotropin levels may even normalize, especially in very young patients (Tauchmanova et al. 2002; Zanetta et al. 2001; Oktay and Sonmezer 2004). This is because developing follicles, which are the main source of steroid production, are invariably damaged during the treatment, and it takes 3–6 months to regrow these follicles from the remaining primordial follicles. Not only may many survivors be infertile despite continuing menstruation, but they are also at high risk of developing premature menopause (Byrne et al. 1992; Larsen et al. 2003; Oktay et al. 2004b). The fact that ovulation and cyclicity may occur despite loss of half of the follicular pool in rodents (Ginsburg et al. 2001) indicates that the indirect assessment of infertility is unreliable.

It is known that AMH is produced by the granulosa cells (Oktay et al. in press; Baarends et al. 1995; Weenen et al. 2004), this production being initiated in primary follicles. Per follicle AMH production declines in late antral stages of follicle development. A recent study found that, compared to estradiol and FSH, anti-Müllerian hormone levels (AMH) showed a more rapid and sustained change after chemotherapy (Anderson et al. 2006). Moreover, the decrease in AMH occurred without a significant decrease in inhibin B or increase in FSH concentrations. Authors concluded that the severity and rapidity of the fall in AMH concentrations compared with the partial decline in inhibin B concentrations might reflect primordial and preantral follicles as the primary site of toxicity. Similarly, another study demonstrated that patients undergoing chemotherapy had diminished AMH levels despite normal baseline FSH levels after chemotherapy

(Azim et al. 2006). Moreover, Reh et al. found that a significant fraction of patients continued to menstruate regularly after chemotherapy, despite biochemical evidence of diminished ovarian reserve (Reh et al. 2006).

In another study by Schmidt et al., despite the fact that all of the eight breast cancer patients regained menstruation after completion of chemotherapy, three had irregular menstrual cycles and five had undetectable inhibin B levels or FSH values >50 IU/ml, suggesting impairment of ovarian reserve (Schmidt et al. 2005). The age of breast cancer patients ranged between 27 and 36, while cumulative dose of cyclophosphamide ranged between 3 and 8 g. The authors claimed that the cumulative dose of cyclophosphamide that was used in the study was not adequate to cause complete ovarian failure in that group of young breast cancer patients. However, in the same study, all of the five patients with leukemia and two with Hodgkin lymphoma undergoing hematopoietic stem cell transplantation, and one receiving high-dose chemotherapy with alkylating agents for Hodgkin disease, had premature ovarian failure after completion of chemotherapy.

These findings support the observation that, even though there may be no clinical signs of ovarian failure, there is always damage to follicular reserve in proportion to the cumulative dose of chemotherapeutic agents, and the compromise in fertility may not be detectable with routinely used laboratory tests (Oktay et al. 2006a). As amenorrhea is the last event to occur in the scheme of menopausal transition and as many women with diminished ovarian reserve still menstruate regularly, previous studies greatly underestimate the extent of chemotherapy-induced infertility. Nevertheless, because no large study with biochemical ovarian reserve assessment is available, risk evaluation on the likelihood of amenorrhea after treatment with each chemotherapy agent or regimen is made based on the likelihood of amenorrhea.

18.2.2 The Impact of Radiotherapy on Ovarian Function

Ionizing radiation is a well-recognized cause of ovarian damage and permanent infertility. Gonadal damage occurs not only by direct exposure, as in the case of pelvic or low abdominal irradiation, but also by scattering even if the gonads are transposed outside of the radiation field. Radiation causes a dose-related reduction in the primordial follicle pool (Gosden et al. 1997). The human oocyte is extremely sensitive to radiation, and irradiation at ovarian dose >6 Gy usually causes irreversible ovarian failure (Howell and Shalet 1998). Wallace et al. (1989a, 2003) demonstrated that <4 Gy is enough to destroy half of the oocyte population (LD_{50} < 4 Gy); however, very recently, using a revised mathematical model, the same authors suggested that the LD_{50} of the oocytes was <2 Gy. Age at the time of exposure to radiotherapy, extent and type of radiation therapy (e.g., abdominal, pelvic external beam irradiation, intracavitary brachytherapy), and fractionation schedule are also important prognostic indicators for development of ovarian failure (Sonmezer and Oktay 2004).

In mice, radiation-induced chromosome damage in the oocytes was more evident in older animals compared with younger ones (Tease and Fisher 1991). In general, irradiation is more toxic when given in a single dose compared to fractionated doses. Stillman et al. (1981) investigated the risk of ovarian failure among 182 long-term survivors of childhood cancers receiving abdominal radiotherapy. The mean follow-up was 16.4 years. Ovarian failure occurred in 68% of the patients when both ovaries were in the irradiation field and in 14% of the patients when both ovaries were at the edge of the treatment field. None of the 122 children developed ovarian failure when one or both ovaries were outside of the abdominal treatment field. In another study, failure in pubertal development or premature menopause was observed in 37 of 38 patients who received external abdominal irradiation in doses ranging from 20 to 30 Gy during childhood for intra-abdominal tumors (Wallace et al. 1989b). Sanders et al. reported the probability of ovarian failure in patients receiving cyclophosphamide and total body irradiation for HSCT as 1.00 at 1 year (Sanders et al. 1988).

Failure in pubertal development may be the first sign of ovarian failure in these patients who received radiotherapy during their childhood. Total body irradiation used in conditioning regimens before HSCT to eradicate the host's pre-existing bone marrow (e.g., leukemias) is commonly associated with ovarian failure (Tauchmanova et al. 2002; Sanders et al. 1988; Thibaud et al. 1988). Although successful full-term pregnancies were reported, the risk of ovarian failure is always high in women who receive high dose abdominal or pelvic irradiation (Giri et al. 1992; Maruta et al. 1995). In addition, if pregnancy is achieved, these patients may have increased risk for pregnancy complications including early pregnancy loss, premature labor, and low birth weight due to impaired uterine growth and blood flow (Critchley et al. 2002; Green et al. 2002a,b).

18.3 Who Are the Candidates for Fertility Preservation?

There is a growing list of indications for fertility preservation ranging from both neoplastic and nonneoplastic diseases treated with cytotoxic therapy to any gynecologic surgery compromising ovarian reserve (Table 18.3). Because each patient presents with a unique clinical situation, a tailored approach to fertility preservation is needed. In our center we developed a comprehensive approach to fertility preservation, depending on the patient's age, presence or absence of ovarian involvement, available time, and the type of cancer.

Table 18.3. Indications for fertility preservation

Cancer in children	
	Hodgkin and non-Hodgkin lymphoma
	Leukemia
	Ewing sarcoma
	Wilms tumor
	Neuroblastoma
	Pelvic osteosarcoma
	Genital rhabdomyosarcoma
Breast cancer	
	Infiltrative ductal histological subtype
	Infiltrative lobular*
	Stage I–III
	Stage IV*
Cancer of the cervix	
	Squamous cell carcinoma
	Adeno/adenosquamous carcinoma*
	Autoimmune and hematological diseases
	Systemic lupus erythematosus
	Behcet disease
	Steroid resistant glomerulonephritis
	Inflammatory bowel disease
	Pemphigus vulgaris
	Rheumatoid arthritis
	Progressive systemic sclerosis
	Juvenile idiopathic arthritis
	Multiple sclerosis
	Autoimmune thrombocytopenia
	Aplastic anemia
	Sickle cell disease
Benign ovarian disease	
	Endometriosis
	Benign ovarian lesions requiring repeated surgeries
Patients receiving pelvic radiation	
	Solid organ tumors presenting in the pelvis
	Ewing sarcoma
	Osteosarcoma
	Tumors of the spinal cord
	Retroperitoneal sarcoma
	Rectal cancer
	Benign bone tumors
Prophylactic oophorectomy**	
	BRCA-I-positive patients
	BRCA-II-positive patients
Hematopoietic stem cell transplantation	
	Malignant diseases
	Genetic, hematological, and autoimmune disorders
Patients undergoing surgery for gynecological cancers***	

* If ovarian cryopreservation is performed, the risk of ovarian involvement should be excluded

** When ovarian cryopreservation is considered, it should be noted that the increased risk of ovarian cancer is not apparent until age 40

*** Fertility-preserving surgery including trachelectomy for early-stage cervical cancer, fertility-preserving surgery for early-stage ovarian and endometrial cancer

18.3.1 Cancer in Children

Cancer ranks as the second leading cause of death in children between the ages of 1 and 14 years (Jemal et al. 2003). Over the past 30 years cure rates have increased dramatically for childhood and adolescent cancers. Currently, when all childhood cancers are combined the 5-year survival rates are over 80%, which is between 80% and 86% for childhood acute lymphoblastic leukemia (ALL), and exceed 90% for Hodgkin disease (Robison and Bhatia 2003; Gurney et al. 1995). Each year almost 2,000 patients are estimated to become long-term survivors of ALL, the most common childhood malignancy (Gurney et al. 1995). Recent studies estimate that by the year 2010 as many as 1 in 640 to 1 in 250 persons will be a survivor of a childhood malignancy (Sonmezer and Oktay 2004). Children who commonly face the risk of ovarian failure due to cytotoxic treatment include those diagnosed with Hodgkin lymphoma, neuroblastoma, non-Hodgkin lymphoma, Wilms tumor, Ewing sarcoma, osteosarcoma of the pelvis, and genital rhabdomyosarcoma.

Although many children survive cancer because of improved treatment modalities, they are not immune to the gonadotoxic effects of various cancer treatments. Unfortunately, it has been shown that only half of pediatric oncologists are knowledgeable of current research and technology in fertility preservation (Goodwin et al. 2007). Since it does not require ovarian stimulation or a partner, ovarian tissue cryopreservation is typically the only practical option for prepubertal or premenarchal girls receiving chemo- and/or radiotherapy.

18.3.2 Breast Cancer

Breast cancer is the most common invasive cancer seen in reproductive-age women, with more than 1 million cases occurring each year worldwide (Avis et al. 2004). In the United States alone, approximately 213,000 new cases of invasive breast cancer are expected to have occurred in 2006. One out of every 228 women develops breast cancer before age 40 years; stated differently ~15% of all breast cancer cases occur during the reproductive years (Oktay and Yih, 2002). Coupled with the increase in the number of women who delay first childbirth beyond the age of 35, the use of adjuvant chemotherapy regimens has resulted in a large proportion of breast cancer patients of reproductive age facing infertility. Studies have shown that reproductive concerns play an important role for young women diagnosed with breast cancer (Avis et al. 2004; Partridge et al. 2004). In a study using a web-based survey, 29% of women stated that infertility concerns influenced their treatment decisions (Partridge et al. 2004). In young women with early-stage breast cancer, the potential benefits of adjuvant cytotoxic treatment should be cautiously weighed against the long-term adverse impact on fertility. Many young breast cancer patients feel that their cancer physicians do not sufficiently inform them about the impact of cancer treatment on their fertility. It is vital to provide the most up-to-date and accurate information on the effects of cancer treatment on fertility to these young women who desire greater involvement in their treatment decision making.

The reported incidence of chemotherapy-induced amenorrhea with polyagent chemotherapy for breast cancer varies widely, mostly because of the nonuniformity of the definition of amenorrhea or menopause as well as variations in age distribution, treatment regimen, and duration of follow-up (Sonmezer and Oktay 2006). The most commonly used chemotherapy regimens for breast cancer, CMF (cyclophosphamide, methotrexate, and 5-fluorouracil) and AC (adriamycin and cyclophosphamide) cause ovarian failure in 14%–86%, and 0%–96% of the patients, respectively. Nevertheless the risk of ovarian failure after chemotherapy is likely to be underestimated, as studies have only looked at amenorrhea incidence as a surrogate for fertility.

In breast cancer, chemotherapy is usually initiated 6 weeks after the surgery, which is adequate for an IVF cycle including ovarian stimulation and oocyte recovery. Because conventional ovulation induction regimens might be detrimental to breast cancer because of the resultant surge in estradiol levels, potentially safer regimens including tamoxifen or aromatase inhibitors have been developed (Oktay et al. 2003, 2005a) (reviewed separately in Sect. 4.1.1). These patients may also be candidates for ovarian tissue cryopreservation, as occult ovarian metastasis is extremely rare in nonmetastatic breast cancer (Oktay and Sonmezer 2004; Oktay et al. 2004b; Gagnon and Tetu 1989; Hann et al. 2000) (discussed in detail below).

18.3.3 Cancer of the Cervix

Cancer of the cervix afflicts 500,000 women each year worldwide. In the year 2002, 13,000 new cervical cancer cases were diagnosed in North America and roughly half of them occurred before the age of 35 years (Waggoner 2003). The risk of ovarian metastasis is extremely rare in squamous cell cervical cancer; however, it may be seen in up to 12% of cases with adenocarcinoma and adenosquamous carcinoma of the cervix (Nakanishi et al. 2001; Yamamoto et al. 2001). Over the past three decades, while the incidence of squamous cell carcinoma of the cervix decreased by 42%, the incidence of adenocarcinoma of the cervix increased by 29% (Smith et al. 2000). Patients with advanced-stage disease and those with early-stage disease that are found to have high risk factors receive pelvic or pelvic/paraaortic radiation therapy. Ovarian transposition can be beneficial in patients receiving pelvic radiotherapy; however, success rates with this procedure vary greatly because of vascular damage and the effect of scatter radiation. If adjuvant radiosensitizing chemotherapy is needed, ovarian cryopreservation is another option. Alternatively, one ovary can be transposed, usually the one on the opposite site of the main tumor, and the remaining ovary cryopreserved (Martin et al. 2007).

18.3.4 Malignant and Nonmalignant Diseases Requiring Pelvic Radiotherapy

Some solid tumors presenting in the pelvis such as osteosarcoma, retroperitoneal sarcomas, Ewing sarcoma, rhabdomyosarcoma, nephroblastoma, tumors of spinal cord, and even some benign bone tumors have been successfully treated with radiation therapy to achieve local tumor control or to improve prognosis (Sonmezer and Oktay 2004; Feigenberg et al. 2001; Bacci et al. 2003). Radiation therapy also plays an important part in the management of colon cancer, which is the third most commonly encountered female cancer (Kapiteijn et al. 2001). These patients can benefit from ovarian, oocyte, or embryo cryopreservation. If only radiation therapy will be implemented, ovarian transposition may be performed, especially if an abdominal surgery is scheduled as part of the treatment of the primary tumor.

18.3.5 Autoimmune Diseases

A growing number of autoimmune diseases are successfully treated with cyclophosphamide-based cytotoxic therapy. The list includes systemic lupus erythematosus, steroid-resistant glomerulonephritis, thalassemia major, Behcet disease, inflammatory bowel diseases, and pemphigus vulgaris (Sonmezer et al. 2005a; Li et al. 2004; Russell et al. 2001; Langford et al. 2003). These patients may resort to embryo or oocyte cryopreservation if there is time available to perform ovulation induction and oocyte collection. When there are time restrictions or if the patient is a child, pieces of ovarian tissue may be frozen for possible future autotransplantation in order to retain fertility.

18.3.6 Hematopoietic Stem Cell Transplantation

Over the past decades various malignant and nonmalignant systemic diseases have been effectively treated with autologous or allogeneic hematopoietic stem cell transplantation (HSCT). In addition to malignant diseases such as leukemia, multiple myeloma, lymphoma, and breast cancer, among the nonmalignant conditions reported to benefit from HSCT are sickle cell disease, thalassemia, aplastic anemia, systemic lupus erythematosus, autoimmune thrombocytopenia, progressive systemic sclerosis, rheumatoid arthritis, juvenile idiopathic arthritis, vasculitis, and multiple sclerosis (Sonmezer and Oktay 2004; Sonmezer et al. 2005a; Burt et al. 2003; Karussis and Slavin 2004; Cohen et al. 2003). Preconditioning with high-dose chemoradiotherapy or radiotherapy before HSTC is extremely gonadotoxic (Couto-Silva et al. 2001). The most commonly used conditioning regimens for HSCT in acute myeloid leukemia (AML) that include cyclophosphamide/total body irradiation or busulfan/cyclophosphamide (Litzow et al. 2002), are extremely gonadotoxic. The risk of developing complete or partial ovarian failure may exceed 80% in children receiving conditioning for HSCT. Child patients can only undergo ovarian tissue cryopreservation, whereas adult patients with a partner may resort to embryo or oocyte cryopreservation.

18.3.7 Benign Ovarian Disease

Some benign ovarian lesions might significantly compromise ovarian reserve either because of their extensive or progressive nature or because of bilateral involvement (Oktay et al. 2001b). In the presence of any benign ovarian lesion, healthy pieces of ovarian cortex can be cryopreserved if the ovarian reserve is deemed to have compromised as a result of repeated surgeries (Oktay 2001). It was previously demonstrated that healthy pieces of ovarian cortical tissue can be found adjacent to ovarian lesions including dermoid cysts, benign serous cysts, and endometriosis (Schubert et al. 2005). If there is a risk of disease recurrence, subcutaneous transplantation of the ovarian pieces might be preferred because of ease of monitoring and the presumed simplicity of removal in the case of recurrence.

18.3.8 Prophylactic Oophorectomy

It has been clearly demonstrated that BRCA 1 and BRCA 2 germ line mutations are responsible for the majority of hereditary breast and ovarian cancers. The cumulative lifetime risk of developing ovarian cancer is about 60% for BRCA-1 and 10%–20% for BRCA-2 mutation carriers (Struewing et al. 1997; Liede and Narod 2002; Carcangiu et al. 2006). Furthermore, the lifetime risk of breast cancer in carriers of BRCA-1 mutation varies from 40% to 85% (Antoniou et al. 2003; Kramer et al. 2005). Even though the risk of peritoneal cancer cannot be eliminated with this strategy, increasing numbers of women are offered the option of undergoing prophylactic salpingo-oophorectomy in order to reduce the future risk of both ovarian and breast cancer after the age of 35–40 and/or when childbearing is completed (Rebbeck et al. 2002; Kauff et al. 2002). BRCA-positive women with a partner can benefit from embryo or oocyte cryopreservation before surgery. When ovarian tissue is cryopreserved, the risk of occult carcinoma should be borne in mind, as it is reported to be between 2% and 18% in mutation carriers undergoing prophylactic oophorectomy (Sonmezer and Oktay 2005). In the future, ovarian tissue should preferably be transplanted to a subcutaneous site to be monitored for any potential malignant transformation.

18.4 Available Options for Fertility Preservation

A number of options are available to preserve fertility in patients facing the risk of imminent ovarian failure. These range from well-established techniques such as embryo cryopreservation to investigational technologies such as oocyte and ovarian tissue cryopreservation. Depending on clinical and social circumstances, a different option may be suitable for each patient (Fig. 18.1).

18.4.1 Assisted Reproductive Technologies to Preserve Fertility

18.4.1.1 Embryo Cryopreservation

Embryo cryopreservation has been used for more than 20 years to store excess number of embryos and to avoid the risk of ovarian hyperstimulation during an IVF cycle. However, an IVF cycle, which typically involves ovulation induction and oocyte retrieval requires at least 2–3 weeks. If treatment cannot be safely delayed, then this is not a suitable option. Embryo cryopreservation is also not suitable for single women not desiring to use donor sperm or for children. With the current freezing technology, the implantation potential of frozen-thawed embryos approaches that of fresh embryos (Veeck et al. 2004). Survival rates

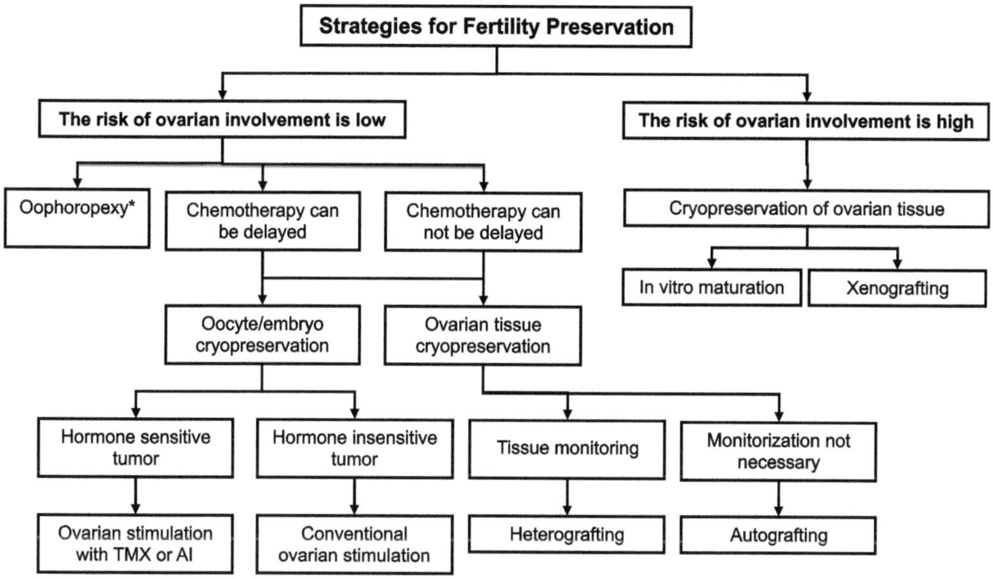

Fig. 18.1 Algorithmic approach for fertility preservation. *The success of oophoropexy is diminished if radiosensitizing chemotherapy is implanted. *TMX*, tamoxifen; *AI*, aromatase inhibitors

per thawed embryo range between 35% and 90% and implantation rates between 8% and 30%, and cumulative pregnancy rates can exceed 60%. Because the effectiveness of IVF diminishes with every round of chemotherapy and because there is a potential for fertilizing a genetically damaged gamete, it is also not recommended to perform IVF after chemotherapy is started (Ginsburg et al. 2001; Dolmans et al. 2005).

Breast cancer patients typically have 4–6 weeks between surgery and chemotherapy initiation and thus have sufficient time to undergo ovarian stimulation. However, the rise in estrogen levels that occurs during ovarian stimulation typically precludes use of standard IVF regimens in breast and other estrogen-sensitive tumors (Sonmezer et al. 2005b). Oocytes can be retrieved during an unstimulated cycle (natural cycle IVF, NCIVF) but the embryo yield is extremely low (Oktay et al. 2003; Ubaldi et al. 2004).

Tamoxifen, a selective estrogen modulator with antiestrogenic actions on breast tissue, is as effective as clomiphene citrate in the treatment of anovulatory infertility. The effectiveness and safety of tamoxifen for ovulation induction in breast cancer patients was studied, and results were compared to a retrospective control group of breast cancer patients who had NCIVF (Oktay et al. 2003). Compared to control subjects, patients stimulated with tamoxifen had fewer cancelled cycles (1/15 vs 4/9) and a higher mean number of mature oocytes (1.6 ± 0.3 vs 7 ± 0.2) and total embryos (1.6 ± 0.3 vs 0.6 ± 0.2). An embryo could be generated in all 12 patients stimulated with tamoxifen; in contrast, NCIVF resulted in embryos in only 3 of 5 patients. Although the peak estradiol levels were higher in the tamoxifen group than in control subjects, cancer recurrence rates were not increased after a mean follow-up of approximately 2 years (Oktay et al. 2005a). It is well known that tamoxifen can block the effects of supraphysiological levels of estrogen on breast tissue and inhibits the growth of breast tumors by competitive antagonism of estrogen at its receptor site. In fact, mean estradiol levels are chronically elevated in breast cancer patients who are on long-term tamoxifen treatment, and can be higher than the levels seen in patients undergoing ovarian stimulation with tamoxifen (Shushan et al. 1996; Klijn et al. 2000).

Letrozole is a potent and highly selective third-generation aromatase inhibitor that competitively inhibits the activity of aromatase enzyme. It significantly suppresses plasma estradiol, estrone, and estrone sulfate levels at doses ranging from 0.1 to 5 mg/day and has a very short a half-life of approximately 48 hours (Pfister et al. 2001). Letrozole was recently shown to be superior to tamoxifen in the treatment of advanced-stage postmenopausal breast cancer (Mouridsen et al. 2003) Aromatase inhibitors alone or in combination with gonadotropins have been recently tested as effective ovulation induction agents. A theoretical advantage of ovarian stimulation with aromatase inhibitors is that the peak estradiol levels are close to or similar to that observed in natural cycles (Oktay et al. 2005a; Fatemi et al. 2003). The letrozole-FSH protocol is preferred in most breast cancer patients undergoing IVF for embryo or oocyte cryopreservation because it results in low estradiol levels and high oocyte recovery. In a prospective study the combination of letrozole plus low-dose FSH (LetFSH-IVF) or tamoxifen plus low-dose FSH (TamFSH-IVF) resulted in a higher embryo yield than IVF performed after stimulation with tamoxifen alone (Tam-IVF) (embryo yield; 5.3±0.8, 3.8±0.8, and 1.3±0.2, respectively) (Oktay et al. 2005a). LetFSH-IVF and Tam-IVF resulted in lower peak estradiol levels lower than TamFSH-IVF (380±57, 419±39, and 1,182±271 pg/mL, respectively). Cancer recurrence rates were similar for IVF and control patients who elected not to undergo IVF (3/29 vs 3/31) over a mean follow-up of 554 days. None of the recurrences occurred in the letrozole-treated patients. Several live births have already occurred as a result of letrozole-FSH stimulation in patients with breast cancer (Oktay 2005).

Very recently, it was demonstrated that letrozole and FSH stimulation resulted in 44% reduction in gonadotropin requirement compared to age-matched retrospective control subjects selected from women who underwent IVF for tubal disease, while the length of stimulation, number of embryos obtained, and fertilization rates were similar. The mean delay from surgery to cryopreservation was 38.6 days, with 81% of all patients completing their IVF cycles within 8 weeks of surgery (Oktay et al. 2006b).

18.4.1.2 Cryopreservation of Mature Oocytes

Oocyte cryopreservation is an investigational procedure that is offered to the single woman who does not desire to use donor sperm to generate embryos for storage. In contrast to embryo and sperm freezing, oocyte cryopreservation has been technically more challenging because oocytes are more sensitive to cryoinjury (Gosden 2005). The meiotic spindle, cytoskeleton, cortical granules, and zonae pellucidae are the structures particularly at risk. However, modifications in the freezing medium and use of intracytoplasmic sperm injection has resulted in improvement in success rates (Porcu and Venturoli 2006). There are two main methods of oocyte freezing: the controlled rate (slow freezing), which is the more established method, and vitrification (fast freezing).

A recent meta-analysis found that fertilization rates and live birth rates per sperm-injected cryopreserved oocyte with the slow-freeze protocol (SF) were 61% and 3.4%, respectively, compared to 76.7% and 6.6%, respectively, for age-matched controls who underwent IVF-ICSI with fresh oocytes (Oktay et al. 2006c). The live birth rates with frozen oocytes were significantly lower compared with those with unfrozen oocytes. For vitrification, fertilization (VF), live birth per injected oocyte, and live birth per embryo transfer rates were 70.6%, 4.5%, and 29.4%, respectively. For the same group, the mean live birth rate per thaw cycle was 24.4%, whereas the implantation rate was 8.8%. Of the 10 live births from vitrification, one involved delivery of twins, whereas the others were singletons. No pregnancy loss was reported. Likewise, the comparison of SF pregnancy rates from 1996–2004 to mean SART data for a similar time period confirmed that the IVF success rates with SF oocytes were lower compared with those with unfrozen oocytes (Table 18.4).

With a slow freezing protocol, a recent study showed a pregnancy rate of 19.2% per transfer and an implantation rate of 12.3% (Borini et al. 2006). A meta-analytic comparison of oocyte vitrification success rates with slow freezing and the SART IVF data with unfrozen oocytes demonstrated that VF success rates were significantly higher compared to SF (Cil et al. 2006). When

Table 18.4. Comparison of success rates of slow freezing procedure with SART data

Variable	SF 1996–2004 (group a; 33 ± 0.24)*	SART (1997–2003) success rates for age 33 years (group b)	P values, group a vs group b	SF 2002–2004 (group c; 31.1 ± 0.6)*	SART 2003 success rates for age 31 years (group d)	P values, group c vs group d
Clinical pregnancies per transfer	27.1 (95/351)	46.6 (14,037/30,109)	<.0001	37.8 (28/74)	54.5 (2,317/4,250)	004
Live births per transfer	21.7 (76/351)	38.4 (11,552/30,109)	<.0001	32.4 (24/74)	47.8 (2,031/4,250)	.009

Note: Data are % (n) unless otherwise indicated

*Age: mean ± SD, SF: slow freezing protocol

compared to age-/year-matched SART data, clinical pregnancy and live birth/ET rates were significantly lower after SF, but there was no difference between the SART data and VF. A higher number of embryos were transferred in VF vs SF groups (3.5 vs 2.5, $p = 0.0001$), resulting in a higher percentage of twins (23.3 vs 19.6) and triplets or more (5 vs 3.5). Vitrification appears to be a promising approach to oocyte cryopreservation; however, the comparative efficiency and safety of this technique should be confirmed in prospective studies. Nevertheless, the improved success rates with oocyte cryopreservation may justify the use of this technique for fertility preservation in cancer patients.

There is limited information on the health of children born from frozen-thawed oocytes. Of the 32 pregnancies in which the perinatal outcome was reported there was one ventricular septal defect (VSD) and one triploid pregnancy (Oktay et al. 2001a; Chia et al. 2000; Porcu 2001). The latter, however, resulted after ICSI of frozen-thawed testicular sperm into cryopreserved oocytes.

18.4.1.3 Ovarian Tissue Cryopreservation and Transplantation

The idea of cryopreserving ovarian tissue is based on the finding that the ovarian cortex is composed of primordial follicles that are more resistant to cryoinjury than mature oocytes. Although the clinical indications for ovarian tissue cryopreservation are almost identical to those for oocyte cryopreservation, there are fewer logistical restrictions in offering this technique. Specifically, the tissue can be obtained without delay since there is no need for ovarian stimulation, and a partner is not required when the tissue is harvested. Furthermore, this is the only fertility preservation technique that can reverse menopause.

After successful animal studies (Gosden et al. 1994; Liu et al. 2001; Salle et al. 2003; Lee et al. 2004), resumption of endocrine function has been reported after orthotopic (Oktay and Karlikaya 2000; Schmidt et al. 2005; Radford et al. 2001) and heterotopic (Oktay et al. 2001b; Callejo et al. 2001) transplantation of frozen-thawed ovarian cortical strips in patients. Recently, an embryo was generated from oocytes retrieved from subcutaneously transplanted ovarian tissue in a breast cancer survivor (Oktay et al. 2004a). Thereafter, two live births were reported after orthotopic transplantation of frozen-banked ovarian tissue in lymphoma survivors (Donnez et al. 2004; Meirow et al. 2005). In the orthotopic transplantation technique, frozen-thawed ovarian cortical pieces can be grafted near the infundibulopelvic ligament or on a postmenopausal ovary. In the heterotopic transplantation method, the tissue is grafted subcutaneously to the forearm or suprapubic area. The advantage of orthotopic transplantation is that natural conception is possible. However, this technique requires general anesthesia. Heterotopic transplantation does not require general anesthesia or abdominal surgery. It is also easy to monitor follicle development, and to remove the transplanted tissue if it becomes necessary.

The life span of ovarian grafts can be limited because of the loss of a fraction of follicles during the initial revascularization (Oktay et al. 2001b; Radford et al. 2001; Wolner-Hanssen et al. 2005). Therefore, the autotransplantation procedure should not be performed until the patient has received a clearance from her oncologist to proceed in attempting pregnancy.

One of the major theoretical concerns when transplanting ovarian tissue after cure is the risk of reseeding the primary tumor. Fortunately, most of the tumors seen during reproductive years, apart from leukemias, have low risk of ovarian involvement (Table 18.5). In breast cancer, occult ovarian involvement is rare, especially if there is no systemic metastasis and if pelvic and ultrasound examinations are normal (Curtin et al. 1994). Previous studies showed that most of the occult metastases belong to the infiltrating lobular histological subtype, which constitutes <15% of all breast cancers and more commonly occurs in postmenopausal women (Curtin et al. 1994; Li et al. 2003; Morrow 2001; Sastre-Garau et al. 1996). Thus early-stage breast cancer is not a contraindication for ovarian tissue cryopreservation and transplantation. However, before ovarian transplantation, a thorough histological assessment of a representative piece is required to rule out occult metastasis. In addition, patients with *BRCA-1* and *BRCA-2* genes are at a higher risk for harboring occult ovarian cancer (Liede and Narod 2002). Even though ovarian cancer is rare before the age of 35, these patients should be counseled about the risk. Incidence of ovarian involvement is high with blood-borne malignancies including leukemias, neuroblastoma, and Burkitt lymphoma. Wilms tumor, Ewing sarcoma, lymphomas, osteosarcomas, and extragenital rhabdomyosarcomas have a low risk of ovarian involvement. In squamous cell cervical cancer, ovarian involvement is <1.0%, whereas it is reported to be between 1.7% and 12.5% in adenocarcinoma of the cervix, (Sutton et al. 1992; Woodruff et al. 1970). Animal studies do not indicate that the likelihood of ovarian involvement is high in Hodgkin lymphoma (Shaw et al. 1996; Kim et al. 2001). A recent study showed that none of 26 patients with lymphoma had evidence of ovarian involvement by histology and immunohistochemistry (Seshadri et al. 2006). The risk of ovarian involvement according to the tumor type is summarized in Table 18.5.

Table 18.5. Malignant diseases and associated risk of ovarian involvement

The risk of ovarian involvement is high
Leukemia
Burkitt lymphoma
Neuroblastoma
Genital rhabdomyosarcoma
The risk of ovarian involvement is moderate
Breast cancer (stage IV, or infiltrative lobular histological subtype)
Colon cancer (includes tumors of rectum and appendix)
Upper gastrointestinal system malignancies
Adeno/adenosquamous carcinoma of the cervix
The risk of ovarian involvement is low
Non-Hodgkin lymphoma
Hodgkin lymphoma
Breast cancer (Stage I–III, or infiltrative ductal)
Ewing sarcoma
Squamous cell carcinoma of the cervix
Nongenital rhabdomyosarcoma
Osteogenic sarcoma
Wilms tumor

Autotransplantation of the fresh ovary to the upper extremity with microsurgical vascular anastomosis could protect ovaries against radiation damage (Leporrier et al. 1987; Hilders et al. 2004). In fact this is by and large a transposition procedure, and it has not been possible to cryopreserve whole ovaries in humans because of the difficulty in devising methods to preserve oocytes, stroma, and ovarian vessels with equal efficiency. Ideally, the ovaries would continue to produce hormones and oocytes, which could be aspirated for IVF. However, this procedure would not be useful if concomitant chemotherapy is also used, and, especially if ovarian cryopreservation is required, transplantation of ovarian cortical strips appears to be a more viable option in most patients. There is a case report of orthotopic transplantation of fresh ovarian tissue from one monozygotic twin sister to the other, who had suffered from premature ovarian failure. The procedure resulted in a live birth (Silber et al. 2005).

Regardless of the magnitude of risk of ovarian involvement, a thorough histological evaluation should be performed on multiple samples taken from the ovarian tissue before and after cryopreservation. When there is a significant concern about ovarian involvement, cryopreservation procedures should not be performed for the purpose of future autotransplantation. Molecular biology techniques and immunohistochemistry can be used to screen for the presence of cancer cells in the ovary (Oktay and Yih 2002). There have been no reports of cancer recurrence in the limited number of cases published in the medical literature, but ovarian cryopreservation and transplantation remains an investigational protocol (Lee et al. 2006).

18.4.1.4 Ovarian Transposition

In case of pelvic/abdominal radiation, ovaries can be moved out of the radiation area in order to avoid direct radiation exposure. Ovarian transposition was first introduced in clinical practice to preserve ovarian function in patients with Hodgkin disease who were to receive pelvic or para-aortic lymph node irradiation (Ray et al. 1970; Nahhas et al. 1971). The degree of ovarian damage depends on the patient's age and the dose of radiation delivered to the ovaries, and can be compounded by the addition of chemotherapy. If the patient will undergo an abdominal surgery, the ovaries can be transposed at that time; otherwise, a laparoscopic transposition can be performed before radiotherapy is given (Tulandi and Al-Took 1998; Morice et al. 2000).

Success rates with this procedure are inconsistent, varying between 16% and 90% (Sonmezer and Oktay 2000).The success rates are affected by various factors such as vascular compromise, scatter radiation, radiation dose, age of the patient, and whether ovaries are shielded during the procedure. The procedure is not completely risk free and can be associated with chronic ovarian pain, infarction of the fallopian tubes, and formation of ovarian cysts. Ovaries can also migrate to the original location in the pelvis. Spontaneous pregnancy may be more difficult, if the uterus was not damaged, and should the patient need IVF, oocyte collection may have to be performed percutaneously unless the ovaries are returned to their original location by a second operation. Spontaneous pregnancies have occurred, however, without repositioning of the ovaries back to their original location. Therefore, ovaries are usually repositioned only if difficulty arises.

A recent study investigated the success of laparoscopic oophoropexy to preserve ovarian function before pelvic irradiation in 10 patients with Hodgkin disease (Williams et al. 1999). The dose of pelvic radiation ranged from 1,500 to 3,500 cGy. All five patients who received minimal or no chemotherapy had evidence of ovarian function, and four conceived. In contrast, four patients who also received multiple courses of chemotherapy, and one who received 3,500 cGy to the femoral lymph nodes and pelvis with little central shielding, had ovarian failure at follow-up.

If attempted, lateral ovarian transposition seems to be superior to medial transposition in limiting ovarian exposure to radiation. It has been suggested that the ovaries be transposed at least 3 cm from the upper border of the radiation field. Performing the procedure close to the time of irradiation also decreases the chance of failure from ovarian migration back to the field of treatment.

18.4.2 Fertility-Sparing Surgery in Gynecologic Cancers

In some gynecologic tumors, patients may benefit from fertility-sparing surgery in which the uterus and contralateral ovary are preserved (Gershenson 2005). Ovarian biopsy is not routinely recommended at the time of surgery if contralateral ovary looks normal on gross inspection. Ovarian tumors of young females usually have a low probability of bilateral ovarian involvement; thus sparing the normal ovary and the uterus may be possible. This is especially true for borderline ovarian cancer, sex cord stromal tumors, and germ cell tumors of the ovary. Furthermore, fertility-sparing surgery may be an option with early-stage epithelial ovarian cancer. Fertility-sparing options for invasive cervical cancer include conization for stage IA_1 and IA_2 disease and abdominal or vaginal trachelectomy for stage IA_2 and IB disease.

18.4.3 Cotreatment with GnRH Analogs to Prevent Chemotherapy-Associated Gonadal Damage

In human ovary, more than 90% of the ovarian reserve is made up of primordial follicles at resting stage containing an immature oocyte. Even though the mechanism of primordial follicle growth initiation is still not understood, it is clearly an FSH-independent process; FSH receptors are not expressed until these follicles initiate growth and reach multilayer stages (Oktay et al. in press, 1997a; Meduri et al. 2003; McNatty et al. 1999) Since GnRH analogs' main mode of action is to suppress pituitary gonadotropin secretion, it does not appear plausible that such a presumed effect is gonadotropin dependent. There are a number of studies investigating the role of GnRH analogs in preventing chemotherapy-related gonadal damage. Many of the studies suffer from small sample size and/or lack of an appropriate control group (Recchia et al. 2006; Somers et al. 2005; Pereyra-Pacheco et al. 2001). In many studies menstrual function was assessed to determine the impact of chemotherapy on ovarian function instead of using more reliable biochemical markers of ovarian reserve such as day 3 FSH, estradiol, inhibin, or anti-müllerian hormone levels (Pereyra-Pacheco et al. 2001; Del Mastro et al. 2006). In some studies the cumulative dose of alkylating agent was either not specified or not sufficient to cause imminent ovarian failure in the age group of patients that was studied (Pereyra-Pacheco et al. 2001; Blumenfeld et al. 1996, 2000). In some studies, follow-up was different among the study and control groups (Somers et al. 2005; Blumenfeld et al. 1996). In the only prospective randomized study reported by Waxman et al., albeit with small numbers, including 30 men and 18 women receiving chemotherapy for Hodgkin disease, GnRHa did not preserve fertility as judged by sperm counts and menstrual function (Waxman et al. 1987). After 3 years of follow-up, all men in both study and control groups became oligo-/azospermic, while four of the eight women treated with GnRHa (50%) and six of nine female control subjects (66.6%) became amenorrheic. There is also no benefit in administering GnRH analogs to protect gonadal function in men and women undergoing hematopoietic stem cell transplantation. Regardless, the majority of these young patients who receive preconditioning treatment will suffer from gonadal failure GnRH.

The safety of use of GnRH analogs has also not also been established. A study on 24 premenopausal breast cancer patients demonstrated that while 23 women who received ovarian suppression with GnRH analogs during chemotherapy regained menstruation, among 11 women who were actively attempting pregnancy, only two delivered healthy children despite six pregnancies in five patients. Three spontaneous abortions were observed, with one elective abortion for a Down syndrome fetus (Fox et al. 2001). Furthermore, since GnRH receptors that mediate several effects such as inhibition of proliferation, induction of cell cycle arrest, and inhibition of apoptosis are expressed in a variety of cancers, one cannot exclude that GnRH agonist therapy concomitant to cytotoxic chemotherapy might reduce the efficacy of the implemented chemotherapy (Vitale et al. 2006; Emons et al. 2003).

18.4.4 Donor Egg and Gestational Surrogacy

IVF with donor oocytes is another alternative in patients who suffer from premature menopause or have diminished ovarian reserve due to cancer treatment (Polak deFried et al. 1998). The success rates with appropriate oocyte donors are now >60% per embryo transfer. Gestational surrogacy can also be employed in patients who have undergone hysterectomy or received pelvic radiation for cervical cancer. Patients with breast cancer who are considered at high risk for recurrence, or who must be on lifelong therapy with aromatase inhibitors, may also resort to gestational surrogacy. However, laws and regulations regarding this procedure vary significantly between countries and between individual states in the United States.

18.5 Future Directions

When the risk of ovarian involvement with cancer cells is high, some other experimental options may be considered in the future. It has been possible to xenograft human ovarian tissue to immunodeficient mice and grow mature follicles in these xenografts (Oktay et al. 1998a,b; Gook et al. 2001). It has also been possible to retrieve oocytes from xenografted human ovarian cortical pieces (Revel et al. 2000). However, the possibility of trans-species viral infections has to be addressed. Primordial follicles can also be isolated from cryopreserved ovarian tissue, and it is theoretically possible to use these follicles for the purpose of in vitro maturation (Oktay et al. 1997b). Even though this has been partially successful in mice, the prospect for success in humans is not clear at the present time. A combination of oocyte and ovarian tissue cryopreservation has also been suggested as a new strategy (Revel et al. 2003). Another possibility is in vitro growth of primordial follicles isolated from cryopreserved ovarian tissue. It has been possible to isolate primordial follicles from human ovarian tissue, but there has been no success in growing them in vitro. Progress has been made in rodents with this technique, including production of oocytes competent for meiotic maturation, fertilization, and preimplantation in vitro from primordial follicle (O'Brien et al. 2003), but whether this will translate to human studies is currently unclear.

It has recently been postulated that the mechanism of age-related as well as chemo- or radiotherapy-induced loss in the ovarian germ cell population is mediated by programmed cell death (Morita and Tilly 1999). Sphingosine-1-phosphate (S1P), a bioactive sphingolipid metabolite formed by sphingosine kinase, is an important lipid mediator and has many actions both inside and outside the cell. Morita et al. showed that wild-type mice treated with S1P resisted both developmental and cancer therapy-induced apoptosis (Morita et al. 2000). Radiation-induced oocyte loss could be completely prevented by S1P therapy in wild-type mice. The same group investigated transgenerational genomic instability and did not detect discernable propagation of genomic damage in mice pretreated with S1P before receiving ionizing radiation (Paris et al. 2002). There have also been recent strides in developing a whole ovary cryopreservation technique. Even though this technique had limited success in animals, it's in infancy in human (Imhof et al. 2004; Revel et al. 2004).

References

Anderson RA, Themmen AP, Al-Qahtani A, et al. (2006) The effects of chemotherapy and long-term gonadotrophin suppression on the ovarian reserve in premenopausal women with breast cancer. Hum Reprod 21: 2583–2592

Antoniou A, Pharoah PD, Narod S, et al. (2003) Average risks of breast and ovarian cancer associated with BRCA1 or BRCA2 mutations detected in case series unselected for family history: a combined analysis of 22 studies. Am J Hum Genet 72: 1117–1130

3. Avis NE, Crawford S, Manuel J (2004) Psychosocial problems among younger women with breast cancer. Psychooncology 13: 295–308

Azim E, Rauch R, Ravich M, et al. (2006) Ovarian reserve is impaired in cancer patients with normal baseline FSH who previously received chemotherapy as determined by response to controlled ovarian stimulation and anti-mullerian hormone measurements: a controlled study. Fertil Steril 86(suppl 1): 123s--124s

Baarends WM, Uilenbroek JT, Kramer P, et al. (1995) Anti-Müllerian hormone and anti-Müllerian hormone type II receptor messenger ribonucleic acid expression in rat ovaries during postnatal development, the estrous cycle, and gonadotropin-induced follicle growth. Endocrinology 136: 4951–4962

Bacci G, Ferrari S, Mercuri M, et al. (2003) Multimodal therapy for the treatment of nonmetastatic Ewing sarcoma of pelvis. J Pediatr Hematol Oncol 25: 118–124

Bahadur G, Steele SJ (1996). Ovarian tissue cryopreservation for patients. Hum Reprod 11: 2215--2216

Bhatia S, Sather HN, Pabustan OB, et al. (2002) Low incidence of second neoplasms among children diagnosed with acute lymphoblastic leukemia after 1983. Blood 99: 4257–4264

Bleyer WA (1990) The impact of childhood cancer on the United States and the world. CA Cancer J Clin 40: 355–367

10. Blumenfeld Z, Avivi I, Linn S, et al. (1996) Prevention of irreversible chemotherapy-induced ovarian damage in young women with lymphoma by a gonadotrophin-releasing hormone agonist in parallel to chemotherapy. Hum Reprod 11: 1620–1626

Blumenfeld Z, Shapiro D, Shteinberg M, et al. (2000) Preservation of fertility and ovarian function and minimizing gonadotoxicity in young women with systemic lupus erythematosus treated by chemotherapy. Lupus 9: 401–405

Borini A, Lagalla C, Bonu MA, et al. (2006) Cumulative pregnancy rates resulting from the use of fresh and frozen oocytes: 7 years' experience. Reprod Biomed Online 12: 481–486

Brewer M, Gershenson DM, Herzog CE, et al. (1999) Outcome and reproductive function after chemotherapy for ovarian dysgerminoma. J Clin Oncol 17: 2670–2675

Brogan PA, Dillon MJ (2000) The use of immunosuppressive and cytotoxic drugs in non-malignant disease. Arch Dis Child 83: 259–264

Burt, R.K., Traynor AE, Craig R, et al. (2003) The promise of hematopoietic stem cell transplantation for autoimmune diseases. Bone Marrow Transplant 31: 521–524

Byrne J, Fears TR, Gail MH, et al. (1992) Early menopause in long-term survivors of cancer during adolescence. Am J Obstet Gynecol 166: 788–793

Callejo J, Salvador C, Miralles A, et al. (2001) Long-term ovarian function evaluation after autografting by implantation with fresh and frozen-thawed human ovarian tissue. J Clin Endocrinol Metab 86: 4489–4494

Carcangiu ML, Peissel B, Pasini B, et al. (2006) Incidental carcinomas in prophylactic specimens in BRCA1 and BRCA2 germ-line mutation carriers, with emphasis on fallopian tube lesions: report of 6 cases and review of the literature. Am J Surg Pathol 30: 1222–1230

Chia CM, Chan WB, Quah E, et al. (2000) Triploid pregnancy after ICSI of frozen testicular spermatozoa into cryopreserved human oocytes: case report. Hum Reprod 15: 1962–1964

Chiarelli AM, Marrett LD and Darlington GA (2000). Pregnancy outcomes in females after treatment for childhood cancer. Epidemiology 11: 161–166

Cil AP, Bang H, Oktay K (2006) A meta-analytic comparison of oocyte vitrification success rates with slow freezing and the SART IVF data with unfrozen oocytes Fertil Steril 86(suppl 1): 126s

Cohen Y, Polliack A, Nagler A (2003) Treatment of refractory autoimmune diseases with ablative immunotherapy using monoclonal antibodies and/or high dose chemotherapy with hematopoietic stem cell support. Curr Pharm Des 9: 279–288

Couto-Silva AC, Trivin C, Thibaud E (2001) Factors affecting gonadal function after bone marrow transplantation during childhood. Bone Marrow Transpl 28: 67–75

Critchley HO, Bath LE, Wallace WH (2002) Radiation damage to the uterus Review of the effects of treatment of childhood cancer. Hum Fertil (Camb) 5: 61–66

Curtin JP, Barakat RR, Hoskins WJ (1994). Ovarian disease in women with breast cancer. Obstet Gynecol 84: 449–452

Del Mastro L, Catzeddu T, Boni L, et al. (2006) Prevention of chemotherapy-induced menopause by temporary ovarian suppression with goserelin in young, early breast cancer patients. Ann Oncol 17: 74–78

Dolmans MM, Demylle D, Martinez-Madrid B, et al. (2005) Efficacy of in vitro fertilization after chemotherapy. Fertil Steril 83: 897–901

Donnez J, Dolmans MM, Demylle D, et al. (2004) Livebirth after orthotopic transplantation of cryopreserved ovarian tissue. Lancet 364: 1405–1410

Emons G, Gründker C, Günthert AR, et al. (2003) GnRH antagonists in the treatment of gynaecological and breast cancers. International Congress on Hormonal Steroids and Hormones and Cancer. Endocr Rel Cancer 10: 291–299

Familiari G, Caggiati A, Nottola SA et al. (1993) Ultrastructure of human ovarian primordial follicles after combination chemotherapy for Hodgkin's disease. Hum Reprod 8: 2080–2087

Fatemi HM, Kolibianakis E, Tournaye H, et al. (2003) Clomiphene citrate versus letrozole for ovarian stimulation: a pilot study. Reprod Biomed Online 7: 543–546

Feigenberg SJ, Marcus RB Jr, Zlotecki RA, et al. (2001) Megavoltage radiotherapy for aneurysmal bone cysts. Int J Radiat Oncol Biol Phys 49: 1243–1247

Fisher B, Sherman B, Rockette H et al. (1979). l-Phenylalanine mustard (l-PAM) in the management of premenopausal patients with primary breast cancer: lack of association of disease-free survival with depression of ovarian function. National Surgical Adjuvant Project for Breast and Bowel Cancers. Cancer 44: 847–857

Fox K, Scialla H, Moore H (2001) Preventing chemotherapy-related amenorrhea using leuprolide during adjuvant chemotherapy for early stage breast cancer. Proc Am Soc Clin Oncol 21: 98a

Gagnon Y, Tetu B (1989) Ovarian metastases of breast carcinoma. A clinicopathologic study of 59 cases. Cancer 64: 892–898

Gershenson DM (2005) Fertility-sparing surgery for malignancies in women. J Natl Cancer Inst Monogr 34: 43–47

Ginsburg ES, Yanushpolsky EH, Jackson KV (2001) In vitro fertilization for cancer patients and survivors. Fertil Steril 75: 705–710

Giri N, Vowels MR, Barr AL et al. (1992) Successful pregnancy after total body irradiation and bone marrow transplantation for acute leukaemia. Bone Marrow Transplant 10: 93–95

Goodwin T, Elizabeth Oosterhuis B, Kiernan M, et al. (2007) Attitudes and practices of pediatric oncology providers regarding fertility issues. Pediatr Blood Cancer 48: 80–85

Gook DA, McCully BA, Edgar DH, et al. (2001) Development of antral follicles in human cryopreserved ovarian tissue following xenografting. Hum Reprod 16: 417–422

Gosden RG (2005) Prospects for oocyte banking and in vitro maturation. J Natl Cancer Inst Monogr 34: 60–63

Gosden RG, Baird DT, Wade JC et al.(1994) Restoration of fertility to oophorectomized sheep by ovarian autografts stored at −196 degrees C. Hum Reprod 9: 597–603

Gosden RG, Wade JC, Fraser HM, et al. (1997) Impact of congenital or experimental hypogonadotrophism on the radiation sensitivity of the mouse ovary. Hum Reprod 12: 2483–2488

Green DM, Peabody EM, Nan B, et al. (2002a) Pregnancy outcome after treatment for Wilms tumor: a report from the National Wilms Tumor Study Group. J Clin Oncol 20: 2506–2513

Green DM, Whitton JA, Stovall M, et al. (2002b) Pregnancy outcome of female survivors of childhood cancer: a report from the Childhood Cancer Survivor Study. Am J Obstet Gynecol 187: 1070–1080

Gurney JG, Severson RK, Davis S, et al. (1995) Incidence of cancer in children in the United States. Sex-, race-, and 1-year age-specific rates by histologic type. Cancer 75: 2186–2195

Hann LE, Lui DM, Shi W, et al. (2000) Adnexal masses in women with breast cancer: US findings with clinical and histopathologic correlation. Radiology 216: 242–247

Hilders CG, Baranski AG, Peters L, et al. (2004) Successful human ovarian autotransplantation to the upper arm. Cancer 101: 2771–2778

Howell S, Shalet S (1998) Gonadal damage from chemotherapy and radiotherapy. Endocrinol Metab Clin North Am 27: 927–943

Imhof M, Hofstetter G, Bergmeister H, et al. (2004) Cryopreservation of a whole ovary as a strategy for restoring ovarian function. J Assist Reprod Genet 21: 459–465

Jemal A, Murray T, Samuels A, et al. (2003) Cancer statistics, 2003. CA Cancer J Clin 53: 5–26

Jemal A, Tiwari RC, Murray T, et al. (2004) Cancer statistics, 2004. CA Cancer J Clin 54: 8-29

Jemal A, Siegel R, Ward E, et al. (2006) Cancer Statistics, 2006. CA Cancer J Clin 56: 106–130

Kapiteijn E, Marijnen CA, Nagtegaal ID, et al. (2001) Preoperative radiotherapy combined with total mesorectal excision for resectable rectal cancer. N Engl J Med 30: 638–646

Karussis D, Slavin S (2004) Hematopoietic stem cell transplantation in multiple sclerosis: experimental evidence to rethink the procedures. J Neurol Sci 223: 59-64

Kauff ND, Satagopan JM, Robson ME, et al. (2002) Risk-reducing salpingo-oophorectomy in women with a BRCA1 or BRCA2 mutation. N Engl J Med 346: 1609–1615

Kim SS, Radford J, Harris M, et al. (2001) Ovarian tissue harvested from lymphoma patients to preserve fertility may be safe for autotransplantation. Hum Reprod 16: 2056–2060

Klijn JG, Beex LV, Mauriac L, et al. (2000) Combined treatment with buserelin and tamoxifen in premenopausal metastatic breast cancer: a randomized study. J Natl Cancer Inst 92: 903–911

Koyama H, Wada T, Nishizawa Y, et al. (1977) Cyclophosphamide-induced ovarian failure and its therapeutic significance in patients with breast cancer. Cancer 39:1403–1409.

Kramer JL, Velazquez IA, Chen BE, et al. (2005) Prophylactic oophorectomy reduces breast cancer penetrance during prospective, long-term follow-up of BRCA1 mutation carriers. J Clin Oncol 23: 8629–8635

Langford CA, Talar-Williams C, Barron KS, et al. (2003) Use of a cyclophosphamide-induction methotrexate-maintenance regimen for the treatment of Wegener's granulomatosis: extended follow-up and rate of relapse. Am J Med 114: 463–469

Larsen EC, Muller J, Schmiegelow K, et al. (2003) Reduced ovarian function in long-term survivors of radiation- and chemotherapy-treated childhood cancer. J Clin Endocrinol Metab 88: 5307–5314

Lee DM, Yeoman RR, Battaglia DE, et al. (2004) Live birth after ovarian tissue transplant. Nature 428: 137–138

Lee SJ, Schover LR, Partridge AH, et al. (2006) American Society of Clinical Oncology. American Society of Clinical Oncology recommendations on fertility preservation in cancer patients. J Clin Oncol 24: 2917–2931

Leporrier M, von Theobald P, Roffe JL, et al. (1987) A new technique to protect ovarian function before pelvic irradiation. Heterotopic ovarian autotransplantation. Cancer 60: 2201–2004

Leung W, Hudson MM, Strickland DK, et al. (2000) Late effects of treatment in survivors of childhood acute myeloid leukemia. J Clin Oncol 18: 3273–3279

Li CI, Anderson BO, Daling JR, et al. (2003) Trends in incidence rates of invasive lobular and ductal breast carcinoma. JAMA 289: 1421–1424

Li CK, Chik KW, Wong GW, et al. (2004) Growth and endocrine function following bone marrow transplantation for thalassemia major. Pediatr Hematol Oncol 21: 411–419

Liede A, Narod SA (2002) Hereditary breast and ovarian cancer in Asia: genetic epidemiology of BRCA1 and BRCA2. Hum Mutat 20: 413–424

Litzow MR, Perez WS, Klein JP, et al. (2002) Comparison of outcome following allogeneic bone marrow transplantation with cyclophosphamide-total body irradiation versus busulphancyclophosphamide conditioning regimens for acute myelogenous leukaemia in first remission. Br J Haematol 119: 1115–1124

Liu J, Van der Elst J, Van den Broecke R, et al. (2001) Live offspring by in vitro fertilization of oocytes from cryopreserved primordial mouse follicles after sequential in vivo transplantation and in vitro maturation. Biol Reprod 64: 171–178

Mackie EJ, Radford M, Shalet SM (1996) Gonadal function following chemotherapy for childhood Hodgkin's disease. Med Pediatr Oncol 27: 74–78

Martin JR, Kodaman P, Oktay K, et al. (2007) Ovarian cryopreservation with transposition of a contralateral ovary: a combined approach for fertility preservation in women receiving pelvic radiation. Fertil Steril 87: 189

Maruta A, Matsuzaki M, Miyashita H, et al. (1995) Successful pregnancy after allogeneic bone marrow transplantation following conditioning with total body irradiation. Bone Marrow Transplant 15: 637–638

McNatty KP, Heath DA, Lundy T, et al. (1999) Control of early ovarian follicular development. J Reprod Fertil Suppl54: 1–16

Meduri G, Touraine P, Beau I, et al. (2003) Delayed puberty and primary amenorrhea associated with a novel mutation of the human follicle stimulating hormone receptor: clinical, histological, and molecular studies. J Clin Endocrinol Metab 88: 3491–3498

Meirow D, Nugent D (2001) The effects of radiotherapy and chemotherapy on female reproduction. Hum Reprod Update 7: 535–543

Meirow D, Lewis H, Nugent D et al. (1999) Subclinical depletion of primordial follicular reserve in mice treated with cyclophosphamide: clinical importance and proposed accurate investigative tool. Hum Reprod 14: 1903–1907

Meirow D, Levron J, Eldar-Geva T, et al. (2005) Pregnancy after transplantation of cryopreserved ovarian tissue in a patient with ovarian failure after chemotherapy. N Engl J Med 353: 318–321

Morice P, Juncker L, Rey A, El-Hassan J, et al. (2000) Ovarian transposition for patients with cervical carcinoma treated by radiosurgical combination. Fertil Steril 74: 743–748

Morita Y and Tilly JL (1999) Oocyte hourglass. Dev Biol 213: 1–17

Morita Y, Perez GI, Paris F, et al. (2000) Oocyte apoptosis is suppressed by disruption of the acid sphingomyelinase gene or by sphingosine-1-phosphate therapy. Nat Med 6: 1109–1114

Morrow M (2001). Breast. In: Greenfield LJ, Mulholland MW, Oldham KT et al., eds. Surgery: Scientific Principles and Practice, 3rd Edition. Philadelphia: Lippincott-Williams & Wilkins, pp. 1334–1372

Mouridsen H, Gershanovich M, Sun Y, et al. (2003) Phase III study of letrozole versus tamoxifen as first-line therapy of advanced breast cancer in postmenopausal women: analysis of survival and update of efficacy from the International Letrozole Breast Cancer Group. J Clin Oncol 21: 2101–2109

Nahhas WA, Nisce LZ, D'Angio GJ, et al. (1971) Lateral ovarian transposition. Ovarian relocation in patients with Hodgkin's disease. Obstet Gynecol 38: 785–788

Nakanishi T, Wakai K, Ishikawa H, et al. (2001) A comparison of ovarian metastasis between squamous cell carcinoma and adenocarcinoma of the uterine cervix. Gynecol Oncol 82: 504–509

O'Brien MJ, Pendola JK and Eppig JJ (2003) A revised protocol for in vitro development of mouse oocytes from primordial follicles dramatically improves their developmental competence. Biol Reprod 68: 1682–1686

Oktay K (2001) Ovarian tissue cryopreservation and transplantation: preliminary findings and implications for cancer patients. Hum Reprod Update 7: 526–534

Oktay K (2005). Further evidence on the safety and success of ovarian stimulation with letrozole and tamoxifen in breast cancer patients undergoing in vitro fertilization to cryopreserve their embryos for fertility preservation. J Clin Oncol 23: 3858–3869

Oktay K, Karlikaya G (2000) Ovarian function after transplantation of frozen, banked autologous ovarian tissue. N Engl J Med 342: 1919

Oktay KH, Yih M (2002) Preliminary experience with orthotopic and heterotopic transplantation of ovarian cortical strips Semin Reprod Med 20: 63–74

Oktay K, Sonmezer M (2004) Ovarian tissue banking for cancer patients. Fertility preservation, not just ovarian cryopreservation. Hum Reprod 19: 477–480

Oktay K, Briggs D, Gosden RG (1997a). Ontogeny of follicle-stimulating hormone receptor gene expression in isolated human ovarian follicles. J Clin Endocrinol Metab 82: 3748–3751

Oktay K, Nugent D, Newton H, et al. (1997b) Isolation and characterization of primordial follicles from fresh and cryopreserved human ovarian tissue. Fertil Steril 67: 481–486

Oktay K, Newton H, Mullan J, et al. (1998a) Development of human primordial follicles to antral stages in SCID/hpg mice stimulated with follicle stimulating hormone. Hum Reprod 13: 1133–1138

Oktay K, Newton H, Aubard Y, et al. (1998b) Cryopreservation of immature human oocytes and ovarian tissue: an emerging technology? Fertil Steril 69: 1–7

Oktay K, Kan MT, Rosenwaks Z (2001a) Recent progress in oocyte and ovarian tissue cryopreservation and transplantation. Curr Opin Obstet Gynecol 13: 263–268

Oktay K, Economos K, Kan M, et al. (2001b) Endocrine function and oocyte retrieval after autologous transplantation of ovarian cortical strips to the forearm. J Am Med Assoc 286: 1490–1493

Oktay K, Buyuk E, Davis O, et al. (2003) Fertility preservation in breast cancer patients: IVF and embryo cryopreservation after ovarian stimulation with tamoxifen. Hum Reprod 18: 90–95

Oktay K, Buyuk E, Veeck L, et al. (2004a) Embryo development after heterotopic transplantation of cryopreserved ovarian tissue. Lancet 363: 837–840

Oktay K, Sonmezer M, Oktem O (2004b), Ovarian cryopreservation versus ovarian suppression by GnRH analogues: primum non nocere': reply. Hum Reprod 19: 1681–1683

Oktay K, Buyuk E, Libertella N, et al. (2005a) Fertility preservation in breast cancer patients: a prospective controlled comparison of ovarian stimulation with tamoxifen and letrozole for embryo cryopreservation. J Clin Oncol 23: 4347–4353

Oktay K, Libertella N, Oktem O, et al. (2005b) The impact of paclitaxel on menstrual function. Breast Cancer Res Treat 94(Suppl 1): 271s–272s

Oktay K, Oktem O, Reh A et al. (2006a) Measuring the impact of chemotherapy on fertility in women with breast cancer. J Clin Oncol 24: 4044–4046

Oktay K, Hourvitz A, Sahin G, et al. (2006b) Letrozole reduces estrogen and gonadotropin exposure in women with breast cancer undergoing ovarian stimulation before chemotherapy. J Clin Endocrinol Metab. 91: 3885–3890

Oktay K, Cil AP, Bang H (2006c) Efficiency of oocyte cryopreservation: a meta-analysis. Fertil Steril 86: 70–80

Oktay K, Sonmezer M, Oktem O et al. Efficacy and safety of gonadotropin releasing hormone analog treatment in protecting against chemotherapy-induced gonadal injury. Oncologist, in press

Paris F, Perez GI, Fuks Z, et al. (2002). Sphingosine 1-phosphate preserves fertility in irradiated female mice without propagating genomic damage in offspring. Nat Med 8: 901–902

Partridge AH, Gelber S, Peppercorn J, et al. (2004) Web-based survey of fertility issues in young women with breast cancer. J Clin Oncol 22: 4174–4183

Pereyra-Pacheco B, Mendez-Ribaz JM, et al. (2001) Use of GnRH analogs for functional protection of the ovary and preservation of fertility during cancer treatment in adolescents: a preliminary report. Gynecol Oncol 81: 391–397

Perrotin F, Marret H, Bouquin R, et al. (2001) Incidence, diagnosis and prognosis of ovarian metastasis in breast cancer. Gynecol Obstet Fertil 29: 308–315

Pfister CU, Martoni A, Zamagni C, et al. (2001) Effect of age and single versus multiple dose pharmacokinetics of letrozole (Femara) in breast cancer patients. Biopharm Drug Dispos 22: 191–197

Poirot C, Vacher-Lavenu MC, Helardot P et al. (2002). Human ovarian tissue cryopreservation: indications and feasibility. Hum Reprod 17: 1447–1452

Polak deFried E, Notrica J, et al. (1998) Pregnancy after human donor oocyte cryopreservation and thawing in association with intracytoplasmic sperm injection in a patient with ovarian failure. Fertil Steril 69: 555–557

Porcu E (2001) Oocyte freezing. Semin Reprod Med 19: 221–230

Porcu E, Venturoli S (2006) Progress with oocyte cryopreservation. Curr Opin Obstet Gynecol 18: 273–279

Porcu E, Fabbri R, Seracchioli R, et al. (1997) Birth of a healthy female after intracytoplasmic sperm injection of cryopreserved human oocytes. Fertil Steril 68: 724–726

Radford JA, Lieberman BA, Brison DR, et al. (2001) Orthotopic reimplantation of cryopreserved ovarian cortical strips after high-dose chemotherapy for Hodgkin's lymphoma. Lancet 357: 1172–1175

Ray GR, Trueblood HW, Enright LP, et al. (1970) Oophoropexy: a means of preserving ovarian function following pelvic megavoltage radiotherapy for Hodgkin's disease. Radiology 96: 175–180

Rebbeck TR, Lynch HT, Neuhausen SL, et al. (2002) Prevention and Observation of Surgical End Points Study Group. Prophylactic oophorectomy in carriers of BRCA1 or BRCA2 mutations. N Engl J Med 346: 1616–1622

Recchia F, Saggio G, Amiconi G, et al. (2006) Gonadotropin-releasing hormone analogues added to adjuvant chemotherapy protect ovarian function and improve clinical outcomes in young women with early breast carcinoma. Cancer 106: 514–523

Reh AE, Oktem O, Lostritto K, et al. (2006) Impact of breast cancer chemotherapy on ovarian reserve: a prospective analysis by menstrual history and ovarian reserve markers. Fertil Steril 86(suppl 1): 97s--98s

Reis LAG, Percy CL, Bunin GR. Introduction. In: Reis LAG, Smith MA, Gurney JG, et al. (eds) Cancer incidence and survival among children and adolescents: United States SEER Program 1975–1995 [NIH Pub. No. 99-4649]. National Cancer Institute, 1999, Bethesda, pp. 1–15

Revel A, Raanani H, Leyland N, et al. (2000) Human oocyte retrieval from nude mice transplanted with human ovarian cortex [abstract]. Hum Reprod 15 (Abstract Book 1): 13

Revel A, Koler M, Simon A, et al. (2003) Oocyte collection during cryopreservation of the ovarian cortex. Fertil Steril 79: 1237–1239

Revel A, Elami A, Bor A, et al. (2004) Whole sheep ovary cryopreservation and transplantation. Fertil Steril 82: 1714–1715

Robison LL, Bhatia S (2003) Late-effects among survivors of leukaemia and lymphoma during childhood and adolescence. Br J Haematol 122: 345–359

Russell AI, Lawson WA, Haskard DO (2001) Potential new therapeutic options in Behcet's syndrome. BioDrugs 15: 25–35

Salle B, Demirci B, Franck M, et al. (2003) Long-term follow-up of cryopreserved hemi-ovary autografts in ewes: pregnancies, births, and histologic assessment. Fertil Steril 80: 172–177

Sanders JE, Buckner CD, Amos D, et al. (1988) Ovarian function following marrow transplantation for aplastic anemia or leukemia. J Clin Oncol 6: 813–818

Sanders JE, Hawley J, Levy W, et al. (1996) Pregnancies following high-dose cyclophosphamide with or without high-dose busulfan or totalbody irradiation and bone marrow transplantation. Blood 87: 3045–3052

Sastre-Garau X, Jouve M, Asselain B, et al. (1996) Infiltrating lobular carcinoma of the breast. Clinicopathologic analysis of 975 cases with reference to data on conservative therapy and metastatic patterns. Cancer 77: 113–120

Schmidt KLT, Andersen CY, Loft A, et al. (2005) Follow-up of ovarian function post-chemotherapy following ovarian cryopreservation and transplantation. Hum Reprod 20: 3539–3546

Schubert B, Canis M, Darcha C, et al. (2005) Human ovarian tissue from cortex surrounding benign cysts: a model to study ovarian tissue cryopreservation. Hum Reprod 20: 1786–1792

Seshadri T, Gook D, Lade S, et al. (2006) Lack of evidence of disease contamination in ovarian tissue harvested for cryopreservation from patients with Hodgkin lymphoma and analysis of factors predictive of oocyte yield. Br J Cancer 94: 1007–1010

Shaw JM, Bowles J, Koopman P, et al. (1996) Fresh and cryopreserved ovarian tissue samples from donors with lymphoma transmit the cancer to graft recipients. Hum Reprod 11: 1668–1673

Shushan A, Peretz T, Mor-Yosef S (1996) Therapeutic approach to ovarian cysts in tamoxifen-treated women with breast cancer. Int J Gynaecol Obstet 52: 249–253

Shusterman S, Meadows AT (2000). Long term survivors of childhood leukemia. Curr Opin Hematol 7: 217–222

Silber SJ, Lenahan KM, Levine DJ, et al. (2005) Ovarian transplantation between monozygotic twins discordant for premature ovarian failure. N Engl J Med 353: 58–63

Smith HO, Tiffany MF, Qualls CR, et al. (2000) The rising incidence of adenocarcinoma relative to squamous cell carcinoma of the uterine cervix in the United States. A 24-year population-based study. Gynecol Oncol 78: 97–105

Somers EC, Marder W, Christman GM, et al. (2005) Use of a gonadotropin-releasing hormone analog for protection against premature ovarian failure during cyclophosphamide therapy in women with severe lupus. Arthritis Rheum 52: 2761–2767

Sonmezer M, Oktay K (2004) Fertility preservation in female patients. Hum Reprod Update 10: 251–266

Sonmezer M, Oktay K (2006) Fertility preservation in young women undergoing breast cancer therapy. Oncologist 11: 422–434

Sonmezer M, Shamonki MI, Oktay K (2005a) Ovarian tissue cryopreservation: benefits and risks. Cell Tissue Res 322: 125-132

Sonmezer M, Akar M, Oktay M (2005b) Strong family history in women who were diagnosed with breast cancer after in vitro fertilization. Fertil Steril 84 Suppl 1: 233s--234s

Speroff L, Fritz MA (2005) The ovary-embryology and development. In: Speroff L, Fritz MA (eds). Clinical Gynecologic Endocrinology and Infertility. 7th edition, Lippincott Williams & Wilkins, Philadelphia, PA, USA. pp. 97–111

Stillman RJ, Schinfeld JS, Schiff I, et al. (1981) Ovarian failure in long-term survivors of childhood malignancy. Am J Obstet Gynecol 139: 62–66

Struewing JP, Hartge P, Wacholder S, et al. (1997) The risk of cancer associated with specific mutations of BRCA1 and BRCA2 among Ashkenazi Jews. N Engl J Med 336: 1401–1408

Sutton GP, Bundy BN, Delgado G, et al. (1992) Ovarian metastases in stage IB carcinoma of the cervix: a Gynecologic Oncology Group study. Am J Obstet Gynecol 166(1 Pt. 1): 50–53

Tangir J, Zelterman D, Ma W, et al. (2003) Reproductive function after conservative surgery and chemotherapy for malignant germ cell tumors of the ovary. Obstet Gynecol 101: 251–257

Tauchmanova L, Selleri C, Rosa GD, et al. (2002) High prevalence of endocrine dysfunction in long-term survivors after allogeneic bone marrow transplantation for hematologic diseases. Cancer 95: 1076–1084

Tease C, Fisher G (1991) The influence of maternal age on radiation induced chromosome aberrations in mouse oocytes. Mutat Res 262: 57–62

Thibaud E, Rodriguez-Macias K, Trivin C, et al. (1988) Ovarian function after bone marrow transplantation during childhood. Bone Marrow Transplant 21: 287–290

Tulandi T, Al-Took S (1998). Laparoscopic ovarian suspension before irradiation. Fertil Steril 70: 381–383

Ubaldi F, Rienzi L, Ferrero S, et al. (2004) Natural in vitro fertilization cycles. Ann NY Acad Sci 1034: 245–251

Veeck LL, Bodine R, Clarke RN, et al. (2004) High pregnancy rates can be achieved after freezing and thawing human blastocysts. Fertil Steril 82: 1418–1427

Vitale AM, Abramovich D, Peluffo MC, et al. (2006) Effect of gonadotropin-releasing hormone agonist and antagonist on proliferation and apoptosis of human luteinized granulosa cells. Fertil Steril 85: 1064–1067

Viviani S, Santoro A, Ragni G et al. (1985) Gonadal toxicity after combination chemotherapy for Hodgkin's disease. Comparative results of MOPP vs ABVD. Eur J Cancer Clin Oncol 21: 601–605

Waggoner SE (2003) Cervical cancer. Lancet 361: 2217–2225

Wallace WH, Shalet SM, Crowne EC, et al. (1989a) Gonadal dysfunction due to cis-platinum. Med Pediatr Oncol 17: 409–413

Wallace WH, Shalet SM, Hendry JH, et al. (1989a) Ovarian failure following abdominal irradiation in childhood: the radiosensitivity of the human oocyte. Br J Radiol 62: 995–998

Wallace WH, Shalet SM, Crowne EC, et al. (1989b) Ovarian failure following abdominal irradiation in childhood: natural history and prognosis. Clin Oncol (R Coll Radiol) 1: 75–79

Wallace WH, Thomson AB, Kelsey TW (2003) The radiosensitivity of the human oocyte. Hum Reprod 18: 117–121

Warne GL, Fairley KF, Hobbs JB, et al. (1973) Cyclophosphamide-induced ovarian failure. N Engl J Med 289: 1159–1162

Waxman JH, Ahmed R, Smith D, et al. (1987) Failure to preserve fertility in patients with Hodgkin's disease. Cancer Chemother Pharmacol 19: 159–162

Weenen C, Laven JS, Von Bergh AR, et al. (2004) Anti-Müllerian hormone expression pattern in the human ovary: potential implications for initial and cyclic follicle recruitment. Mol Hum Reprod 10: 77–83

Williams RS, Littell RD, Mendenhall NP (1999) Laparoscopic oophoropexy and ovarian function in the treatment of Hodgkin disease. Cancer 86: 2138–2142.

Wolner-Hanssen P, Hagglund L, Ploman F, et al. (2005) Autotransplantation of cryopreserved ovarian tissue to the right forearm 4(1/2) years after autologous stem cell transplantation. Acta Obstet Gynecol Scand 84: 695–698

Woodruff JD, Murthy YS, Bhaskar TN, et al. (1970) Metastatic ovarian tumors. Am J Obstet Gynecol 107: 202–209

Yamamoto R, Okamoto K, Yukiharu T, et al. (2001) A study of risk factors for ovarian metastases in stage Ib-IIIb cervical carcinoma and analysis of ovarian function after a transposition. Gynecol Oncol 82: 312–316

Zanetta G, Bonazzi C, Cantu M, et al. (2001) Survival and reproductive function after treatment of malignant germ cell ovarian tumors. J Clin Oncol 19: 1015–1020

19 Psychooncologic Care in Young Women Facing Cancer and Pregnancy

J. Alder, J. Bitzer

Recent Results in Cancer Research, Vol. 178

19.1 Introduction

During the past decades the lives of many women in developed countries have undergone essential changes. After a longer and more specialized professional formation many women follow a career before starting a family. Therefore, births to women 30 and older continue to rise, which is associated with increased maternal and fetal risks during pregnancy (Nabukera et al. 2006). Moreover, as the risk of developing breast cancer increases with age, more women are confronted with breast cancer during their childbearing years.

The concept "critical life event" refers to the stimulus-based perspective of stress with particular attention to the characteristics of a stressor. Each critical episode has its unique demands that challenge the individual's coping resources, thus triggering a particular stress response. Holmes and Rahe (1967) attempted to measure life stress by assigning numbers (life-change units) to a list of 43 critical life events that includes illness as well as pregnancy. The use of average weights to define the magnitude of life events has several shortcomings: From a cognitive-transactional process perspective, stress is defined as a particular relationship related to the person's appraisal of the stressfulness of the event as exceeding his or her (coping) resources and therefore endangering well-being (Lazarus 1966, 1991). Consequently, the awareness that a pregnant woman with cancer has to face and adjust to two life events at the same time is important in understanding the manifold (coping) reactions of the patient.

Most studies have found a delay particularly in the diagnosis of breast cancer during pregnancy. The focus of the woman may be entirely on her pregnancy, and changes in breast tissue may be attributed to normal physiological breast changes. On the other hand, physical examination is mostly concentrated on the abdomen and imaging during pregnancy is more difficult. Once the diagnosis has been made the process of deciding on treatment options may be delayed because of the complexity of the situation, with two beings involved in the treatment. However, treatment delay increases the risk for lymph node involvement in dependence of doubling time (Nettleton et al. 1996). Hence, the complicating issues of cancer during pregnancy relate to medical, bio-/medicoethical (Oduncu et al. 2003), and personal/psychological aspects. Support of women facing cancer during pregnancy must consider the complexity of the life situation, being confronted with two critical life events that symbolize the beginning and the end of life at the same time. From a psychodynamic point of view the situation for some women may reflect a classic conflict between the instincts of self-preservation and breed preservation. The decision making process is complex and has a special focus on the autonomy of the woman and the balance of best possible treatment for the woman with least harm to the fetus. Special communication skills facilitate shared decision making (Elwyn 2001). The woman and her family often have a special need for psychooncologic care during the adjustment process of having cancer and requiring treatment at the same time as being pregnant (which often extends from pregnancy into the postpartum period). This chapter therefore focuses on the complexity of understanding the meaning of the diagnosis, the challenging adjustment process, and what professionals can do to support the woman during this life phase.

19.2 Adjustment to Pregnancy and Cancer

19.2.1 Adjustment to Pregnancy

Pregnancy is not only associated with physiological changes in a mother's body. Psychological changes refer to the developmental process or tasks that prepare the mother for her new responsibilities. Failure to achieve these tasks during this period may lead to a lack of emotional response to the infant at delivery and limited maternal-neonatal attachment (Attrill 2002). Gloger-Tippelt (1988) describes the transition to parenthood within a developmental psychological model with four different stages during pregnancy. The parents' desire for a child increases steadily during pregnancy. Each of the stages puts specific demands of adjustment on physical, cognitive, emotional, and behavioral levels. The first stage of uncertainty during the first trimester is characterized by physical discomfort, ambivalence, and insecurity about the progress of the pregnancy. Then, after the 12th week of gestation, a stage of adjustment follows with a reduction in anxieties and, therefore, cognitive and emotional adjustment that leads to an increase of positive valence of the pregnancy. The third stage begins with the second half of the pregnancy and is characterized by a change in perception of the child due to noticeable fetal movements. The mother starts to perceive the child as being separate from herself. In addition, the increased perceptibility of the pregnancy leads to change in the social role of the pregnant woman. During the last 10 weeks of pregnancy, the stage of anticipation and preparation, expectant mothers actively imagine the appearance and behavior of their baby and what it will be like to care for it. The perception of time changes to counting weeks or days until delivery instead of counting gestational weeks or months. With a worsening of mood and enhanced discomfort, the readiness to end the pregnancy increases.

Adjustment to pregnancy naturally is multifaceted and depends on intrapersonal, interpersonal, social, and somatic factors among others. The model of developmental stages during pregnancy as described by Gloger-Tippelt (1988) therefore must be understood as a general framework that will not apply to all pregnancies.

19.2.2 Adjustment to Cancer

Adjustment to cancer is influenced by three main factors (Rowland 1990): (1) disease-related factors such as site of the disease, stage, treatment, and course; (2) individual factors such as values and beliefs, personality characteristics, and social support (in addition, the specific life phase in which the cancer illness affects the patient is relevant for understanding the adjustment process, with pregnancy demanding completely different developmental tasks from the person than, e.g., the postmenopausal life phase); (3) sociocultural factors such as stigma or resources available from the health care system. In addition, the patient's relationship with doctors and nurses and experience with the medical system influence the adaptation process as well as compliance with treatment.

Table 19.1 summarizes the most common emotional reactions evoked when the cancer diagnosis is received (Barraclough 1999). During pregnancy, these reactions most often are more pronounced because of the unexpectedness of the diagnosis and because of fears of not being able to meet the demands of motherhood and or to continue the pregnancy (see below). The early work by Kübler-Ross (1969) offers a useful framework for understanding adjustment to cancer. The model assumes the following four adjustment stages: (1) the stage of denial, usually lasting not more than a few days with shock, disbelief, or numbness; (2) the stage of acute distress, often lasting several weeks with the most prevalent reactions of anxiety, anger, bargaining, and protest; (3) the stage of chronic distress, which again may last several weeks and is characterized by sadness and despair; and (4) gradual adjustment and acceptance, often taking several months. The model is not understood as a rigid formula, and one stage does not strictly follow the one before. Adjustment is not a normative process. However, it can be understood as heuristic and can give a broad orientation and understanding to professionals and patients. Mostly, it is important to consider that adjustment to cancer calls for a long-term view with periods of distress often being a necessary prelude to positive adaptation. This process is highly individual and is based on a multifactorial environment-person interaction (Filip and Aymanns 1987).

Table 19.1 Emotional reactions to cancer diagnosis

Shock
Fear and anxiety
Sadness and despair
Anger
Guilt or shame
Relief (after a period of diagnostic uncertainty)
Sense of challenge
Acceptance

Barraclough (1999) emphasizes the reaction to or threat of loss in the context of cancer. Adjusting to loss of physical strength, loss of or change in role, loss of interpersonal relationships, loss of physical integrity, loss of life expectancy, loss of control, or loss of mental integrity may seem overwhelming at first. In the case of cancer during pregnancy, the patient is additionally confronted with the prospect of losing a wished-for child.

During the adjustment process to illness the patient will demonstrate a wide variety of coping strategies. Coping refers to the different patterns of thought, belief, emotions, and behavior observed in response to the illness. Adaptive coping does not mean being free of emotional distress but rather not being overwhelmed by it and demonstrating flexibility in adapting to new circumstances while maintaining one's own sense of self-worth and relationships with others. There have been many attempts to classify coping styles (Lazarus 1966, 1991; Heim et al. 1991). A widely recognized categorization refers to problem-focused coping, appraisal-focused coping, and emotion-focused coping (Moos and Schaeffer 1984; Folkman and Lazarus 1980). The individual's appraisal of the situation determines the coping style. In situations that are appraised as being changeable, active, problem-focused coping strategies are employed. For example, cancer patients who search the Internet, adhere to treatment, or undertake changes in their lifestyle demonstrate a problem-focused coping style. On the other hand, appraisal-focused and emotion-focused coping styles occur more often when the situation is appraised as uncontrollable or not changeable, as is frequently the case during cancer illness. The strategies then focus on finding the best possible attitude toward an encumbering situation or doing anything to be more comfortable in bearing and tolerating the situation. Typically, talking about emotions or relaxation but also blaming others or consumption of psychoactive substances fall into this coping style. For health care professionals it is sometimes difficult to understand the individual reactions of the patients. Coping strategies may seem wrong or bad or right or good. However, as Haan (1977) states "The person will cope if he can, defend if he must, and fragment if he is forced, but whichever mode he uses, it is still in the service of his attempt to maintain organization." Thus, reactions may be adaptive and supportive of well-being or maladaptive and contributing to additional distress.

From a psychodynamic point of view, experiences and relationships of early childhood and instinctual drives continue to influence a person's feelings and behavior in adulthood. For many women pregnancy reflects a time period in which memories of their own childhood are being reactivated and relationships with parents are changing. Psychodynamic models of reaction to cancer conceptualize mental or ego defense mechanisms as unconscious processes designed to protect against anxiety. Defense mechanisms include, among others, denial, repression, projection, regression, or intellectualization. While true denial is rare among cancer patients, intellectualization with an emphasis on reason and factual knowledge and at the same time denial of emotional aspects is more common.

19.2.3 Adjustment to Cancer During Pregnancy

Women with cancer during pregnancy are not only faced by the challenge to adjust to two critical life events at the same time. More importantly, for many people these two events lie on two opposite ends of the continuum of life. Pregnancy is associated with the beginning of a new life, and cancer for most people is still associated with the end of life. In addition, decision making becomes much more complicated and emotionally loaded because at least two perspectives must be involved, that of the mother and that of the fetus.

The following section highlights the cognitive-emotional and ethical complexity of this situation, which has been referred to as maternal-fetal conflict (Oduncu et al. 2003).

Many women first react with lifestyle changes as soon as they know about their pregnancy. This may affect eating habits, intake of vitamins, smoking and drinking behavior, or physical activity. Thus, a sense of responsibility toward the growing child is often assumed as early as in the first trimester. A cancer diagnosis during pregnancy challenges this sense of responsibility in various ways.

First, the decision whether to continue with the pregnancy or not weighs up the life of the mother against the life of the fetus. No mother would sacrifice the life of a living child to save her own life, and for some women this is true from the earliest days of pregnancy. Psychodynamically speaking, some women develop a conflict between the instinct of self-preservation and the instinct of breed preservation.

Second, the decision about treatment options in the case of continuing the pregnancy may be a decision for a second-best possible treatment. In terms of Beauchamp and Childress' (2001) medicoethical approach, conflicts within the ethical principles of beneficence and autonomy may develop. The conflict between the beneficence for the mother and the beneficence for the child relates to the fact that the optimal therapy for the mother may harm the child and delay of maternal treatment for the best of the child may harm the mother. The physician's perspective on fetal beneficence additionally may not be shared by the mother, and opinions on acceptance of potential risks to the fetus may differ. The conflict between maternal autonomy and the physician's perspective on what is best for the patient and the fetus may stress the physician-patient relationship (Zanetti-Dällenbach et al., accepted for publication).

Yet another area that leads to high emotional distress is the threat to the woman's self-concept when she is confronted with cancer during pregnancy. In the same body a beloved and wished-for child is growing and at the same time a life-threatening disease has to be stopped from growing. Especially in the case of breast cancer, where breast feeding will not be possible because of mastectomy or systemic therapy, this may lead to loss of the sense of self-worth in fulfilling the role of a good mother. This offense is further supported by fears of not being able to take care of the child because of the treatment or the course of the illness. The mother may also be confronted with a preterm child as a result of early caesarean section. Furthermore, the strong emotional distress will lead to a dysregulation of the hypothalamic-pituitary-adrenal axis (HPA) (Vedhara et al. 2006; Porter et al. 2003). Several studies have associated chronic distress in pregnant women with a suboptimal intrauterine environment, which may negatively affect fetal development and pregnancy outcome (Wadhwa 2005).

In the case of continuation of pregnancy, the joy about being pregnant and the pleasant anticipation of becoming parents may be restricted because of preoccupations with the illness, and some women will need support for maternal-fetal attachment comparable to women with enhanced levels of depression during pregnancy (Lindgren 2001).

19.3 Supporting the Pregnant Woman with Cancer

For most women the situation of being diagnosed with cancer during pregnancy is absolutely unexpected and overwhelming. The woman has no previous knowledge on how to deal with the situation and therefore will be very insecure about what to ask and what she can expect from the medical team. Often she is being counseled by more than one specialist, and especially when talking to obstetricians and oncologists, she will be confronted with different opinions. A multidisciplinary approach to the patient lies in the nature of this clinical situation. The patient has to feel safe in this network of team members, and experts should practice regular exchange of opinions and views. In this complex context the importance of the use of specific counseling skills by the physician cannot be emphasized enough. In addition, more specialized psychooncologic care may support the patient and her partner in the complex decision making process, during mourning after termination of pregnancy, for promoting maternal-fetal attachment, in adjusting to the diagnosis, during treatment, and during aftercare.

19.3.1 Communication Skills in Oncology

The terminology of counseling has been widely used in oncology and it refers to specific communication skills as in breaking bad news or information giving until professional psychooncologic treatment can be applied. Communication skills are regarded as the cornerstone of comprehensive cancer care. Pregnant women who are confronted with cancer often are in special need of support when receiving the diagnosis, during the decision making process, and during treatment. The following section first takes into consideration these initial stages of counseling before expanding the psychooncologic care of pregnant cancer patients.

Table 19.2 Guidelines for breaking bad news

Ensure privacy and adequate time
Assess and reassess understanding
Provide information (diagnosis) simply and honestly
Encourage patients to express feelings and thoughts; be empathetic
Give broad time frame
Arrange review, if possible within 48 hours
Discuss treatment options
Offer assistance in telling others
Provide information about support services
Document information given

19.3.1.1 Breaking Bad News

Because of its rarity (Smith et al. 2001), a cancer diagnosis during pregnancy always is a great unexpected shock to the patient and her partner. Because this is an obstetric and an oncologic event at the same time, these patients need to be seen and counseled by an interdisciplinary team of experts to reassure the patient that optimal treatment from the perspective of different disciplines is being recommended (Jenkins et al. 2001). Breaking bad news to these patients should be performed by a person skilled in communication with a high biomedical and psychological competence (Girgis and Sanson-Fisher 1995, 1998). Receiving bad news is painful to any patient in this situation; it is a challenging situation and necessitates good communication skills. A patient-centered approach when communicating the diagnosis should be applied. Table 19.2 summarizes the essential steps in breaking bad news (Girgis and Sanson-Fisher 1998).

In the context of cancer during pregnancy, breaking bad news always has to include information on the actual pregnancy situation. Summarizing age, position, approximate size, and developmental status of the fetus, by adding information on what the specific cancer illness means for fetal well-being, helps to relativize possible unrealistic concepts.

Because of the high emotional activation it is important to consider that the information-processing capacity of the patient will be very limited. It is therefore recommended to limit the information provided and to arrange a new appointment shortly thereafter. Also, the patient can be supported by making notes about the diagnosis, the next steps, and treatment options or by drawings of localization of the tumor. The principle of hope is of great importantance in this overwhelming situation (Schmid Mast et al. 2005). The identification of the *patient's* concerns by direct questioning ("Which questions are most important to you at the moment?") helps the physician to understand what information the patient will most probably be ready to process and to structure the great amount of information that must be delivered in this situation. In this way, patient-centered information giving reassures and supports the patient in better understanding investigations, prognosis, risks, and treatment options (Maguire and Pitceathly 2002).

The physician's dilemma in the situation of cancer during pregnancy can be viewed as what has been called being a lawyer of two worlds (Hepp 1996), the maternal and the fetal world. An additional difficulty may be the frequently found delay in diagnosis (Smith et al. 2001; Woo et al. 2003), which may stress the establishment of a trustful patient-physician relationship. Questions and reproaches referring to the diagnostic process should be answered in an open, nondefensive way, and the patient's great emotional distress should always be understood in her reactions. As mentioned above, anger is a normal phase in the adjustment to a cancer diagnosis, and some patients obtain a release through free expression of this anger. The following don'ts summarize unhelpful behavior in the context of breaking bad news. *DO NOT* feel obliged to keep talking when the patient falls silent, assume that you know what is troubling the patient, eliminate emotional reactions with treatment offers, give false reassurance, hide behind medical jargon, criticize, make judgments, give direct advice about psychological matters, or overload with information (Barraclough 1999).

Table 19.3 Steps for patients to share in the decision making process (Towle 1997)

Establish a context in which patient's views about treatment options are valued and necessary
Elicit patient's preferences so that appropriate treatment options are discussed
Transfer technical information to the patient on treatment options, risks, and their probable benefits in an unbiased, clear, and simple way
Help the patient to conceptualize the process of weighing risks versus benefits, and ensure that her preferences are based on facts and not misconceptions
Share the treatment recommendation with the patient, and/or affirm the patient's treatment preferences

19.3.1.2 Information Giving and Shared Decision Making

Information giving on diagnosis, prognosis and, especially, treatment options in the context of cancer during pregnancy is most complex and always includes the maternal and the fetal perspective. A comprehensive process of informational exchange in which the patient's values as well as expert knowledge on treatment options are considered is the basis of the shared decision making process. Without this process the patient often is not able to come to an informed decision regarding termination or continuation of pregnancy and cancer treatment. The shared decision making process therefore, can be viewed as a process between experts: The physician is the expert on disease and its treatment, and the patient is the expert on herself and her values, beliefs, and priorities in life.

Information must be given in a simple and clear but not blunt language. The information should be simple, specific, and relevant, taking into account the social context and general knowledge of the patient. Information should be categorized, with the most important information being presented first. Repetitions and short words and sentences further support understanding and processing of the information (Morrow et al. 1983; Godolphin 2003; Edwards 2003; Alaszewski and Horlick-Jones 2003; Paling 2003). Table 19.3 outlines the steps, as suggested by Towle (1997), that must be taken in order to involve patients in the decision making process.

In her review, Hopwood (2005) emphasizes the lack of validated approaches to communicating risk and the need for communication skills training in this area. Some studies in women with high genetic risk for breast cancer have evaluated communication strategies, and they underline the importance of facilitating understanding over verbal and written information in reducing depression and anxiety (Lobb et al. 2004).

O'Connor (2003) distinguishes two different kinds of clinical decisions. The first is effective decisions where scientific evidence of benefits and harms is known, with minimal harm in relation to the benefit. Counseling in such a situation of standard care can be brief, and the decision to be made by the patient is usually easy. This is not so in the case of preference-sensitive decisions. Here, the scientific evidence might not be clear, there could be important harms expected, the benefit might be questionable, and the decision therefore strongly depends on the person's values. This applies to situations like the management of menopausal symptoms, antenatal screening, or cancer during pregnancy. Often, physicians underestimate the patient's preferences for a shared decision making process. In particular for a young woman with cancer her wish regarding her part in the decision making process should be clarified and she should be provided with evidence-based information to come to a decision based on her values, objectives, wishes, and fears.

In summary, the specific difficulties in counseling a woman and her partner in order to come to an informed consensus on how to proceed are at least fourfold. First, because of the rarity of cancer during pregnancy, there is still a lack of evidence-based information and some uncertainty regarding optimal treatment during pregnancy. Second, risk calculation and risk counseling in this context are complex and therefore prone to professional biases. Third, counseling and decision making are happening in a situation that is highly emotional, for the patient as well as for her physician. It is a special challenge and yet of critical importance to ascertain that the patient is able to process, understand, and evaluate the information instead of being simply overwhelmed and letting someone decide for her. Fourth, consideration of the personal values, experiences, and life perspectives of the patient in the evaluation of the different possibilities is of importance. While time constraints of the clinical encounter often limit the possibilities of a profound analysis, these individual aspects are of great importance, especially for the following adjustment process.

19.3.1.3 Adherence to Emotions

Despite of the increased awareness of the importance of communication skills in oncology and the implementation of training courses for teaching these skills over the past decade, cancer patients continue to have unmet communication needs. Communication outcomes are positively associated with physicians' attendance to the emotional needs of patients (Hack et al. 2005). However, emotionally charged consultations may also trigger clinicians' defense mechanisms, protecting them from painful emotions. These so-called distancing techniques may hamper the recognition of patients' suffering (Favre et al. 2006).

Communication of emotion is especially related to nonverbal communication. The emotion-related communication skills, including sending and receiving nonverbal messages and emotional self-awareness, are regarded as critical elements of high-quality care (Roter et al. 2006). Some women appear very analytical and without affect and describe physical symptoms in depth and discuss laboratory data at length. Instead of simply going into the presented topics, the physician can take the opportunity to inquire about the underlying emotions and to open discussion of the personal dimension: "So, that's what has happened to you in recent days. How has that affected you personally?" The mnemonic NURS aids in recalling emotion-handling skills: naming or labeling the emotion of the patient ("That frightens you"), understandability or legitimation ("I can imagine that must have been overwhelming"), respect ("You have been coping really well with that"), and support or partnership ("Together, I think we'll find some solutions for the next steps") (Smith and Hoppe 1991).

19.3.2 Psychooncologic Care During Pregnancy and Postpartum

As several specialists are involved in caring for the patient it is of utmost importance to ensure the flow of information and to have intermittent briefing sessions among the specialists to share information and views. It is very supportive for the patient to feel that all involved professionals are caring for the mother-baby unit as a whole. She should not have to deal with the impression that the oncologist does not know or support what the obstetrician says and vice versa since the situation is difficult enough for her.

During pregnancy there are different ways to provide additional support for the woman. The different approaches of psychooncologic care in practice often add to an integrative approach including client-centered, supportive, psychodynamic, cognitive-behavioral, and, especially during pregnancy, systemic elements. Relaxation techniques and guided imagery have been shown to be effective to deal with treatment side effects and reduce anxiety. The decision on the introduction of different interventions depends largely on the situation the patient is in and on personal variables of patient and partner.

19.3.2.1 Dealing with the Diagnosis

In a first phase of adjustment to the diagnosis, the psychooncologist supports the understanding of the meaning of the diagnosis in the context of being pregnant. Having to deal at the same time with emotions such as fear of death and hopelessness and with the joy of being pregnant and becoming a mother can be very challenging, not only for the patient and her partner but for the caregiver as well. Cancer patients in general are tormented with many questions that sometimes are hard to answer, and this applies even more to pregnant cancer patients. In this stage interventions such as ventilation of emotions, thought-stopping, or the planning of concrete steps and activities as well as activating the social support system can be important. The consultation in which no further results or therapeutic suggestions are introduced and no decisions have to be discussed provides room to sort information and associated emotions and thoughts. In the context of the preference-sensitive decision on treatment, it is of great importance to consider the patient's values, beliefs, and ideas on life ambitions. Intermediate counseling sessions during this process can clarify and balance these concepts.

If the patient decides for a termination of pregnancy, she will be confronted with having to detach from her child and from the idea of becoming a mother and at the same time undergoing a stressful treatment such as radiation or chemotherapy after/before surgery. Some women will not be able to cope with both processes in parallel. A mourning process can, consciously or unconsciously, be suspended and become an encumbrance later on. Supporting the patient to deal with side effects, for example, through relaxation techniques and relief in daily life can release power and energy to confront the mourning process earlier. Also, it can be helpful to sort out the issues that sooner or later will be confronted during the adjustment process. The patient can be counseled that she doesn't have to deal with everything simultaneously and that handling and confronting one pile after another is for some women a good way of managing the adjustment process.

19.3.2.2 Supporting Maternal-Fetal/Neonatal Bonding During Treatment

Women who continue with pregnancy have the challenge of being very ill and—often—receiving treatment and being pregnant at the same time. This situation can have consequences for maternal-fetal bonding. The patient is dealing with treatment side effects and body image changes due to breast surgery, has appointments with the oncologist, and has much less time and peace to adjust to pregnancy and to get emotionally prepared for her role as mother. In addition, she may have toddlers at home to take care of. Psychooncologic support, therefore, has to focus on the illness and associated treatments *and* should leave room for the theme of pregnancy and feelings toward the child and motherhood. Feelings of guilt toward the fetus' possible exposure to therapy may arise, and the patient may need support in developing an attitude that helps her to follow the treatment.

It can be advisable to split consultations, leaving time to discuss anxieties regarding illness and leaving time and space to talk about pregnancy-associated feelings and preparing for birth and the postpartum period. Regular sonography and palpation can enhance maternal-fetal bonding and give reassurance regarding fetal well-being. Three-dimensional ultrasound may be especially helpful because it allows more easy perception of the fetus' features. The mother can be supported in developing a more concrete image of the child by assigning perceptions of the fetus such as level of activity to imagined behavior ("active child," "has its own will"). Guided imagery can be an additional strategy to enhance bonding. For example, a picture of the fetus softly embedded in the uterus or of the mother cuddling the newborn can be developed with the patient, and in a relaxed state she will be accompanied through the imagery. In addition, the patient needs time and room to get prepared emotionally for birth and the postpartum period. Some women with a strong wish for natural birth will have difficulties in accepting an early cesarean section and need support in dealing with anxieties and disappointment. The postpartum period for many women is associated with additional treatments. Preparation for and anticipation of this period is very important. The patient will need practical and emotional help and relief for the situation of having a newborn at home and at the same time being on therapy for a life-threatening illness.

Patients who undergo adjuvant treatments in the postpartum period most likely will have less time to spend with their neonate. They are dealing with strong side effects and for some days are not able to do the household chores. Thus, they may have less emotional and physical capacity to build up a relationship with the child and to take care of it, which sometimes leads to feelings of guilt. At the same time, having a newborn the mother has an obvious reason for undergoing treatment for this life-threatening disease. Some women also develop a fighting spirit from the experience of childbirth. Practical support should be organized early enough for the patient and her partner. It must be guaranteed that the couple can spend quality time with the newborn without having to worry about household tasks or running errands. The parents may need help and assistance in parenting. In most cases the patient will not be able to breast-feed. While providing some relief because of the ease of having significant others take care of the child, these circumstances can also be disappointing to the patient. Additional interventions such as a baby massage course may strengthen the maternal-neonatal attachment. Regular visits to the pediatrician also give reassurance about the child's well-being, especially after exposure to chemotherapeutic agents during pregnancy.

19.3.2.3 Supporting Coping

Ambivalent and negative feelings can be very normal in these circumstances. However, after a first shock at diagnosis the patient will be confronted with people in her environment or even her partner who tell her to think and feel positive about the pregnancy and the child. Simply thinking positive is not only difficult but sometimes can be quite dangerous for physical and mental health. Not being able to think positive can lead to a sense of guilt toward the child and to the impression of failing. The patient may need to talk with a neutral person about her ambivalence and her negative feelings.

Having cancer treatment during pregnancy and in the postpartum period and dealing with anxieties and doubts regarding the future challenge the patient's coping strategies to a great extent. The counselor reviews her coping behavior and helps to distinguish helpful from unhelpful behavior. Cognitive-behavioral interventions will help to identify unhelpful, irrational thinking (e.g., "I will never be able to deal with this.") and to elaborate more realistic thinking (e.g., "There may be things that will be hard to cope with and for which I will need support. On the other hand, I have already been doing quite well with reacting to the diagnosis, which shows that I am able to deal with some things."). Enhancing a sense of control is very important and prevents the development of depressive symptoms. The patient must be assisted in identifying situations in which she is in control and in which she can actively contribute. On the other hand, she might have to be supported in finding strategies to deal with and withstand situations that are not controllable at the moment (such as waiting for results). Relaxation techniques, distraction, or emotional catharsis can be introduced and planned.

In some cases, it is advisable to develop a plan for crisis intervention early in the treatment. Crises develop during chemotherapy, because of environmental factors or in the context of relationship difficulties. The elaboration of an emergency plan that tells the patient what she has to do and who she can consult when upset is an important intervention for patients who have limited coping ability or an unstable environment.

Some patients with maladaptive coping strategies or a predisposition are at increased risk of developing a postpartum depressive disorder. About 5%–10% of patients develop a depressive disorder soon after first-time diagnosis of cancer, while adjustment disorders are being diagnosed more often (Mehnert and Koch 2006; Okamura et al. 2005; Kissane et al. 2004). During pregnancy and in the first year postpartum, the combined point prevalence estimated for major and minor depression ranges from 6.5% to 12.9% (Gavin et al. 2005). No data exist so far on the prevalence of mental health disorders in patients with cancer in the peripartum period. The medical team should be familiar with the detection of psychopathologic symptoms, and specialized treatment should be initiated as soon as a mental health disorder is diagnosed.

19.3.2.4 Inclusion of the Partner/Family

Cancer threatens the whole family with separation and loss. Such threats can seriously divert the life course of the family. In the case of cancer in a first-time pregnancy, the family system is only developing and the diagnosis may disrupt this important process. The family system develops from the time during pregnancy to the first months postpartum. If the newborn is an addition to a family with children, the places and positions especially among the siblings have to be reallocated. Sometimes older siblings react strongly to the addition to the family, which requires a lot of patience from the parents.

Optimally, the partner has an active part in the decision making process and should explicitly be invited to attend consultations by the medical team.

The family plays a critical role for the pregnant woman with cancer, in both the early detection of cancer and its treatment. Social support in general but more specifically provided by the partner or the family is a resource for the patient and in the best circumstances reinforces the patient in her efforts to stay healthy. However, social support from the family differs from support from friends and colleagues and can also have a negative impact. Family members often are emotionally closer to the patient and will have their own fears and concerns, which may reduce their effectiveness in assistance with the situation (Bloom 2000).

The prospective father is being confronted with the chance of becoming an only parent. He can be ambivalent but will hesitate to openly talk about his anxieties in order to protect his partner. The woman is bearing his child, and he may have a strong wish for this child. On the other hand, he wants the best for his wife and wants her to live. This conflict is not easily communicated. A change in roles of the couple can be an additional burden. The woman, who up to was pregnant and healthy, is now pregnant and ill while her partner is not pregnant and not ill. He might feel the pressure of responsibility, but, again, in the present situation this is not easily communicated. Single sessions with the partner sometimes help to elaborate these conflicts. However, optimally the couple is being counseled together and supported in the dyadic adjustment process to this difficult situation. The couple is tormented with many questions and worries regarding the future. Especially in the postpartum period it therefore may be very helpful to help the couple to concentrate on the moment.

Oncology professionals may assume an important role in safely accompanying the cancer patient from a previous life phase without illness to a new life phase with different signs and limits. The new life phase often is characterized by a change in concerns and problems. Preoccupations with prognosis, changes in body image, sexuality, and fertility, frustration of life plans, increased vulnerability, transition to an early menopause, change in social roles, and changes in the family system are just some of the issues patients have to adapt to. To satisfy the needs of cancer patients optimally requests a multidisciplinary approach. This is especially true for the highly emotional situation of cancer during pregnancy. Concurrently, the strain on the physician who is confronted with a pregnant cancer patient can be considerable. The possibility of regular exchange and consultation with other involved professionals ultimately may support the caregivers in meeting the high demands of their profession.

References

Alaszewski A and Horlick-Jones T (2003) How can doctors communicate information about risk more effectively? BMJ 327: 728–731

Attrill B (2002) The assumption of the maternal role: a developmental process Aust J Midwifery 15: 21–25

Barraclough J (1999) Cancer and emotion. John Wiley and Sons, New York.

Bloom JR (2000) The role of family support in cancer control. In Cancer and the family, Baider L, Cooper CL, Kaplan De-Nour A (eds). John Wiley and Sons, New York

Edwards A (2003) Communicating risks. BMJ 327: 691–692

Elwyn G (2001) Shared decision making. Ponsen and Looijen, Wageningen

Favre N, Despland JN, de Roten Y, Drapeau M, Bernard M, Stiefel F (2007) Psychodynamic aspects of communication skills training: a pilot study. Support Care Cancer 15: 333–337

Filip SH, Aymanns P (1987). Die Bedeutung sozialer und personaler Ressourcen in der Auseinandersetzung mit kritischen Lebensereignissen. Z Klein Psychol 16: 1–14

Folkman S, Lazarus RS (1980) An analysis of coping in a middle-aged community sample. J Health Social Behav 21: 219–239

Gavin NI, Gaynes BN, Lohr KN, Meltzer-Brody S, Gartlehner G, Swinson T (2005) Perinatal depression: a systematic review of prevalence and incidence. Obstet Gynecol 106: 1071–1083

Girgis A, Sanson-Fisher RW (1995) Breaking bad news: consensus guidelines for medical practitioners J Clin Oncol 13: 2449–2456

Girgis A, Sanson-Fisher RW (1998) Breaking bad news. 1: Current best advice for clinicians. Behav Med 24: 53–59

Gloger-Tippelt G (1988) Schwangerschaft und erste Geburt. Psychologische Veränderungen der Eltern. Kohlhammer, Stuttgart

Godolphin W (2003) The role of risk communication in shared decision making. BMJ 327: 692–693

Haan N (1977) Coping and defending. Processes of self-environment organization. Academic Press, New York

Hack TF, Degner LF, Parker PA, SCRN Communication Team (2005). The communication goals and needs of cancer patients: a review. Psychooncology 14: 831–845

Heim E, Augustiny KF, Blaser A, Schaffner L (1991) Berner Bewältigungsformen (BEFO) Handbuch. Huber, Bern

Hepp H (1996) Medizinische und ethische Aspekte der Pränatal- und Frühgeburtsmedizin. Stimmen der Zeit 214: 651–669

Holmes TH, Rahe RH (1967) The social adjustment rating scale. J Psychosom Res 11: 213–218

Hopwood, P (2005) Psychosocial aspects of risk communication and mutation testing in familial breast-ovarian cancer. Curr Opin Oncol 17: 340–344

Jenkins VA, Fallowfield LJ, Poole K (2001) Are members of multidisciplinary teams in breast cancer aware of each other's informational roles? Qual Health Care 10: 70–75

Kissane DW, Grabsch B, Love A, Clarke DM, Block S, Smith GC (2004) Psychiatric disorder in women with early stage and advanced breast cancer: a comparative analysis. Aust N Z J Psychiatry 38: 320–326

Kübler-Ross E (1969) On death and dying. Touchstone, New York

Lazarus RS (1966) Psychological stress and the coping process. McGraw-Hill, New York

Lazarus RS (1991) Emotion and adaptation. Oxford University Press, London

Lindgren K (2001) Relationship among maternal-fetal attachment, prenatal depression, and health practices in pregnancy Res Nurs Health 24: 203–217

Lobb EA, Butow PN, Barratt A, Meiser B, Gaff C, Young MA, Haan E, Suthers G, Gattas M, Tucker K (2004). Communication and information-giving in high-risk breast cancer consultations: influence on patient outcomes.Br J Cancer 90: 321–327

Maguire P, Pitceathly C (2002) Key communication skills and how to acquire them. BMJ 325: 697–700

Mehnert A, Koch U (2007) Prevalence of acute and post-traumatic stress disorder and comorbid mental disorders in breast cancer patients during primary cancer care: a prospective study. Psychooncology 16: 181–188

Moos RH, Schaefer JA (1984) The crisis of physical illness: an overview and conceptual approach. In Moos RH (ed) Coping with physical illness. Plenum, New York, pp. 3–25

Morrow BM, Hoagland AC, Carpenter PJ (1983) Improving physician-patient communications in cancer treatment. J Psychosoc Oncol 1: 93–101

Nabukera S, Wingate MS, Alexander GR, Salihu HM (2006) First-time births among women 30 years and older in the United States: patterns and risk of adverse outcomes. J Reprod Med 51: 676–682

Nettleton J, Long J, Kuban D, Wu R, Shaeffer J, El-Mahdi A (1996) Breast cancer during pregnancy: quantifying the risk of treatment delay. Obstet Gynecol 87: 414–418

Oduncu FS, Kimming R, Hepp H, Emmerich B (2003) Cancer in pregnancy: maternal-fetal conflict. J Cancer Res Clin Oncol 129: 133–146

Okamura M, Yamawaki S, Akechi T, Taniguchi K, Uchitomi Y (2005) Psychiatric disorders following first breast cancer recurrence: prevalence, associated factors and relationship to quality of life. Jpn J Clin Oncol 35: 302–309

Paling J (2003) Strategies to help patients understand risks. BMJ 327: 745–748

Porter LS, Mishel M, Neelon V, Belyea M, Pisano E, Soo MS (2003). Cortisol levels and response to mammography in breast cancer survivors: a pilot study. Psychosom Med 65: 842–848

Roter DL, Frankel RM, Hall JA, Sluyter D (2006) The expression of emotion through nonverbal behaviour in medical visits. Mechanisms and outcomes. J Gen Intern Med 21 Suppl 1: S28–S34

Rowland JH (1990) Intrapersonal resources: coping. In: Holland JC, Rowland JH (eds) Handbook of psychooncology. Oxford University Press, New York, pp. 44–57

Schmid Mast M, Kindlimann A, Langewitz W (2005) Recipients' perspective on breaking bad news: how you put it really makes a difference. Patient Educ Couns 58: 244–251

Smith LH, Dalrymple JL, Leiserowitz GS, Danielsen B, Gilbert WM (2001) Obstetrical deliveries associated with maternal malignancy in California, 1992 through 1997. Am J Obstet Gynecol 184: 1504–1512

Smith RC, Hoppe RB (1991) The patient's story: integrating the patient- and physician-centered approaches to interviewing. Ann Intern Med 115: 470–477

Towle A (1997) Physician and Patient Communication Skills: Competencies for Informed Shared Decision-Making. Informed Shared Decision-Making Project: Internal Report. Vancouver, Canada: University of British Columbia

Vedhara K, Stra JT, Miles JN, Sanderman R, Ranchor AV (2006) Psychosocial factors associated with indices of cortisol production in women with breast cancer and controls. Psychoneuroendocrinology 31: 299–311

Wadhwa PD (2005) Psychoneuroendocrine processes in human pregnancy influence fetal development and health Psychoneuroendocrinology 30: 724–743

Woo JC, Yu, T, Hurd TC (2003) Breast cancer in pregnancy: a literature review. Arch Surg 138: 91–98

Zanetti-Dällenbach R, Tschudin S, Lapaire O, Holzgreve W, Wight E, Bitzer J (accepted) Psychological management of pregnancy related breast-cancer.

20 Counseling Young Cancer Patients About Reproductive Issues

A. Surbone

Recent Results in Cancer Research, Vol. 178

20.1 Introduction

Counseling our young female cancer patients and survivors faced with fertility and pregnancy issues requires specific knowledge and expertise, as well as respect, humility, and compassion. Reproductive choices are extremely personal, and they are especially difficult for a cancer patient and her family at times of great distress and vulnerability. Young women may be weighing their natural desire to maintain their childbearing potential against the need to start cancer treatments; they may wonder about the best timing for conceiving after chemotherapy; they may be troubled by uncertainties of their children's future if they should experience a recurrence; or they may be exploring alternatives such as adoption.

Many women tend to postpone childbearing until later in their reproductive life, while treatments for early-stage cancers, including adjuvant treatments, may induce iatrogenic infertility. For example, it has been estimated that 10%–15% of women presently diagnosed with breast cancer in the United States are younger than 40 years of age. Many of these women have not had children and may still wish to do so (SEER 2007).

The medical, psychological, ethical, and social implications of carrying and raising a child are magnified after cancer. Reproductive issues are a primary cause of late morbidity in cancer survivors, potentially involving all physical, psychological, and social dimensions of our patients' well-being. Potential treatment-related reproductive dysfunctions should be addressed with all young patients in order to provide them with timely and adequate information and education (Lee 2006). The existing literature, however, suggests that only half of cancer patients of childbearing age receive the information they need from their health care providers about cancer-related infertility at the time of diagnosis and treatment planning (Hewitt 2005). Oncologists often find it difficult to counsel their patients about reproductive issues when they have just been diagnosed with cancer and are already overwhelmed with information and decision making about cancer therapies, especially since options for preserving fertility during cancer treatments are still under evaluation. Oncologists should thus try to refer their patients to other experts, including reproductive endocrinologists and psychologists. However, even in developed countries with efficient health care systems, it may be difficult, outside large urban contexts, to have access to a fertility specialist, or to an OB/GYN or neonatologist with expertise in managing cancer patients (Davis 2006; Partridge and Winer 2005; Thewes et al. 2003).

In the case of subsequent pregnancy after cancer treatment, published retrospective data indicate that pregnancy is safe, and several prospective studies are ongoing. (Gelber et al. 2001; Sankila et al. 1994; Surbone and Petrek 1997) The feasibility, safety, and success rate of fertility treatments and techniques are still under evaluation. Oncologists face the delicate task of counseling their patients by reviewing and discussing existing evidence with them, by providing their expert opinion with full respect of their patients' autonomy, and by referring interested women to specialized fertility centers, when appropriate (Lee et al. 2006).

With respect to the occurrence of any cancer during pregnancy, the concomitance of these two events poses acute and dramatic dilemmas for the patient, her family, and her physician

(Chervenak 2004). As discussed extensively in this volume, the management of cancer during pregnancy requires a collaborative team effort among oncologists, gynecologists, obstetricians, neonatologists, psychologists, and social workers to provide the best medical care for the mother and her fetus and to ensure adequate psycho-social support for the patient and her partner and family throughout the course of the pregnancy and in the years to follow. It is essential to understand the key role played in the care of cancer patients and survivors by their families and other support and caregiving systems (Surbone 2002).

20.2 Counseling About Fertility and Pregnancy: Definition, Scope, and Limitations

In this chapter, based on my clinical experience and research with breast cancer patients and survivors, I describe the salient aspects of a global approach to counseling young cancer patients with fertility and pregnancy issues within the context of oncology clinics. The word counseling is used here broadly to indicate the process of providing our young patients with appropriate information, referrals, and support within the context of their regular visits to oncology clinics for the diagnosis, treatment and follow-up care of various forms of cancer. To better understand its scope and limitations, it may help to consider the example of cancer genetics, where counseling is a well-defined structured activity, performed by dedicated specialists. A cancer genetic counselor generally meets his or her clients at different times of their lives, when they may or may not already have an illness or may never develop one. The cancer genetic counselor investigates the family and personal history, interprets information about existing cancer(s), analyzes inheritance patterns and risks of recurrence, and reviews available options with the client and her family. The cancer genetic counselor provides information and facts to facilitate the client's decision-making process, while refraining from being directive (Lerman et al. 1995). As the basic information shared in cancer genetic counseling is common to most sessions, genetic counselors make frequent use of written or audiovisual material that can benefit their clients, while allowing more time for them to address the specific needs and questions of each individual during their sessions (Axilbund et al. 2005; Chapman et al. 1995; O'Connor 1999). In some cases, genetic counseling is accompanied by additional professional counseling to explore the specific family dynamics and the possible psycho-social impact of genetic information.

The pregnancy and fertility and counseling that oncologists provide to young women of childbearing age who must undergo cancer treatments or have undergone them in the past is less structured than that which women receive from genetic counselors, for several reasons. First, it generally occurs within the context of regular patients' visits to their oncologists, often taking place at times of particular vulnerability of the patient, when she may be already overwhelmed with the cancer diagnosis and the treatment choices. Second, most oncologists work under major time constraints, and oncology clinics do not generally have enough dedicated spaces to provide consultations that frequently involve also partners or families. Third, oncologists are rarely qualified to provide psycho-social support, and yet, in many contexts, they may be the only source of emotional support for their patient. Finally, medical schools and postgraduate oncology education do not usually cover these aspects of cancer care, and there is no specific training for oncologists in dealing with reproduction-related issues.

Ideally, for example, oncologists should review with all young breast cancer patients requiring adjuvant treatment the reproductive effects of various regimes and illustrate alternatives that may allow them to retain their childbearing potential. This may help the individual patient in her decision-making process about immediate treatment for breast cancer, while also taking into account her hopes and expectations about future reproduction. Oncologists should then illustrate specific fertility preservation treatments and measures to interested women (Partridge and Winer 2005; Lee et al. 2006). Oncologists should also take time to understand their patients' motivations, and they should explore with their patients different alternatives, including adoption, and make appropriate referrals (Surbone and Petrek 1997).

In most cases, counseling a patient of childbearing age regarding reproduction involves one or more discussions with her partner or entire family, and ideally any oncology clinic should have dedicated spaces where extended meetings can take place (Thewes et al. 2003). The use of written material or audiovisual tools may facilitate communication between doctors, patients and families, especially about those issues that could take a longer time to be processed and absorbed (Axilbund et al. 2005; Chapman 1995). This form of counseling clearly requires expertise, time, and dedication of oncologists, nurses, and their teams, as well as economic resources and institutional commitment (Tables 20.1 and 20.2).

Table 20.1 Counseling young female patients about reproductive issues

Oncological aspects
OB/GYN aspects
Psychological aspects
Social and economic aspects
Ethical and legal aspects

Table 20.2 Obstacles to counseling young female patients about reproductive issues

Lack of oncologists' education about reproductive issues and ways to minimize them
Lack of patient information at time of cancer diagnosis and treatment
Lack of proper consideration of patients' personal preferences and values
Lack of communication and coordination between oncology and fertility experts

20.3 Role of Individual and Cultural Differences in Counseling

In counseling young women about reproductive issues, oncology teams need to consider each patient and her individual, religious, and cultural beliefs, as well as the ethical and legal requirements of their countries. The complexity of clinical consultations involving counseling about fertility and pregnancy issues is magnified by cross-cultural differences with respect to truth-telling attitudes and practices and decision making styles. Despite the universal value of each person's autonomy as a guiding ethical principle and its priority in western societies, there are, in fact, still persisting differences in the extent and modalities of truth—telling to cancer patients throughout the world (Mystadikou et al. 2004) While in industrialized countries patients are fully informed of their diagnosis, prognosis, and treatment options, in other contexts patients are still shielded from bad news and they are not involved in the decision making process. (Authors Various 1997) In many cultures, doctors and families still consider full disclosure to be overwhelming for the cancer patient, and issues related to reproduction may be considered especially sensitive and consequently excluded from clinical consultations. Cross cultural differences deeply influence communication between patients and doctors and they also affect decision making with respect to information and treatment. For example, the extent of involvement of families in medical decisions varies in different cultures, as does the symbolic meaning that fertility and childbearing may have not only for the woman, but also for her family and community. Even in western hospitals it is not uncommon for relatives of cancer patients to ask oncologists to withhold the truth or for family members to have a dominant role in making treatment decisions. Oncologists should thus be especially aware of cultural differences in counseling their young patients about fertility and pregnancy issues. (Surbone 2002 and 2006)

Not withstanding the recent evolution of truth-telling practices for cancer patients worldwide, oncologists at times still make unilateral paternalistic decisions to postpone the discussion of reproductive issues until the patient has completed the prescribed cancer treatment. However, research shows that reproductive concerns rank among the first for cancer patients and survivors (Carde 2004, Ganz 2003, Hewitt 2006). It is thus a requirement for oncologists to deliver information about late sequelae of cancer treatments in an early phase of the illness trajectory (Gradishar and Schilsky 1988; Lamb 1991; Fosså 2005).

For example, in a large western urban context, a 40-year-old highly educated cancer survivor was recently told for the first time, 10 years after diagnosis and treatment and after having undergone multiple failed IVF attempts, that her chances of success with IVF were much lower because she had received chemotherapy, which made her ovarian function several years older. This case illustrates a lack of coordination of care between oncologists and fertility centers and a failute to deliver timely information to cancer patients. Respect for patient autonomy in a spirit of cultural sensitivity, should be the leading principle in oncology practice, and disclosure of the potential risks and benefits to female cancer patients of childbearing age must become part of standard communication between oncologists and their patients. The American Society for Clinical Oncology has recently published guidelines to assist oncologists worldwide in this difficult task (Lee et al. 2006).

20.4 Counseling Women with Cancer During Pregnancy

The issues involved in counseling a pregnant cancer patient are many, and the medical aspects of cancer during pregnancy have been reviewed elsewhere in this volume. Ideally, every individual pregnant cancer patient should be approached by a multidisciplinary team involving oncologists, gynecologists and obstetricians, neonatologists, psychologists, social workers, and family counselors. When such multidisciplinary teams are not available, oncologists should refer pregnant patients to large centers with more expertise. In those countries, however, where specialized centers are not accessible for geographic and economic reasons, oncologists may find help by asking for the opinion and advice of colleagues with special expertise or by accessing online dedicated websites.

In counseling a woman with pregnancy-associated breast cancer, many psycho-social and ethical issues need to be considered, along with the increased medical risks for the mother-patient and for the fetus (Surbone et al. 2000; Chervenak et al. 2004; Giacatone et al. 1999; Ring et al. 2005; Hahn et al. 2006). The availability and accessibility of specialized referral centers for pregnant cancer patients should always be taken into consideration. The oncology team and the mother and family may find themselves faced with the dilemma of choosing between mother and child. As many chapters of this volume illustrate in reference to specific cancers, this choice is not always necessary. Evidence is growing to suggest that in many cases it is possible for the mother to give birth without compromising her own chances of being treated successfully and of surviving. The oncology team must evaluate the individual medical situation and review existing published data, in order to base their recommendations on the most solid evidence and to ensure the best possible outcome to both the mother and the fetus.

In those cases, however, where major ethical dilemmas arise, the physician's primary obligation is toward the patient, including respect for her values and autonomy of choice. A comprehensive ethical framework has been recently published to guide physicians treating cancer-associated pregnancy. This model is based on the western bioethics principles of autonomy and beneficence, as applied not only to the mother but also to the developing fetus, and it may not be applicable to all cultural settings (Chervenak et al. 2004).

In pregnancy-associated cancer, the decision making process involves not only the oncologist and the sick mother, but also the entire family, as partners and relatives will likely share immediate and long-term child care and child-raising responsibilities. (Chervenak et al. 2004; Surbone and Petrek 1997, Thewes et al. 2003) Given the particular vulnerability of the young pregnant cancer patient, establishing a trusting relationship with her and her loved ones, in a spirit of individual and cultural sensitivity, assumes a special relevance.

20.5 Counseling Female Cancer Survivors About Reproductive Concerns

Endocrine and gonadal dysfunctions are common consequences of anticancer treatments in young cancer patients (Gradishar and Schilsky

1988). Cancer survivors are rapidly increasing in number because of earlier cancer diagnosis, aging of society, and improvements in cancer treatments. There are now over 10 million cancer survivors in the US, representing approximately 3.5% of the US population. (Hewitt 2006, Jemal et al. 2005). The number of cancer survivors continues to increase also in developing countries. The definition of cancer survivorship extends from the patient's cancer diagnosis to death, and increasing attention is now being paid to the well-being and age-specific concerns and needs of cancer survivors, including reproductive issues (Connell et al. 2006, Ganz et al. 2003, Surbone and Peccatori 2005).

Until recently, fewer than 50% of western women of childbearing age appear to have received information and counseling about fertility issues, even though studies show that younger women have greater psychological morbidity and poorer quality of life after breast cancer diagnosis when compared to older women. (Hewitt 2006, Lee 2006) The concerns of younger premenopausal and older postmenopausal breast cancer patients differ both quantitatively and qualitatively. (Ganz et al. 2003) Young women are especially preoccupied with changes in their body image, relationships with actual or potential partners, treatment-induced loss of fertility, and children's care and psychosocial well-being in the immediate and distant future (Dunn and Steginga 2000; Partridge et al. 2004).

When feasible and when the clinical situation is appropriate, oncologists should discuss reproductive issues with their female patients before initiating chemotherapy or radiation. For example, for women with early-stage breast cancer, oncologists should discuss the risks and benefits of adjuvant treatments. In addition, they should address the likelihood of treatment-induced amenorrhea or iatrogenic menopause and infertility, which are also related to a woman's age and prior reproductive history (Partridge and Winer 2005; Walshe et al. 2006) The need for adjuvant therapies and the choice between chemotherapy or hormonal therapy should be weighed against the risk of infertility for any individual patient. For example, in clinical practice it is not infrequent to encounter women older than 40 years whose first instinct may be to refuse adjuvant therapy for early-stage breast cancer because of the risk of infertility. The first step in counseling these women is to explain that an age-related decline in fertility already exists and then to review published evidence on benefits and risks of different adjuvant therapies. Oncologists should also present to their patients the available options for fertility preservation, including experimental ones, when available (Lobo 2005; Marholm and Cohen 2006; Nisker et al. 2006; Oktay et al. 2004; Sonmezer and Oktay 2004). Cell and tissue banking should be offered, as recently highlighted in ASCO guidelines (Lee et al. 2006).

For proper counseling, the oncologist and the patient need to evaluate costs, time, and potential alternatives, such as adoption. For many patients, the financial costs associated with in vitro fertilization and subsequent embryo cryopreservation are prohibitive. Patients and physicians also need to consider each patient's individual, religious, and cultural beliefs, as well as the ethical and legal requirements of different countries. (Whitworth 2006) Pregnancy outcomes after assisted reproductive technology must be assessed for the magnitude of their benefits, but also for their harms and costs, as recently outlined in the guidelines by the Canadian Genetic Committee and Reproduction and Infertility Committee (Allen et al. 2006). Good counseling may, in fact, not always translate into clinical success, and patients may suffer additionally. For example, failures after repeated attempts of in vitro fertilization may carry severe negative effects in terms of the psychological well-being of the woman and of the couple and family dynamics. Discussing failures and helping patients decide when to stop is beyond the oncologist's expertise and referrals should be made to professionals with specific knowledge and skills (Santiago-Delefosse et al. 2003).

20.6 Counseling Women About Subsequent Pregnancy After Cancer Treatment

The safety of subsequent pregnancy after cancer treatment is supported by solid evidence, as discussed elsewhere in this volume. While most data have been obtained through retrospective analysis and may be subject to potential biases, ongoing prospective studies also indicate that a subsequent pregnancy has no detrimental effect on the woman's health (Blakely et al. 2004. Gelber et al. 2001; Ives et al. 2007; Sankila et al. 1994; Surbone and Petrek 1997). Women treated with cytotoxic chemotherapy who remain fertile do not seem to be at an increased risk of birth defects (Reichman and Green 1994). Additional data are now being collected on the safety of assisted reproductive techniques, especially when they involve the use of ovarian hyperstimulation in young women with hormone-responsive cancers.

In addition to medical issues, young survivors who consider whether or not to attempt a subsequent pregnancy after cancer treatment face different psycho-social and ethical concerns, which should be recognized and addressed in counseling by skilled trained professionals (Baider et al. 2003; Bloom et al. 2004; Canada and Schover 2005). Concerns about recurrence and death, about the risk of being a sick mother, about the repercussions of a subsequent pregnancy on the family dynamics, and about child care and child-raising responsibilities are among the most common ones. Ideally, counseling should be provided before anticancer treatments start, and all interested patients should be referred to fertility specialists (Table 20.3).

20.7 Future Directions

Studies show persisting discordance between patients' concerns regarding the negative impact of cancer treatments on reproduction and oncologists' perceptions and attitudes toward their patients' concerns (Ganz et al. 1998; Carde 2004). In many cultural contexts, it is still common for oncologists to believe that their only duty is to treat the cancer effectively and in a timely manner, and that discussion of possible side effects should be limited to acute ones. In some cases, oncologists appear to be concerned about overwhelming their patient with too much information at a time when patients should concentrate on their cancer treatment. While this concern can be a legitimate one, especially in those cultural settings where patients and doctors are not used to sharing the decision making process, oncologists should explore and respect the importance that reproductive issues have in the lives of their patients and provide effective and sensitive care to women of childbearing age. (Table 20.3)

In 2005, the Institute of Medicine (IOM) issued a report that details a plan for cancer survivors, including how to address their reproductive concerns (Hewitt et al. 2006). The American Society of Clinical Oncology (ASCO) has established programs dedicated to survivorship issues, and it has published guidelines for fertility preservation in young cancer patients undergoing oncologic treatments (Lee et al. 2006) The Multinational Association for Supportive Care in Cancer (MASCC) has endorsed extending supportive care to cancer survivors. National and international organizations have joined in the commitment to cancer survivors and their quality of life (Pollack et al. 2005; Rowland et al. 2006).

These projects will require considerable personal and community efforts and resources. Education and training of all oncology professionals and of general practitioners regarding reproductive issues is necessary. Oncologists should also be knowledgeable about the reproductive issues of special patient populations, such as very young women or BRCA-positive women, and about new fertility preservation treatments and fertility enhancement techniques (Davis 2006). In view of the increasing number of cancer survivors, most of whom are still young, medical schools and oncology curricula must include communication skills and cultural competence (Betancourt 2003; Kagawa-Singer 2003; Seibert et al. 2002;). Basic knowledge about the key psychosocial aspects of cancer care should be integrated in the education of all oncologists, to enable them to recognize the immediate and delayed stress of the woman and her partner and family in relation to

Table 20.3 Proper counseling of young female patients about reproductive issues

Discuss fertility issues with all young patients at diagnosis.
Monitor ovarian function and reproductive events in all young breast cancer patients.
Be available to counsel each patient at different stages of treatment and follow-up.
Refer interested women to fertility specialists or dedicated centers.

the decision making process when facing cancer during pregnancy, or when deciding whether or not to undergo a subsequent pregnancy, or when dealing with fertility treatment failures. Recognition of signs of patient distress or of altered family dynamics should prompt referral to trained psychooncology professionals.

Supplemental tools to educate and facilitate communication are important, given the high demands and lack of time that characterize most oncology clinics. Adequate written and audiovisual material should be designed in a culturally sensitive way. While this will never become a substitute for direct interpersonal communication between the oncologist and the woman and her partner or family, such information should be made easily available to all young cancer patients in any oncology clinic.

Multidisciplinary teams with expertise in addressing fertility and pregnancy issues in cancer patients should be established, and, whenever possible, dedicated clinics should be created where patients and their families can meet different specialists in the same building or center. Rigorous studies to collect data on cancer treatment-related endocrine and gonadal dysfunctions, as well as on all reproductive events and on the safety and efficacy of fertility preservation therapies and enhancement techniques, are of paramount importance. Patients and advocates should be involved in the design and evaluation of all prospective studies. Funding should be allocated to dedicated research and clinical activities in this field.

References

Allen VM, Wilson RD, Cheung A et al. (2006) Joint SOGC-CFAS guideline. Pregnancy outcomes after assisted reproductive technology. JOGC 173: 220–233

Authors Various (1997) In : Surbone A, Zwitter M. (Eds) Communication with the Cancer Patient: Information and Truth. Ann NY Acad Sci 809

Axilbund JE, Hamby LA, Thompson DB, Olsen SJ, Griffin CA (2005) Assessment of the use and feasibility of video to supplement the genetic counselling process: a cancer genetic counselling perspective. J Genet Counsel 14: 235–243

Baider L, Andritsch E, Uziely B et al. (2003) Effects of age on coping and psychological distress in women diagnosed with breast cancer: a review of literature and analysis of two different geographical settings. Crit Rev Oncol Hematol 46: 5-16

Betancourt JR. (2003) Cross-cultural medical education: Conceptual approaches and frameworks for evaluation. Acad Med 78: 560–569

Blakely LJ, Buzdar AU, Lozada JA, Shullaih SA, Hoy E, Smith TL, Hortobagyi GN (2004) Effects of pregnancy after treatment for breast carcinoma on survival and risk of recurrence. Cancer 100: 465–469

Bloom JR, Stewart SL, Chang S et al. (2004) Then and now: quality of life of young breast cancer survivors. Psycho-Oncol 13: 147–160

Canada AL, Schover LR (2005) Research promoting better patient education on reproductive health after cancer. J Natl Cancer Inst Monogr 34: 98–100

Carde P (2004) Risks of infertility and early menopause from anticancer and immunosuppressive programs: methods of fertility preservation and palliation. ASCO Educational Book, p. 400

Chapman GB, Elsetin AS, Kostbade Hugehs K (1995) Effects of patient education on decisions about breast cancer treatments: A preliminary report. Med Decis Mak 15: 213–239

Chervenak FA, McCullough LB, Knapp RC, Caputo TA, Barber HR (2004) A clinically comprehensive ethical framework for offering and recommending cancer treatment before and during pregnancy. Cancer 100: 215–222

Connell S, Patterson C, Newman B (2006) A qualitative analysis of reproductive issues raised by young Australian women with breast cancer. Health Care Women Int 27: 94–110

Davis M (2006) Fertility considerations for female adolescents and young adult patients following cancer therapy: a guide for counselling patients and their families. Clin J Oncol Nurs 10: 213–222

Dunn J, Steginga SK (2000) Young women's experience of breast cancer: defining young and identifying concerns. Psychooncology 9: 137–146

Fosså SD, Magelssen H, Melve K et al. (2005) Parenthood in survivors after adulthood cancer and perinatal health in their offspring: a preliminary report. J Natl Cancer Inst Monogr 34: 77–82

Friedman LC, Kramer RM (2005) Reproductive issues for women with BRCA mutations. J Natl Cancer Inst Monogr 34: 83–86

Ganz PA, Greendale GA, Petersen L, et al. (2003) Breast cancer in younger women: Reproductive and late health effects of treatment. J Clin Oncol 21: 41 84-41 93

Ganz PA, Rowland JH, Desmond KA et al. (1998) Life after breast cancer: understanding women's health-related quality of life and sexual functioning. J Clin Oncol 16: 501–514

Gelber S, Coates AS, Goldhirsch A et al. (2001) Effect of pregnancy on overall survival after the diagnosis of early stage breast cancer. J Clin Oncol 19: 1671–1675

Giacatone P-L, Laffargue F, Benos P (1999) Chemotherapy for breast carcinoma during pregnancy. A French National Survey. Cancer 86: 2266–2272

Gradishar WJ, Schilsky RL (1988) Effects of cancer treatment on the reproductive system. Crit Rev Oncol Hematol 8(2): 153–171

Hahn KME, Johnson PH, Gordon N et al. (2006) Treatment of pregnant patients and outcomes of children exposed to chemotherapy in utero. Cancer 107: 1219–1226

Hewitt M, Greenfield S, and Stovall E, eds. (2006) From Cancer Patient to Cancer Survivor: Lost in Transition. Committee on Cancer Survivorship: Washington, D.C.: The National Academies Press

Ives A, Saunders C, Bulsara M et al. (2007) Pregnancy after breast cancer: population based study. BMJ 334: 194-199,

Jemal A, Murray T, Ward A et al (2005) Cancer statistics, 2005. CA Cancer J Clin 2005: 55: 10-30

Kagawa-Singer M (2003) A strategy to reduce cross-cultural miscommunication and increase the likelihood of improving health outcomes. Acad Med 78: 577-587

Lamb MA (1991) Effects of chemotherapy on fertility in long-term survivors. Dimens Oncol Nurs 5 (4): 13–16

Lee SJ, Schover LR, Partridge AH et al. (2006) American Society of Clinical Oncology recommendations on fertility preservation in cancer patients. J Clin Oncol 24: 2917–2931

Lerman C, Lustbader E, Rimer B et al. (1995) Effects of individualized breast cancer risk counselling: a randomized trial. J Natl Cancer Inst 87: 286–292

Lobo RA (2005) Potential options for preservation of fertility in women. N Engl J Med 353: 64–73

Marholm E, Cohen I (2006) Fertility preservation options for women with malignancies. Obstet Gynecol Surv 62: 58–72

Mystadikou K, Parpa E, Tsilika E et al. (2004) Cancer information disclosure in different cultural contexts. Support Care Cancer 12: 147–154

Nisker J, Baylis F, McLeod C (2006) Choice in fertility preservation in girls and adolescent women with cancer. Cancer 107 (7 Suppl): 1686–1689

O'Connor AM (1999) Decision aids for patients considering options affecting cancer outcomes: evidence of efficacy and policy implications. J Natl Cancer Inst 25: 67–80

Oktay K, Buyuk E, Veeck L et al. (2004) Embryo development after heterotopic transplantation of cryopreserved ovarian tissue. Lancet 363: 837–840

Partridge AH, Gelber S, Peppercorn J et al. (2004) Web-based survey of fertility issues in young women with breast cancer. J Clin Oncol 22: 4174–4183

Partridge AH, Winer EP (2005) Fertility after breast cancer: questions abound. J Clin Oncol 23: 4259–4261

Pollack LA, Greer GE, Rowland JH et al. (2005) Cancer survivorship: a new challenge in comprehensive cancer control. Cancer Causes Control 16: 51–59

Reichman BS, Green KB (1994) Breast cancer in young women: effect of chemotherapy on ovarian function, fertility, and birth defects J Natl Cancer Inst Monogr 16: 125-9

Ring AE, Smith IE, Jones A et al. (2005) Chemotherapy for breast cancer during pregnancy: an 18-year experience from five London teaching hospitals. J Clin Oncol 23: 4192–4197

Rowland JH, Hewitt M, Ganz PA (2006) Cancer survivorship: a new challenge in delivering quality cancer care J Clin Oncol 24: 5 101 -5 104

Sankila R, Heinavaara S, Hakulinen T (1994) Survival of breast cancer patients after subsequent term pregnancy: „healthy mother effect". Am J Obstet Gynecol 170: 818–823

Santiago-Delefosse M, Cahen F, Coeffin-Driol C (2003) The analysis of physicians' work: announcing the end of attempts at in vitro fertilization. Encephale 29: 293–305

Seibert PS, Stridh-Igo P, Zimmermann CG (2002) A checklist to facilitate cultural awareness and sensitivity. J Med Ethics 28: 143–146

Sonmezer M, Oktay K (2004) Fertility preservation in female patients. Hum Reprod Update 10: 251–266

Surbone A Cultural aspects of communication in cancer care. In: Communication in cancer care. Recent Results in Cancer Research. Stiefel F (Ed) Heidelberg: Springer Verlag 2006; 168: 91-104

Surbone A, Petrek JA (1997) Issues in childbearing in breast cancer survivors. Cancer 79: 1271–1278

Surbone A, Petrek JA, Currie VE (2000) Treatment of breast cancer during pregnancy. In Dixon JM, Sacchini V, eds. Breast Cancer: Diagnosis and Management. pp. 385–393

Surbone A (2002) The role of the family in the ethical dilemmas of oncology. In Cancer and the Family. Baider L, Cooper CL, Kaplan De-Nour A (eds). John Wiley and Sons pp. 513–534

Surbone A, Peccatori F (2006) Unmet needs of cancer survivors: supportive care's new challenge. Editorial. J Supp Care Cancer 15: 397–399

Surbone A (2006) Telling truth to patients with cancer: what is the truth? Lancet Oncol 7: 944–950

Surveillance, Epidemiology, and End Results (SEER), available at www.seer.cancer.gov, accessed September 25th 2007

Thewes B, Meiser B, Rickard J, Friedlander M (2003) The fertility and menopause-related information needs of younger women with a diagnosis of breast cancer: a qualitative study. Psychooncology 12: 500–511

Walshe JM, Denduluri N, Swain SM (2006) Amenorrhea in premenopausal women after adjuvant chemotherapy for breast cancer. J Clin Oncol 24: 5769–5779

Whitworth A (2006) Freezing embryos-A woman's best option, but is it legal? News J Natl Cancer Inst 98: 1359

21 Psychosocial Issues in Young Women Facing Cancer and Pregnancy: The Role of Patient Advocacy

Stella Kyriakides

Recent Results in Cancer Research, Vol. 178

21.1 Introduction

The psychosocial issues facing young women confronting a cancer diagnosis are extremely complex. A diagnosis of cancer finds any individual unprepared. The realities that one was accustomed to in everyday life change overnight, and many uncertainties enter into this new life scenario. It is a frightening and complicated new world with difficulties at psychological, social, and emotional levels, the key concern, however, being that of individual survival.

There are, of course, many different types of cancer, and diagnosis can occur at different points in one's life, in different circumstances. The nature of the cancer, the stage at which it is diagnosed, the type of treatment required, and the factors pertaining to prognosis are just some of the issues that are involved in the diagnosis.

Women can be diagnosed with different types of cancer and at different points in their life.

The life situation in which the individual woman finds herself, her age, her support system, her family status, and the perceptions in the family of a cancer diagnosis are all factors that will affect the way in which she will respond and determine her coping mechanisms.

A cancer diagnosis is in itself a traumatic and painful process. A cancer diagnosis that is related in any way to the stage in a woman's life that is associated with pregnancy and childbearing is traumatic at a different level, in a different way.

However, there are also many common threads running through the issues facing a young women when confronted with a cancer diagnosis and pregnancy. For example, issues arise that have to do with ethics and with different assessments of needs, possibly even conflicting needs between mother and baby. Dilemmas are faced that add to the anxiety and fear that the cancer diagnosis itself brings about, dilemmas that need to be addressed not only by the individual woman and her family but by medical and other health professionals as well.

In a changing world, where the realities of cancer diagnosis and treatment constantly require new information and education, new challenges to be met, and constant adjustments made, this is possibly one of the most complicated subjects that we need to address today.

21.2 The Cancer Diagnosis

A diagnosis of cancer finds no individual, man or woman, prepared. This is what is often heard from patients, and one of the reasons they may need significant time of adjustment to the diagnosis on hearing the news.

When individuals are diagnosed with cancer it is not only the patients themselves who are affected but also those around them. In women, their childbearing and caretaking role has a set of different repercussions.

Frequently, before diagnosis there were no overt symptoms, or at least no attention was given to possible indications that there was a serious problem. Even in the most common type of cancer in women, breast cancer, and even though much emphasis has been placed upon the importance of early diagnosis, screening, and awareness in young women this is often not seen to be directly relevant as we associate the occurrence of this disease with older age groups.

The history of the perceptions surrounding a cancer diagnosis shows marked changes. In the past, cancer was associated with stigma and there was often silence about the diagnosis. The stigma in many parts of the world was such that cancer patients were shunned or avoided. There was the misconception that it was even a contagious disease, and even more prevailing was the belief that any cancer diagnosis meant sure death.

There is an inherent fear associated with this disease, and in many parts of the world it is still difficult to encourage women and men to attend early detection and screening programs as their fear of being diagnosed with cancer is by far greater than the advocated value of early diagnosis.

As scientific knowledge and understanding on the causes and biology of cancer have increased, the perceptions surrounding the disease and the diagnosis have gradually changed. There has been a gradual differentiation between the types of cancer, the staging, the prognostic factors, and the guidelines pertaining to treatment involving not only the medical procedures but also the need for multidisciplinarity in order to address the needs of the cancer patient. The complexity of this diagnosis, not only in terms of its medical realities but also because of the psychological, emotional, and social turbulence it brings, has slowly been recognized.

Many cancer patients describe the traumatic experience of having to tell loved ones of their diagnosis, and especially the anxiety of having to tell children. This is once again related to the perceptions that exist concerning this disease, that this is a six-letter word that is associated in people's minds with the fear of death. When the cancer diagnosis affects a woman, if she has a family, this experience is transmitted in a traumatic way throughout the family.

A cancer diagnosis is experienced as a direct threat to life. Many patients and their families require counseling and specialized support in order to cope not only with the diagnosis but also with the treatment. So there is in itself a paradox, a sense almost of irony, when we need to discuss and negotiate two different life situations—a diagnosis of cancer and a pregnancy.

21.3 Cancer and Pregnancy

Pregnancy is associated with the beginning of life. It is a stage in a woman's life that often leads to fulfillment; it marks the continuation of life, of the building of the family unit to completion, as often is imagined, at least.

Pregnancy has been called a miracle, a gift, a very special time in a woman's life.

Today, the time for bearing children is often later in life because of the changing roles of women in society who are not only an important part of the working force but today often have careers before they decide to have children.

This means that a cancer diagnosis in a young woman may find her at a stage in her life when she either has no children or has young children; she may be in a relationship or not. In any case, the consequences of the diagnosis of a life-threatening disease are of paramount importance in terms of their impact on the woman and her family.

In the instance when pregnancy occurs after a woman has had children and after a diagnosis of cancer, the issues that are involved are different from those involved when a pregnancy occurs before the diagnosis, if the diagnosis comes during a pregnancy, or if a woman has not yet had children. Therefore, one can only discuss the issues involved from the broader sense, based on many personal stories from women in the younger age groups, that is, under 40 years, and how this has impacted on their life realities. There are psychological, moral, social, medical, and cultural perspectives to this question, and all must be given due attention when discussing the questions involved in cancer and pregnancy.

21.4 Ethical Issues

The bioethical issues involved when considering how to manage and advise a young women with a cancer diagnosis where pregnancy issues are involved are extremely complex. Ethics are, of course, involved in terms of the choices given to the woman and the decisions she has to make involving, on some occasions, her unborn child. Younger women facing cancer have a different set of issues that are of relevance to them than women in older age groups. And this is not only related to their childbearing realities, but also to the young age of their family, their career stage, their level of energy, and the dreams they have set out before them.

Ethics involve principles that govern decision making in questions of health. From the time of Hippocrates, medicine has always been governed by principles and values that protect patients and take into account the social norms.

There are a number of such ethical issues involved when discussing cancer and pregnancy in the case of the cancer patient who decides to proceed with having children.

Some of the questions involve the principle of autonomy, that is, the right to make decisions for oneself as long as others are not affected and the right of equal access to the best possible care. Decisions are measured as right or wrong according to the result they bring. In the case of the female cancer patient, decisions of whether she will become a mother or not become more complicated, as what she decides will directly affect the life of another human being, her child. She has the right to bear children even if she has been through cancer, and questioning this would be infringing on her rights. She must not be made to feel that she does not have the rights of other patients. However, she must be made aware of all possible ethical issues that may be involved because of the risks to the health of her child.

A woman who is a cancer patient is without doubt more emotionally vulnerable than other pregnant women. Her child may or may not be at risk itself in the future, and that is related to a number of factors. What is relevant, though, is her prognosis in relation to the raising of her child.

To this end, allowing a cancer patient to have the choice and freedom to proceed with a pregnancy is possibly one of the most fundamental ways of safeguarding freedom of rights. On the other hand, one must consider the fact that the unborn child does not have a choice, and also consider the amount of pain and suffering that may be involved. So how are the child's rights safeguarded?

These are all questions that need to be carefully discussed with the parents, and it needs to be ensured that any decisions taken are taken responsibly. In order to do so, the most important factor is that of availability of information. If this is provided and explained, then one can be more certain that the correct decisions are taken, taking into account all the ethical and societal factors mentioned above. For information to be absorbed and assimilated, the woman must be emotionally able to do so, and she often requires counseling in order to reach this stage of emotional and even cognitive stability.

21.5 Motherhood

Motherhood is a role that many young girls dream of.

Motherhood is possibly the most fundamental role that women feel they have to fulfill. Pregnancy is the beginning of a journey that is associated with new life, with creation, with the future of the species. There is almost something deep within the soul of a women to nurture children.

From the beginning of puberty, young women begin to imagine themselves as mothers, and the maternal instinct has often been described, with young girls role playing this role in various contexts. Puberty brings the sexual maturity that prepares women for this role, although today their changing roles in many Western societies may mean this role of motherhood is delayed.

The way in which women view themselves during pregnancy is often determined not only by their own psychology but also by the way society views pregnancy and motherhood—there are societies in which pregnant women are viewed with special respect and protection.

Of course, some women look forward to this part of their lives and show no anxiety about their changing body image as many others do.

The stability in a woman's life and the way in which her partner views the pregnancy are also important factors. However, there are also additional changes today in the way pregnant women feel about their baby, because today for many parents the sex of the child is known before the birth. This results in different emotions and expectations as one now identifies with an unborn baby that has its own very specific characteristics.

21.6 Cancer Diagnosis During Pregnancy

A diagnosis of cancer during pregnancy is an especially difficult medical and ethical dilemma. All decisions automatically involve two beings, the mother and the embryo, while the partner is usually involved as well. These are, of course, rare medical situations, but the do raise social, psychological, medical, ethical, and moral issues that need to be addressed. It may be the case that the mother will need urgent treatment that may put the embryo's life or health in danger. Exactly because these cases are infrequent, there is not as much information and expertise as one would like in this area, and not all doctors have been exposed to such cases.

The question of what constitutes a human being and the beginning of life is a question that not only involves science but morals, ethics, and, of course, religion. The cultural and religious beliefs will determine the way in which a cancer diagnosis during pregnancy is experienced and, of course, managed.

Not all pregnancies, however, are wanted or desired. There are occasions in which the pregnancy is not wanted by the mother, or by the parents, the changes that come to the body are experienced in a negative way, and there is often hidden aggression toward the unborn baby, which must be realized and confronted in any case of a concurrent cancer diagnosis.

21.7 The World of Uncertainty

No matter whether the pregnancy was desired or not, a diagnosis of cancer will throw the woman into emotional turmoil—there will be feelings of distress, sadness, ambivalence, and even guilt involved. The woman will need a great deal of not only emotional but also professional support in this decision making process. A diagnosis of cancer in any case is a source of great stress and anxiety, evoking fear and confusion. Many cancer patients have described this stage of diagnosis, saying they feel they have been thrown into a world of uncertainty, where their lives change from one moment to the next and where they often feel numb. The stages of emotions they go through have been described, and the range from fear to depression, from anger to denial. This situation is rendered even more complicated when the diagnosis of cancer comes at a time when the woman is emotionally vulnerable, and with all the idiosyncrasies of a pregnancy.

It is well recognized that the way individuals deal with stress is associated with previous life experiences, personality, predispositions, and genetics.

A cancer diagnosis is a source of massive stress. Patients are faced with new medical terminology that they have to understand at a period of great stress, and they not only must do so but also must make important life decisions that affect not only themselves but also the embryo. It's an extremely complicated situation both in terms of emotions and in terms of the science involved. with the diagnosis of cancer comes at a time when the focus of the woman and her family most often has been on the positive, creative, and exciting time of bringing a new life into the world. Suddenly, what in fact is most often a part of family and personal growth and development is suddenly associated with a disease that means life risk.

The approach to the woman and her family needs to be individualized, as, of course, in the case of every patient but in this case it is even more complex because it involves another life. There are many variables that need to be taken into consideration—the age of the woman, the presence of other children in the family, whether it was a wanted or unwanted pregnancy, the stage of the pregnancy, the type of cancer.

Decisions pertaining to whether the woman will continue with the pregnancy, whether she will commence treatment while pregnant, what the side effects may be, and how her partner feels about this situation must all be taken, while she must be encouraged to express her feelings and to be given the opportunity to work through them.

This can only be done with the care and support of a multidisciplinary team.

The role of the multidisciplinary team is recognized as part of optimal cancer care. The diagnosis of cancer in itself is, as has been mentioned, a source of stress that requires the attention of a wide variety of disciplines and team work. A cancer patient needs psychological and social support and a team of experts to consult. This is even more imperative where there are ethical, religious, social, and moral issues, as in the case of a pregnancy during a cancer experience.

21.8 Role of the Doctor Team

The role of the doctor in this process of providing the correct amount and type of information so the cancer patient and her partner can make the right decision is of paramount importance. Doctors need to be specially equipped to do this with communication skills that will allow them to convey this information in an objective way without allowing their own ethical and societal beliefs to affect their communication. Often, personal prejudices affect the type of communication, and this is very dangerous in this case, in either encouraging or discouraging a cancer patient to proceed with a pregnancy. Doctors and health team professionals may need special training in order to perform their role effectively.

The health team need this in order to deal with their own feelings as well in a very emotionally loaded situation. Access to team discussions is also important in order to gather as much expertise as possible, which not only will make the woman feel safer but will also make the health team feel safer when advising in difficult life circumstances.

In many clinic settings, the doctors are supported by specialized nursing staff who have the role of ongoing provision of information. Doctors are accustomed to giving clear and definite answers in order to allow decisions to be reached. In the case of cancer and pregnancy, it may be impossible to so; all one can do is advise in a specific direction and provide the woman and her family with the information to reach a decision that respects her and her family's ethos and philosophy and that safeguards her health.

Doctors are also trained to preserve life, and in the case of cancer in young women they have to weigh up the risks to the mother and to the baby and whether the mother will have all the factors on her side that will allow her to bring up her child.

The provision of optimal services can only be achieved if there are consensus guidelines in effect so that the health care team has set objectives and no one member of the team is forced to shoulder such an emotional burden alone.

21.9 The Role of Advocacy

Advocacy is the act of arguing on behalf of a particular issue, idea, or person. Individuals, organizations, businesses, and governments can engage in advocacy. Advocating for an idea can include a wide range of subjects as broad as social justice.

Over the last decades, cancer advocacy has succeeded in changing many of the realities for cancer patients. A cancer advocate is someone who becomes the voice for others, who puts forward the cause, who is in fact the supporter of rights, and upholder of principles. Advocates have developed as voices in many fields, of course, and not just the medical world—advocates for children's rights, for women's rights, for animal rights, etc.

The provision of accurate information concerning a cause is what in effect brings about the raising of awareness of the cause and thus can bring or promote change or protect rights. Advocacy has been one of the most powerful tools in used by patient groups. Around the globe, patient advocacy groups have without a doubt had such an impact that they have led to changes of medical systems and of the safeguarding of rights.

The use of organized patient groups has helped to raise awareness concerning the needs of cancer patients, but more than that, it has helped to promote the rights of patients, to highlight the needs of patients and families.

It has helped to put pressure on governments to implement policies that will help ensure a better quality of life, to allow access to the best possible diagnosis and treatment. It has also allowed the promotion of awareness of what constitutes optimal care and has brought respect into the lives of patients.

Over time and with the changing world of information, advocates have become better informed and educated, thus ensuring the best possible access to information.

Advocacy has also helped put the personal experience across as a political voice; it has helped promote guidelines in cancer care, in partnership with the scientific and medical worlds.

Personal experience with any disease does not in itself mean that one can be a successful or even effective advocate.

In order to be a successful advocate one needs to have a broader understanding of the situation—in the case of cancer advocacy, this has changed the way in which many types of cancer are approached.

A fundamental principle that must always be upheld is the protection of patients' rights: the right to information, the right to optimal care, the right to prevention, diagnosis, and palliative care. Fundamental patients' rights like, for example, the right to be treated with respect, the right to privacy, the right to confidentiality, and the right to dignity. Advocating for these is the foundation of patient protection, and many cancer patient organizations have been established exactly to achieve this in societies where it was lacking.

One way to ascertain the responsible way of informing patients is to always uphold their rights as stated in the Charters of Patients' Rights. These ensure that cancer patients are given access to all available information and are allowed to have freedom of choice. Freedom of choice, justice, autonomy, are all principles that form the basis of bioethics, that allow freedom of choice.

But, in order to make choices, one must have access to correct and accurate information. Advocacy has this important role to play in that through its voice information is spread and shared.

However, the role of advocacy in terms of disseminating information is a complicated one when the scientific evidence is not clear in order to give a direction in which a decision can be made.

This is the case in many instances when cancer and pregnancy are concerned.

Young women facing a cancer diagnosis before, during, or after a pregnancy need very clear and specific information that will allow correct decision making. This is often not available, so advocates need to promote the right of women to have access to multidisciplinary teams so that the best possible sources of information are available and so that their multiple needs are met: medical, psychological, social, and emotional needs.

Advocacy in the instance of cancer and pregnancy can do exactly what is most needed—ensure that given the many difficult realities, women are approached and advised in centers that are able to give the latest information, that have counseling services available, and, most importantly, that promote the development of guidelines so that health professionals are able to implement these in all parts of the world and women can look to these centers in order to feel safe and reassured.

And, in this relatively new field, with so many uncertainties, only through responsible and educated advocacy can one hope to pool all the information together in order to gain a better understanding of what ethical and other issues are involved.

Suggested Reading

Love S (2000) Breast book (3rd edn). Perseus Publishing

Murphy B (2003) Fighting for our future. McGraw-Hill

Pavlides N (2006) Cancer and pregnancy. Iatrikes Ekdosis P. Pashalides

MIX
Papier aus verantwortungsvollen Quellen
Paper from responsible sources
FSC® C105338

If you have any concerns about our products,
you can contact us on
ProductSafety@springernature.com

In case Publisher is established outside the EU,
the EU authorized representative is:
Springer Nature Customer Service Center GmbH
Europaplatz 3, 69115 Heidelberg, Germany

Printed by Libri Plureos GmbH
in Hamburg, Germany